Intensive Family Therapy

MEDICAL DEPARTMENT
HARPER & ROW, PUBLISHERS
HAGERSTOWN, MARYLAND
NEW YORK, EVANSTON, SAN FRANCISCO, AND
LONDON

Intensive

Family Therapy

Theoretical and

Practical Aspects

---

by 15 authors

edited by
IVAN BOSZORMENYI-NAGY, M.D.

Director of Family Therapy Project, Eastern Pennsylvania Psychiatric Institute;
Associate Professor of Psychiatry, Jefferson Medical College; Psychiatrist,
Philadelphia Psychiatric Center, Philadelphia

and
JAMES L. FRAMO, Ph.D.

Medical Research Scientist, Department of Clinical Research, Eastern
Pennsylvania Psychiatric Institute; Instructor in Psychiatry, Jefferson Medical
College, Philadelphia; Consultant, Delaware County Juvenile Court, Media,
Pennsylvania

For our families, personal and professional

INTENSIVE FAMILY THERAPY

Theoretical and Practical Aspects

Library of Congress catalog card number: 65-17591

Table of Contents

v

List of Authors

Nathan W. Ackerman, M.D.

Clinical Professor of Psychiatry, Columbia University; Director of Professional Program, Family Institute of New York; Supervising Psychiatrist, Family Mental Health Clinic, Jewish Family Service, New York City

Ivan Boszormenyi-Nagy, M.D.

Director of Family Therapy Project, Eastern Pennsylvania Psychiatric Institute; Associate Professor of Psychiatry, Jefferson Medical College; Psychiatrist, Philadelphia Psychiatric Center, Philadelphia

Murray Bowen, M.D.

Associate Clinical Professor of Psychiatry, Georgetown University School of Medicine, Washington, D.C.; Consultant in Family Psychotherapy, University of Maryland School of Medicine, Baltimore; Consultant in Family Psychotherapy, Medical College of Virginia, Richmond

Richard E. Felder, M.D.

Psychiatrist, Atlanta Psychiatric Clinic, Atlanta, Georgia

Raymond D. Fogelson, PH.D.

Assistant Professor of Anthropology, University of Washington, Seattle

James L. Framo, PH.D.

Medical Research Scientist, Department of Clinical Research, Eastern Pennsylvania Psychiatric Institute; Instructor in Psychiatry, Jefferson Medical College, Philadelphia; Consultant, Delaware County Juvenile Court, Media, Pennsylvania

Paul F. Franklin, M.D.

Psychoanalyst, American Institute for Psychoanalysis, and Karen Horney Clinic; Psychiatrist, Jewish Family Service, New York City

Ronald D. Laing, M.B., CH.B.

Chief Investigator, Schizophrenia and Family Research Unit, Tavistock Institute of Human Relations; Director, Langham Clinic, London

vii

David Rubinstein, M.D.

Assistant Professor of Psychiatry, and Staff Psychiatrist, Institute for Psycho therapy, Temple University Medical School; Medical Research Scientist, Eastern Pennsylvania Psychiatric Institute, Philadelphia

Harold F. Searles, M.D.

Supervising and Training Analyst, Washington Psychoanalytic Institute, Washington, D.C.; Consultant in Psychotherapy, Sheppard and Enoch Pratt Hospital, Towson, Maryland; Clinical Professor of Psychiatry, Georgetown University School of Medicine, Washington, D.C.

Anthony F. C. Wallace, PH.D.

Medical Research Scientist, Eastern Pennsylvania Psychiatric Institute; Professor and Chairman of Department of Anthropology, University of Pennsylvania, Philadelphia

John Warkentin, M.D., PH.D.

Psychiatrist, Atlanta Psychiatric Clinic, Atlanta, Georgia

Carl A. Whitaker, M.D.

Professor of Psychiatry, University of Wisconsin College of Medicine, Madison

Lyman C. Wynne, M.D., PH.D.

Chief, Adult Psychiatry Branch, and Chief, Section on Family Studies, National Institute of Mental Health, Bethesda, Maryland; Faculty, Washington Psychoanalytic Institute and Washington School of Psychiatry, Washington, D.C.

Gerald H. Zuk, PH.D.

Medical Research Scientist, Department of Clinical Research, Eastern Pennsylvania Psychiatric Institute, Philadelphia

Preface

The chapters of this volume were written for the purpose of surveying the field of intensive family therapy. The book is not a compilation of previously published articles; all of the chapters are original
contributions written at the request of the editors. The structure of
the volume was determined by the editors' experience with
family therapy and their continuous exchange with other workers
in the field through symposia, personal discussions, and, in most
cases, direct observation of their work. In our search for contributors
we first turned to investigators whose clinical work we respected
and assigned them problem areas which we thought were most relevant to their interests and expertness. We have represented in this
volume nearly every major family therapy worker who operates
in a psychoanalytically oriented manner based on psychodynamic
principles with the goal of deep reconstructive change, both in the
family group and its individual members.

The term "*intensive* family therapy" was selected in an attempt
to characterize the distinctive quality shared by the schools of family
therapy represented in this volume. It was the editors' belief that
there is a need to distinguish between two kinds of family therapy:
intensive and supportive. By classifying other family therapies as
supportive we do not wish to minimize the contribution of an approach which aims to clarify communication, change interaction
patterns, and help the family to cope with concrete stress situations;
these supportive approaches have their valid indications. Too often,
however, we have heard professional psychotherapists refer to
all family therapy as a kind of supportive, counseling procedure (e.g.,
which helps the family to understand and cope with the designated
patient). The *intensive* family therapy described in this volume
aims toward the working through of unconscious transference dis-

tortions which pervade close family relationships. Intensive individual therapy and intensive family therapy do share depth goals but contrary to the view that deep intrapsychic change can only occur in one-to-one psychotherapy, the therapists in this volume maintain that certain transference problems can be explored and affected more advantageously in conjoint family sessions. In long-term, intensive family therapy the family members are helped to work through their transference distortions *with each other*, as well as with the therapists.

We have given the contributors considerable leeway in presenting their own points of view and have restricted our editing to points of clarity rather than to statements with which we might disagree. The book is oriented around the traditional dimensions of psychotherapy with certain relevant elaborations peculiar to the family therapy approach also included. We have envisioned a volume which transmits clinical experience on the one hand and projects a conceptual viewpoint on the other. Each of the clinicians is, in his own right, a thoughtful and penetrating theoretician and, hopefully, each has succeeded in integrating the practical and the theoretical, the abstract and the concrete.

In Chapter 1 the authors, Drs. Gerald H. Zuk and David Rubinstein, present a review of the literature which led to the development of family therapy and attempt to elucidate in critical fashion some of the significant issues and concepts in the field. Dr. Zuk has published articles in the field of family relations of retarded children and of family therapy observations. Dr. Rubinstein has contributed to the literature on family therapy as therapist, investigator and reviewer. He has had a long-standing interest in intensive psychotherapy of schizophrenics.

Chapter 2 is a theoretical chapter by Dr. Ivan Boszormenyi-Nagy which attempts to place family process concepts in a broad-based relationship framework, aimed at the integration of psychoanalytic-psychiatric and humanistic-existential outlooks. Dr. Boszormenyi-Nagy has published works on various research aspects of schizophrenia, and, in more recent years, in the field of family therapy. His publications range from conceptual and therapeutic issues in family therapy to problems of patient and staff "family transferences" in psychiatric programs. His long-standing interest in the psychopathology and psychotherapy of schizophrenia led to the establishment in 1957 of the Family Therapy Project of the Department of Clinical Research of the Eastern Pennsylvania Psychiatric Institute.

In Chapter 3 Dr. Boszormenyi-Nagy applies theoretical concepts from the previous chapter to certain key issues of the family therapy situation and, in particular, illustrates his concepts of family system and process with excerpts from sessions of an actual family in treatment. Of special importance in this chapter is the documentation of how intrapsychic, structural change in the individual members paralleled critical change in the system of the family.

In Chapter 4 Dr. James L. Framo describes a broad spectrum of conceptual and technical issues as they have emerged from his years of therapy experience in the Family Therapy Project at the Eastern Pennsylvania Psychiatric Institute. One of the few writers on technique of family therapy, he attempts to delineate the rationale and stages of the therapy process, as well as such special problems as resistance, marriage problems, the "well" sibling, transference/countertransference, co-therapy team relationship, termination problems, and a clinical evaluation of family therapy. His publications range from systematic research in the areas of perception, dreams, and rating scales of psychopathology to clinical papers on schizophrenia, family-oriented hospital organization, family dynamics, and family therapy.

In Chapter 5 Dr. Murray Bowen integrates his knowledge of theory of family dynamics with his experience in the hospitalization of entire families and the treatment of families in private practice. He illustrates how society, medical practice, hospital structure, and laws governing mental illness, which are all based on the individual concept of illness, may fit in with the "family projection process." This point of view is an extremely significant one which may have wholesale implications. Dr. Bowen, a psychoanalyst, is widely known for his study of the treatment of hospitalized families of schizophrenics conducted at the National Institute for Mental Health. He is the originator of some of the important concepts of family pathology.

In a verbatim transcript of an entire family therapy session Drs. Nathan W. Ackerman and Paul F. Franklin demonstrate in Chapter 6 their intuitive and imaginative interpretation of the treatment of a family. The reader can sense in this transcript the importance of the therapist's sensitivity to non-verbal interaction, a much more vital element in family therapy than in individual or group therapy. An interesting complement to this chapter is the film "In and Out of Psychosis," based on the treatment of this same family. In this case study the authors show how an apparently malignant illness can be treated effectively when dealt with as an illness which is embedded in the family relationships.

Dr. Ackerman, a psychoanalyst, is one of the earliest pioneers of the family therapy approach and is probably the person most identified with the field. His publications range from child psychiatry, psychosomatic research, and social prejudice to international relations. He is the author of *The Psychodynamics of Family Life* and *Exploring the Base for Family Therapy* (Editor) plus several other books and numerous articles. Dr. Franklin is a psychoanalyst and psychiatrist, who for many years has been interested in family dynamics, with special emphasis on "schizophrenic" families.

In Chapter 7 Dr. Lyman C. Wynne addresses himself to the practical question of indications and contraindications for family therapy. Although many practitioners may feel that an attempt to spell out indications and contraindications for family therapy as a treatment of choice may be premature because of the lack of fully developed knowledge, no one can dismiss the courageous views of one of the most experienced family therapists in the country. Besides being a psychiatrist and a psychoanalyst, Dr. Wynne has a doctorate in Social Psychology. He is the originator of several of the key theoretical concepts of transactional family dynamics. His thorough and broad conceptual background enables him to be one of the most profound scientific workers in the field of family dynamics, personality dynamics, thought disorders, and cross-cultural family studies.

Drs. Carl A. Whitaker, Richard E. Felder, and John Warkentin are especially qualified to write Chapter 8 on countertransference in family therapy. They have developed a truly experiential approach to the therapy process in individual as well as family therapy. This chapter is also a documentation of the complex interrelationships of personal and professional aspects of therapy for which the authors are so noted. Dr. Whitaker is a well-known contributor to the field of intensive psychotherapy. He is author (with Thomas P. Malone) of the *Roots of Psychotherapy*, editor of *Psychotherapy of Chronic Schizophrenia*, and author of many articles and book chapters. He has been interested in the therapist-patient relationship and, together with his colleagues at the Atlanta Psychiatric Clinic, he is responsible for the development of the "multiple therapy" approach. Dr. Felder is a psychiatrist who has collaborated with his colleagues at the Atlanta clinic in producing papers on experiential psychotherapy. Dr. Warkentin, a psychiatrist who also has a doctorate in psychology, is known for his perceptive contributions to the experiential aspects of psychotherapy and has had an enduring interest in family therapy.

Chapter 9 by Dr. Ronald D. Laing, a psychoanalyst from England, introduces the concept of mystification for the study of pathogenic communication patterns in families. He illustrates how family members manipulate, confuse, and exert power over one another through mystifying communications. Dr. Laing has been known for his broad interests in existential and psychoanalytic orientations. He is the author of *The Divided Self*, *The Self and Others*, and *Sanity, Madness, and the Family*. Recently he has been studying "normal" families.

In Chapter 10 Drs. Anthony F. C. Wallace and Raymond D. Fogelson, anthropologists, utilize their systematic observation of work at the Family Therapy Project at the Eastern Pennsylvania Psychiatric Institute for the explication of what they designate as the "identity struggle." They attempt to integrate psychoanalytic-psychiatric and anthropological concepts of identity and to highlight the ubiquitous cultural implications of the identity struggle. Dr. Wallace is the author of *Culture and Personality* and of many publications dealing with the cultural aspects of psychiatry. Dr. Fogelson has had a long-standing interest in the anthropological aspects of social psychiatry.

In Chapter 11 Dr. Framo attempts to examine some of the problems involved in doing systematic research on family dynamics by reviewing the contribution of the small-group discipline, critically evaluating systematic studies done on the interacting family unit, focusing on methodological problems in measuring family interaction, and, finally, developing a point of view about research in family dynamics which is intended to orient the researcher in the direction of the most meaningful variables.

In Chapter 12 Dr. Harold F. Searles, one of the foremost contributors to the literature on intensive psychotherapy, particularly of schizophrenia, is especially qualified to write the concluding chapter in this volume. His distinction between intrapsychic and interpersonal processes keynotes what will probably be the major theoretical issue of psychopathology for some time to come. The integration of these two major vantage points will be needed in the development of a complete theory of personality and treatment. Dr. Searles, a training analyst, and formerly associated with Chestnut Lodge, is noted for his original contributions on the subjective experience of the therapist as part of the process of psychotherapy. The International Universities Press has recently published a collection of his papers. He is also the author of *The Nonhuman Environment, in Normal Development and in Schizophrenia*.

During the course of putting together a book such as this, one accumulates many obligations to other people. We could begin with our wives and immediate families and families of origin who helped provide the emotional context and family experience out of which grew, probably, our interest in family in the first place. More concretely, our wives did read over our own manuscripts and helped in the role of sympathetic critics.

We are certainly indebted to our contributors who agreed to go through all the pain and labor of writing a chapter in an edited book. When they had completed their own chapters they helped us work through our own resistances in finishing our work.

Our gratitude to our co-workers on the Family Therapy Project of the Eastern Pennsylvania Psychiatric Institute is expressed in our individual chapters.

The editors and contributors are grateful to the various publishers and authors of books and articles from which material has been quoted in this book.

We owe a debt of appreciation to Mr. Paul Hoeber, our publisher, for his faith and encouragement. Thanks are also due to his staff members Miss Claire Drullard and Mrs. Mitsi Sundvall for their helpfulness.

In the early phases of designing the composition and scope of this volume we received helpful suggestions for contributors from Drs. Harold F. Searles, Norman Elrod, and Lyman C. Wynne.

We are grateful to Rita M. Tocci, not only for typing our manuscripts and other sections of the volume, but also for handling numerous other clerical details.

IVAN BOSZORMENYI-NAGY, M.D.
JAMES L. FRAMO, PH.D.

Philadelphia, Pa.

Introduction

The publication of this book ushers in the depth family transactional approach to psychopathology and treatment. Impetus for editing this volume evolved from our desire to communicate the accumulated experiences and findings of the various pioneers of the relatively new field of family therapy—findings which may have far-reaching implications about the interactional nature of personality dysfunction and its therapeutic handling. The entire spectrum of our current, individual-based concepts will have to be re-examined from the vantage point of observing the individual in the context of his most intimate relationships, the family. In conjoint or unit family therapy the whole family is considered to be the patient, and this "mutation" of traditional approaches to psychopathology introduces not only a new technique of therapy and a new outlook on mental illness, but a new perspective of man.

Family therapy was initially undertaken for both investigative and practical therapeutic management considerations. Workers in the field of intensive family therapy at least implicitly agreed upon a need for redefining illness, i.e., that family relationships are *constituents* of the designated psychiatric condition rather than only environmental factors which influence or historically cause it.

Most of the innovators of this unique approach came from the field of intensive individual psychotherapy of schizophrenic patients; they found, while treating these severe ego disturbances, that they were treating the patients in a vacuum. Treatment progressed only up to the point where insight had to be translated into lasting behavioral changes, then the whole endeavor would collapse, primarily because of regressive unconscious collusion between the family and the patient. These invisible but powerful outside influences, it was reasoned, could only become palpable and manageable if they were integrated into the treatment program. But psychologic investigation and treatment of the whole family had been a long-standing cultural and professional taboo; people had always regarded, almost instinctively, that family matters were private, personal and sacrosanct. Although the genius of Freud led to profound understanding of the intrapsychic world of the individual, his discouragement of involvement of family members in the treatment process of individuals and his view of the individual as a closed system established the practice of exclusion of the family in most forms of psychotherapy. It is understandable, then, that certain early family therapists were reluctant to report publicly their experiences to the professional community and that their experimenting with seeing families together was disclosed surreptitiously to their colleagues. Puzzling treatment failures led to re-examination of the exclusion principle as other therapists began to realize that when they treated a single individual a part of the total problem was not visible, that treatment was often undermined by the family, that it was the unusual patient who could make lasting progress if his family did not change, and that individual therapy often bogged down because the primary emotional investments lay outside the treatment situation.

The thinking of family therapists progressed from seeing the illness in the patient, to seeing it in the relationship between the patient and mother, to realizing that father and "well" siblings were involved in the shared psychopathology and that the patient was not so much a victim but an agent who helped maintain the family pathology, to finally wondering whether the family, aside from being considered the noxious agent, contained the potential for possible change which could be capitalized upon. For many years therapists have had to rely on the reports of patients *about* families or on interviews of family members seen separately; it was only when families were observed interacting together that new and unexpected findings began to emerge. Family therapy offered family members the opportunity to express warded off feelings which had heretofore been expressed indirectly or symbolically, often in hurting ways. The actual, physical presence of the family members within the therapeutic milieu in which co-therapists made explicit that which had been implicit, facilitated the emotional exchanges; the family members were all helped to say things to each other which they had never been able to say before. What began as a practical treatment consideration, however, yielded surplus dividends. The family when intensively studied was found to have its own unique rules, underground, myths, communication network, secrete alliances, loves, and hates. It was learned that no matter how mature some people seemed to be in ordinary social relationships, certain childish features of their personality emerged only when they were in the presence of members of their family. Not only did the most incomprehensible symptoms of the designated patient begin to make sense when seen embedded in the family matrix, but maladaptive motivations seemed to be present not only in the designated patient but subclinically in all the family members. One family member would deal with his own irrationality by projection and then handling the "sickness" in another family member. A turning point in psychiatric thinking was achieved when it was realized that symptoms served to balance forces within the family as well as intrapsychic forces. A deep, unconscious, multiperson motivational structure was found to exist in every family. Behavior, rather than being determined solely by an individual's own psychic forces, was found to be determined, in part, by the motive systems of important others who could gratify or frustrate. It was learned that there is always cross-complicity in what people do to each other, and that the giving, getting, and withholding is reciprocal. Family therapists began to get some inkling of the interlocking, homeostatic system of the family and how, in extremely intricate fashion, the intrapsychic struggles were blended into a transactional whole. If one family member got better, another one had to balance the system and get sick. The reality of the family relationships did not, as feared, contravene dealing with transference; on the contrary, the essence of the family system was found to consist in unitary, hidden interpersonal forces derived in part from the individual members' past intrapsychic conflicts acted out in the present. It was learned, further, that conjoint family therapy arouses the ghosts of the therapists' own internal, relational expectations in a way which is not encountered in individual or conventional group psychotherapy.

Utilizing the insights gained from treating families of schizophrenics, family therapists began to apply family system principles to families with a wide variety of emotional difficulties in living— thus reflecting the transition which this volume underwent during the course of its development in broadening from the area of schizophrenia to the entire range of psychiatric conditions. We could have related the book to concepts of individual psychiatric conditions such as schizophrenia, but we believe that the time has come to replace individual diagnostic thinking with transactional diagnostic thinking.

When books of this type are advertised the cliche-like statement is usually made that "This book is intended for psychiatrists, clinical psychologists, social workers . . . etc." In our judgment it would be more useful if we delineated some examples of the types of concrete situations where the family concept could be productively applied. The entire range of possible application of this approach is far from known. The direct exploration of intimate, close relationships may be the key to many elusive psychotherapeutic problems. The traditional child guidance approach of treating the child with the parents being seen separately may have to be re-evaluated in the light of the family approach. The community mental health centers now being established throughout the country may move more in the direction of family mental health centers. Probation officers dealing with delinquency, suicide prevention centers, family social service agencies, marriage counselors, practitioners in private practice, mental hospitals, rehabilitative centers for the aged and the handicapped, those handling problems of school dropouts and unemployment, etc.—these are only some of the groups which may find the family diagnostic intake interview especially useful in determining the meaning of the presenting problem, even if formal family therapy is never undertaken.

Those who conduct training programs for medical and psychology students have long been concerned about how to counteract an intellectual, de-humanizing approach to man which academic courses often impart; observation of family therapy sessions would provide a direct avenue to an appreciation of real emotional difficulties in living. Psychoanalytic candidates, by becoming familiar with family therapy, will become aware of a whole new dimension of personality disturbances and may be better able to do analysis on an individual basis. Once having seen the individual patient, where he lives, in the fabric of his closest relationships, one can never again look upon psychopathology or even one's own family relationships in the same way.

Exposing intimate family relationships to direct observation and intensive therapeutic scrutiny is bound to lead to new hypotheses about psychopathology, personality, relationships, and society. We do have some words of caution, however. At the present time no one is in a position to scientifically prove that the family transactional method of treatment is preferential to other approaches to any given psychiatric problem, even in those cases where it is feasible. We are only beginning to explore the indications, limits, and safeguards of this form of treatment. The family therapy movement is growing and gaining adherents in almost unprecedented fashion among the mental health professions. We feel it necessary, however, to warn against misuses which over-enthusiasm and lack of knowledge can bring about. Besides, resistance to family therapy can take the form of a negative evaluation of the approach based on the experimentations of the novice. The readers of this book will recognize that competence and experience in individual or group therapy is not sufficient for the undertaking of family therapy; specialized training is necessary. Only time will tell whether or not family therapy truly signifies a major turning point or breakthrough in psychiatric thought and method. All the implications of the family concept are far from full development, and we shall be satisfied to know that our volume has made at least one distinct step in that direction.

IVAN BOSZORMENYI-NAGY, M.D.
JAMES L. FRAMO, PH.D.

1

GERALD H. ZUK

DAVID RUBINSTEIN

A Review of Concepts in the Study and Treatment of Families of Schizophrenics

Nearly a decade of experience has been gained in doing conjoint psychotherapy with families. This chapter aims to establish a sense of order in the historical development of work in family psychotherapy with particular reference to the problem of schizophrenia. Intended as an orientation to this relatively new area rather than as an exhaustive review of the literature, it is divided into three parts: (1) a review of concepts in selected studies which have dealt primarily with dyadic family relationships and in which family psychotherapy itself was not employed as a therapeutic and investigatory technique; (2) a review in greater depth of concepts in selected studies in which the family system was itself the object of therapeutic attention; (3) and, finally, a summary of some assumptions and general characteristics of studies on family systems. Throughout the chapter, the emphasis will be on the establishment of conceptual trends rather than on a critical evaluation of these trends or on a methodologic critique, both of which at this stage in the study of family systems might be premature.

Clinical experience and research in the family system has not yet reached a point of sophistication at which comprehensive and integrated theories are available. It may be said, however, that there is an extensive and active theorizing currently taking place which should eventually produce the desired integration of understanding. To date, psychoanalysis has provided the richest single source of theory, although recently existential theory has been playing an increasing role (see, for example, the study by Whitaker, Felder, Malone, and Warkentin, 1962). Four types of approaches have been made in the formulation of family process, by (1) communication theorists, who have been especially concerned with the relations and levels of meanings of verbal and nonverbal behavior; (2) role theorists, who have explored the effect of role development and assignment on identity formation; (3) intrapsychically-oriented ego theorists, who have investigated the more primitive emotional levels and attempted to define such concepts as self-nonself boundaries and individuation versus symbiosis; and (4) game or strategy theorists (see Haley, 1963) who have addressed themselves to the definition of those networks of relationships in which human beings place themselves and to the definition of the reciprocating behavior in the networks.

There have been three recent reviews presented, describing the stages which have led to the development of family psychotherapy as a method of treatment and psychological study. One by Parloff (1961) describes historical stages. The first stage occurred at the height of orthodoxy in psychoanalytic thinking: contact between therapist and family was discouraged, for it was thought to be poor technique to involve the family because disturbances in the patient-therapist transference and countertransference would be antitherapeutic. In the second stage, certain negative effects of caretaking persons (for example, mothers) were believed worthy of study. The third stage was ushered in with the development of the psychoanalytically oriented positions of Sullivan, Horney, Fromm, Erikson, and others, which gave increasing weight to the influence of culture and current life stress on personality. During the latter part of the second and in the third stage, new therapeutic techniques were tried out: Slavson paved the way for group psychotherapy and Moreno for psychodrama. Favorable experience with these techniques tended to diminish somewhat the anxiety about the effect on transference and countertransference of the presence of more than two persons, namely, the patient and the therapist, in the psychotherapeutic situation.

A review by Jackson and Satir (1961) cites several factors believed to be responsible for the current interest in family treatment of schizophrenia. Among these were the impact of psychologic and sociologic studies which showed differential rates of schizophrenia among social, ethnic, and other subcultural groups in the United States; the established practice of child guidance clinics of treating family members and the child concurrently; and the development of interpersonal theories, such as Sullivan's, which gave greater weight to intercurrent difficulties in patients' lives.

A neat summarization of the historical background of family treatment has been given by Haley (1959). He says that, "A transition would seem to have taken place in the study of schizophrenia; from the early idea that the difficulty in these families was caused by the schizophrenic member, to the idea that they contained a pathogenic mother, to the discovery that the father was inadequate, to the current emphasis upon all three family members involved in a pathological system of interaction" (p. 358).

Family Pathology Studies in the 1940's and 1950's: The "Pathogenic" Mother and "Inadequate" Father

David Levy was one of the first to clearly establish a relationship between a supposedly pathogenic trait in the mother and disturbed behavior in the offspring.

As aptly noted by Spiegel and Bell (1959), Levy's (1943) study of maternal overprotection was a classic of the 1940's. It showed a correlation between an overprotective attitude in mothers and deprivation of love in the mothers' own childhood. The mothers' own deprivation apparently set up a pattern in which they sought to obtain from their children what they had not obtained from their mothers. Levy distinguished between types of overprotectiveness: one type of mother was dominatingly overprotective, another indulgently overprotective. The children of mothers of the first type were submissive at home but had difficulty making friends at school and in the neighborhood; these children tended to have eating problems, but had a relative absence of difficulties relating to sleep or toilet training. Children of mothers of the second type were disobedient at home but were well-behaved at school and got good grades.

Exploratory studies of the pathogenic parent-child relationship were begun as early as the mid-1930's (see, for example, the study of Kasanin, Knight, and Sage, 1934), but a pattern of results did not emerge until studies originated in the mid-1940s were completed. The so-called schizophrenogenic mother, a term first used apparently by Fromm-Reichmann (1948), was described as aggressive, domineering, insecure, and rejecting; by contrast, the father came to be described as inadequate, passive, and rather indifferent. One study (Reichard and Tillman, 1950) classified parents in three ways: schizophrenogenic mother—overtly rejecting type; schizophrenogenic

4 INTENSIVE FAMILY THERAPY

mother—covertly rejecting type; and schizophrenogenic father—domineering and sadistic type. A study of 25 mothers (Tietze, 1949) of schizophrenic children resulted in a broad description of the mothers as rigid and rejecting. In a study by Gerard and Siegel (1950), exclusive attachment to the mother was found in over 90 percent of the cases observed. Thomas (1955) studied the mother-daughter relationship of 18 Negro schizophrenics and concluded that the mothers could not tolerate verbal expression of hostility. The mothers were excessively punitive with the patients after puberty. Interestingly, the majority of the fathers in these families had either died or separated from or deserted the mother. Galvin (1956) found that maternal overcontrol, which is not readily admitted by mothers of schizophrenic patients, is exerted by appeals to pity, shame, and guilt.

A few studies done in the middle and late 1940's and early 1950's dealt with the general adequacy of the families in which one of the members was schizophrenic. Lidz and Lidz (1949) found only 5 patients in a hospitalized sample of 50 who were considered to have had an adequate home life. In the case of 40 percent of these patients, one or both of the parents had died before the patient was 19 years old. Rosenzweig and Bray (1943), in a study based on a sample of 356 male hospitalized schizophrenics, found that 39 percent had experienced the death of a sibling. The authors suggested that intense feelings of hostility toward a sibling who subsequently died may have caused a sense of pervading guilt which triggered a psychotic episode. Ellison and Hamilton (1949) found in more than 30 percent of a sample of 100 cases that the stability of the family was disturbed by the early death of a member or by a divorce or separation. Three-fifths of the mothers in the sample were found to be excessively overprotective. One-third of the fathers were found to be overaggressive. Johnson, Griffin, Watson, and Beckett (1956) noted frequent instances of physical or psychological assault by parents on children who later became schizophrenic. Studies by Wahl (1954, 1956) give support to the suggestion that loss of a parent in childhood or adolescence may be a precipitating factor in schizophrenia. In a study often cited as a landmark in establishing the concept of transmission of psychopathology from parents to children, Johnson and Szurek (1954) pointed out that antisocial behavior in children was based on a superego defect which corresponded with superego defects in their parents.

A number of writers have called attention to the deficiencies in experimental control in the studies of the 1940's and 1950's. Sanua (1961), in his review, points to the need for caution in drawing firm conclusions from these studies. Important variables were often uncontrolled, such as, for example, social class, educational level, and ethnic and religious origin. A few investigators carefully described some of the limitations of their work. Kohn and Clausen (1956), in their study of experiences recalled from early adolescence by schizophrenic patients, took pains to present their results as suggestive rather than firm. They noted that their results were based on small numbers of patients and social class was not rigorously controlled. A positive feature in their experimental design, however, was that they did have a control group of subjects who had gone to the same schools as the schizophrenic patients being investigated. Their main finding was that schizophrenic patients, more frequently than normal controls of comparable background, reported that their mothers played a comparatively strong authority role in the family.

Also in the late 1940's and early 1950's some interesting new experiments in therapy technique were being undertaken. Among others, Ross (1948), Bauer and Gurevitch (1952), and Kirby and Priestman (1957) used the technique of group psychotherapy with schizophrenic patients and their parents. Abrahams and Varon (1953) studied the relationship between mothers and schizophrenic daughters in conjoint group psychotherapy. The mothers' own great emotional dependence on the daughters was revealed in the sessions. The need of the mothers to feel superior was maintained at the cost of the daughters feeling worthless. Acute maternal anxiety was precipitated when the daughters refused to conform to expectations. On these occasions, some of the mothers reported that they had lost their sense of being alive, or of being a separate person. In 1956, Szurek and Berlin reported positive results in the simultaneous psychotherapy of more than 100 schizophrenic children and their parents.

At about the same time novel therapy techniques were being applied to marital couples one of which was neurotic or psychotic. Oberndorf (1938) and later Mittelman (1956) described numerous patterns of neurotic interaction between marriage partners, including the description, by Mittelman, of the couple one of whom is emotionally detached while the other has strong needs for affection. Bychowski (1956) has described the interaction in marriages in which the partners are psychotic or pre-psychotic. He was pessimistic about a good therapeutic outcome in the case of schizophrenic marital partners, since he believed the marital choice was based on pathologic motives in the first place. Neubeck (1954), Wolf (1950), Moreno (1954) and Whitaker (1958b) have also worked with marriage partners concurrently. The book edited by Eisenstein (1956) reports some interesting studies of the psychotherapy of marriage partners.

(Reference is made in this section to authors of several chapters in the book by Eisenstein). A major concept underlying the work with neurotic and psychotic married couples was that the marriage was based on pathologic needs and expectations and that even the choice of the mate was determined in large part by prior pathology originating in a nuclear family situation.

The concept "symbiotic tie," referring particularly to a pathogenic relationship between mother and child, came into currency in the 1950's. The phrase was one of those which helped usher in a new period of greater attention to the pattern of pathogenic relationships within families rather than concern only with the isolation of an array of negative traits of individual family members. In children Mahler (1952) described the "symbiotic syndrome." Of this condition she said that it aimed at restoring the symbiotic-parasitic fantasy of oneness with the mother. In the syndrome of "infantile autism," Kanner (1949) stated that the child was unable to utilize the symbiotic relation with the mother to orient himself to the inner or outer world.

Limentani (1956) studied the symbiotic tie between adult schizophrenic patients and their mothers and found strong unconscious wishes to return to the infantile states, to remain attached to the mother or to the therapist in the fashion of small children. The passivity which the patients expressed protected them from the danger of opposing their mothers' demands and acknowledging their own feelings of worthlessness. When the patient could accept the therapist as a person with whom he could establish a relationship similar to that with his mother, Limentani believed that the patient could recover from the overt part of the psychosis.

Hill (1955) gave considerable attention to the symbiosis between mother and child in cases of schizophrenia. He held that the mother is a living, internalized presence in the patient's ego. He pointed out that the mother of the schizophrenic gives love excessively but conditionally. The patient believes that if he gets well, his mother will get sick. By staying sick, he preserves his mother's mental, as well as physical, sense of well-being. But by meeting her conditions, the patient forfeits development of an independent personality. Hill's description of the symbiotic tie goes in some respects beyond the usual interpretation of that concept by positing a two-way interdependency between mother and child. His formulation is more attuned to the current interest in the gestalt of relationships among family members, that is, in the interlocking and reciprocity of mutual needs.

In summarizing this section briefly, it can be said that a sizable number of studies about pathologic family interactions appeared in the 1940's and 1950's. Some stressed theoretical conceptualizations; others reported experiences, observations, and statistics. A major effort was made to relate certain abnormal traits in parents with the same or other abnormal traits in offspring; emphasis was on dyadic relationships. Parallel developments in therapeutic technique were taking place which made it practicable to consider an approach in which the pathologic family *system* would itself become the central object of attention, rather than pathology in the individual family member or in the dyadic relationship between family members.

Family Pathology and Treatment in the 1950's and
Early 1960's: The "Pathogenic" Family

Spiegel and Bell (1959) have commented on the relatively late emergence of interest in the functioning of the family as a biosocial unit in relation to mental illness. They point out that, "Isolated aspects of the total picture—selected traits of the relationship of the parents and child, or of siblings, selected situational or psychodynamic factors—have been extensively investigated, but such relationships are almost always dealt with out of context, as if the family-as-a-whole did not exist" (p. 114). The authors note, however, that within the past decade a new approach has been gaining adherents, an approach still largely based on psychoanalytic theory but attempting to avoid those aspects of the theory which experience has shown to be unsatisfactory. This approach seeks to avoid a rigid dichotomy between organism and environment, substituting the focus of the patient-in-the-family. One assumption of this approach is that the patient is a *symptom* of the family pathology. Accordingly, work with the patient in isolation from the family gives inadequate results. The family must be treated as a biosocial unit in order to establish a new equilibrium in which the patient as well as other family members can improve their psychological functioning. Richardson's book (1948) was an early contribution to the evolving concept of the family as a biosocial unit of study and treatment, as was an article by Josselyn (1953).

Midelfort (1957) was one of the early workers in the family treatment approach to the problem of schizophrenia, stating that, "Family therapy is an example of group therapy, and it utilizes the assets in the family group to make real and external, or objective, those activities that satisfy the person's social and cultural needs" (p. 12). (It should be noted that Handlon and Parloff [1962] have pointed out some major differences between family therapy and regular group psychotherapy.) Midelfort believes that the family unit is strengthened by bringing together the various members and he encourages constant attendance at therapy sessions by relatives. He believes that beneficial therapeutic results follow when the family members interact in an affectionate and loving way with the patient, and he presents data which seem to substantiate his impression that patients with families who give this type of support do better than patients with families who do not.

Midelfort stresses the importance of a community of cultural factors between the patient and the therapist, believing that a similar ethnic and religious background enhances the possibility of a successful course of treatment. The therapist who comes from a different ethnic or religious background may be perceived as an intruder who wishes to deprive the family of its unique standards and values.

Midelfort suggests that the so-called sick member is one who has experienced excessive pressure to maintain the subculture of the family; or he is the one who has undergone a crisis which threatens his sense of belonging to the family. The person may actually wish to continue as a member but feels isolated and unable to relate himself meaningfully to other people. In Midelfort's opinion, a change in the behavior of family members can increase the likelihood of a beneficial change in the patient. The patient, of course, is the symptomatic member of the family, but his behavior merely reflects the existence of a general family pathology. Disturbance in other family members who appear conforming may be perceived upon close perusal of their behavior.

Midelfort's work, impressionistic as it was, was a stimulus in focusing attention on the problem of family pathology in schizophrenia. He was one of the first workers to show the promise of family treatment. At about the same time, others began a more methodologic exploration of family relationships in family therapy in order to assess the value of family therapy not only as a method of treating schizophrenia but also as a means of exploring multiple levels of personality functioning.

One of these others was Bowen (1959, 1960). He began his study with the working hypothesis that the basic character disturbance out of which schizophrenia developed was an unresolved symbiotic attachment to the mother. But after a year's work with several mothers and their schizophrenic daughters in a milieu treatment program, he was forced to revise his hypothesis. He now considered the schizophrenic reaction of the patient as a symptom of a larger pathology in the family, and he revised his treatment plan so that as many of the family members as possible could be included. He arranged to have several families, consisting of patient, mother, and father, live in a hospital ward for periods up to two and a half years. The parents were given the principal responsibility for care of the patients, but it was found that the parents asked for and even demanded the intervention of staff at troublesome times in family interaction. Bowen observed that each family member had his own conception of what the family stood for. Also, each member exhibited different behavior while "inside" and while "outside" the family setting. These families were in serious emotional tumoil. Bowen comments on the character of the tense emotional climate as follows: "A nonparticipant observer might aspire to scientific objectivity, but, in the emotional tension that surrounds these families, he begins to participate emotionally in the family drama just as surely as he inwardly cheers the hero and hates the villain when he attends the theatre" (p. 351).

Bowen became interested in the three-generation hypothesis to account for the development of a schizophrenic process. This hypothesis was originally formulated by Hill (1955), who wrote that: ". . . mothers of schizophrenics almost uniformly report their respect for their mothers . . . through their mothers they have come to idealize motherhood—they believe in the divinity of motherhood" (p. 113). Hill noted that the grandmothers of schizophrenics tended to rule the roost at home, and the mothers learned the technique of domination from them. They skillfully created a sense of pervading guilt in their children.

Bowen's version of the three-generation hypothesis runs as follows: "The grandparents were relatively mature but their combined immaturities were acquired by one child who was most attached to the mother. When this child married a spouse with an equal degree of immaturity, and when the same process repeated itself in the third generation, it resulted in one child (the patient) with a high degree of immaturity, while the other siblings were more mature." (1960, p. 354). Those interested in current studies which bear on the three-generation hypothesis should see the reports by Mendell and Fisher (1958), Fisher and Mendell (1956), and Sivadon (1957).

The concept of emotional divorce is used by Bowen to explain an important feature of the married life of parents of schizophrenic offspring. This term encompasses a wide range of behavior: it may signify a relationship in which the marital partners seem to have few overt differences and live conforming lives but in which highly charged personal feelings are not shared; on the other hand, it may describe a marital relationship in which the partners appear congenial in ordinary social settings but cannot tolerate each other when alone together. Both parents are immature, but one may deny the immaturity and function with a facade of overadequacy, while the other functions as the overtly inadequate person. The overadequate parent seems to make the major decisions affecting the family, but in reality is unable to do so. Circumstances compel decisions or appeal to outside authorities is made. It should be noted that the level of adequacy is not fixed but may shift back and forth between parents.

Bowen conceives of projection as having major psychological importance in the mother-child relationship in schizophrenia. By this he means that the mother projects onto the child her own sense of inadequacy or helplessness, which the child accepts. The mother then cares not for the child for himself but for the image of herself which she has projected onto the child. Bowen has observed instances ". . . in which the soma of one person reciprocates with the psyche of another person" (1960, p. 361). By this he implies a transfer of basic feelings and anxieties between persons, for example, mother and child. In this facet of projection he describes a process similar to that described earlier by Harry Stack Sullivan (1948) in his term "anxiety induction." Sullivan believed that is was possible for anxiety to flow between persons, especially when there pre-existed a relationship of high emotional charge.

The major threat to the mother in the mother-child symbiosis, according to Bowen, is growth of the child. The passage from one developmental level to another can drive the mother to increased demands, threats, or even retaliations. The emotional equilibrium established in the first few years of the child's life is disturbed by the child's growth. Adolescence is a particularly critical stage because of the numerous physiologic, social, and psychological developments in this period. A move toward independence by the child at this stage brings a sharp response from the mother to force the child back into the helpless position. Bowen reports one patient who became psychotic at 15 years of age after failing in efforts to free himself in some degree from a domineering mother. Others succeed in attaining some independence at adolescence only to fail at a later stage, perhaps as a result of stress upon entering college, taking a first job, or getting married.

Bowen believes that loosening of fixed family patterns occurred in a few of the cases he treated. He observed that the patient could improve when the parents became more emotionally responsive to each other. The patient could then even tolerate some criticism by the parents and could also accept management from them. If an improved relationship between the parents later deteriorated, however, it was found that the patient's condition would also deteriorate.

Brodey (1959) has reported on the families seen in the project directed by Bowen. He formulates the type of relationship observed in the families as a circular or feedback system in which ". . . what is produced by the cause simultaneously affects the causal force" (p. 379). He comments on the difficulty the staff and families had in working with one another. Staff members became "stand-in" parental figures, and clashes occurred between these "stand-in" figures and the actual parents when one group attempted to test the vulnerability of the other.

Brodey contends that the potentially schizophrenic child is the battleground on which the parents attempt to work out serious conflicts. However, in focusing their attention on himself rather than on themselves, the patient makes it more difficult for his parents to resolve their differences. They seek a resolution through him, and thus the nuclear family unit is bound in a circular situation in which there is a high narcissistic investment by all parties.

Although they did not investigate the process of family psychotherapy itself, Lidz, Cornelison, Fleck, and Terry (1957a) did study the intrafamilial environment of 14 families with a schizophrenic member. Family members were interviewed over periods ranging from six months to two years. In this study the requirement was that the mother be living and available for therapeutic as well as general interviews and also that one other sibling be living who could be compared with the patient. Records of family interaction were kept, and home visits were made by various staff members. Diaries and other personal effects were studied and projective testing was carried out.

The father in the family in which one member is schizophrenic was a major focus of the study by Lidz *et al.* (1957a) referred to above. In a prior study (Lidz and Lidz, 1949), it was concluded that the influence of the father was often as noxious as that of the mother. Had some of the fathers been more stable figures, it was thought, the potentially schizophrenic child might not have become so embroiled in the pathologic symbiosis with the mother. In studies by Hajdu-Gimes (1940), Ellison and Hamilton (1949), and Frazee (1953), it was revealed that a proportion of the fathers of schizophrenics were cruel and rejecting.

In the follow-up study on fathers of schizophrenics, Lidz *et al.* (1957a) discussed five types of fathers. A first group was composed of fathers of some female patients who were in serious conflict with their wives. These men tried to undercut their wives' authority by seeking to align the daughters on their side. Having been disappointed in their marriages, they sought to mold their daughters to satisfy their needs. They tended to be somewhat paranoid, unreasonable in their demands, and generally distrustful. The fathers' hostility to their wives could be observed in their, at times, overt sexual seductiveness toward their daughters.

A second group of fathers was described as turning hostility toward their children rather than toward their wives. This group was comprised of fathers of male patients. They behaved as might jealous older siblings and experienced a sense of rivalry with sons for their wives' attention. They belittled the sons and sabotaged their self-confidence. Confused by the jealous demands of the husbands, the wives tended to turn to the sons for affection. The sons, in turn, sensing the ineptness of the fathers in filling their role as husbands, sought to fill the vacuum in their mothers' lives. These fathers were intensely narcissistic, showed paranoid ideation and suspiciousness, and were subject to violent temper tantrums.

A third group of fathers was characterized as having an exalted concept of themselves. Although some did exhibit real capacities and achievements, these they regarded as nothing compared to their grandiose estimate of themselves. The fathers were aloof and distant from their children. The children were impressed from an early age with the idea that they could not attain the heights of their fathers. Wives supported their husbands' fantasies about their omnipotence, at the same time depriving the children of attention. The children may have recognized that the fathers' self-glorification existed only in fantasy, yet this merely contributed to the childrens' distrust of people and to their faulty superego formation.

A fourth group of fathers were described as failures in life. They scarcely concerned themselves with care for the children since they were so absorbed in their conviction of personal worthlessness. They were pathetic figures, without prestige in the family, scorned by their wives. A fifth group of fathers were very passive men, totally accepting the dominant role of their wives in the marriage. They gave passive support to their wives but never made major decisions affecting the family. They were inadequate male identification figures, although in some cases they were pleasant men and affectionate with the children.

Recently, Lidz and Fleck (1960) critically reviewed their work on the intrafamilial environment of families with schizophrenic members. In this paper they focussed attention on pathology in the marriage relationship, stating that, "The anxieties conveyed to the child by the mother may have less to do with her concerns about the child than with her concern about her husband. Rejective behavior by a parent may reflect the wish to be rid of the marriage to which the child binds" (p. 335). The authors stress the failure of schizophrenic families to differentiate clearly between the two generations most directly involved in nuclear family relationships. They have used the terms marital schism and marital skew (see the study by Lidz, Cornelison, Fleck, and Terry, 1957b) to characterize the disturbed relationship. In both these processes there is a mutual failure of the marital partners to meet each other's deep dynamic needs: in the first case, families stay together despite overt scrapping; in the second, overt harmony masks covert disagreement. Marital schisms and marital skews pave the way for a seduction of children by one parent or the other into a pathologic alliance.

Lyman Wynne has been interested in the development of concepts which might explain underlying pathogenic processes in families. A paper by Wynne, Ryckoff, Day, and Hirsch (1958) reports on work with families of hospitalized schizophrenics begun as part of a major project on family therapy. Patients received intensive psychotherapy in the hospital and parents were seen concurrently twice weekly on an outpatient basis. Data were collected from other family members, the nursing staff, and the ward administrator. This particular paper is based on very intensive concurrent psychotherapy with patients and families, although the authors are also experienced in conjoint family psychotherapy.

The authors describe some forms of interpersonal group relationship. One is pseudomutuality, a form of relationship believed to be particularly pathogenic. Pseudomutuality is a type of relatedness in which there is a preoccupation of family members with a fitting-together into formal roles at the expense of individual identity. While in true mutuality family members can experience a sense of personal identity and separateness, in pseudomutuality divergence is forbidden. Family members strive to maintain an outward appearance of uniformity. The authors contend that ". . . the pseudomutual relation involves a characteristic dilemma: divergence is perceived as leading to disruption of the relation and therefore must be avoided; but if divergence is avoided, growth of the relation is impossible" (p. 207).

Wynne *et al.* (1958) suggest that the typical organization of the family with a schizophrenic member is one in which there are a limited number of fixed roles, but the family members may shift in these fixed roles and there may even be competition for certain roles. In one case that the authors describe, two daughters exchanged roles during adolescence: the one who had been the "good" child became wild and rebellious and had a psychotic episode; the "bad" child became meek, passive, and obedient.

In families in which there is a potential schizophrenic member, the authors state, divergence is not merely excluded from awareness but mechanisms are applied by which future threats to uniformity may be aborted. Despite this, divergence is an omnipresent threat, if for no other other reason than that almost anything that happens to the family can be interpreted as a source of possible divergence.

When they talk about mechanisms to reduce divergence, the authors make it clear that they mean not only conscious concealment of information but a more basic and unconscious process: "The problem is a more primary failure of the ego in articulating the meaning of experience and participation, not so much a defense by the ego against the conscious recognition of particular meanings" (Wynne et al., 1958, p. 210).

In families which practice a high degree of pseudomutuality, the members act as if they were truly in a self-contained unit. The pseudomutual structure is supported by a variety of means, among which are myths and ideologies about the family. Children are rewarded when they behave with uniformity and dependently toward the family, but they are punished when they behave independently. In one case reported, the authors discovered that right up until the time a son was hospitalized the parents seemed oblivious of the changes that were taking place in him. They seemed quite unaware of the disturbed, anxious state expressed in letters he had written. His disturbance had become acute as a result of ambivalence about efforts to become more independent of the family. In other cases, secrecy was used as a means of forestalling divergence. The potentially schizophrenic member was denied important information; or the patient's activities were secretly investigated by the family, although they strenuously supported the view that the patient's life was his own affair.

Pathologic family relationship as a major causative factor in schizophrenia is espoused by Wynne et al. (1958) in a statement in which they contend that: "The fragmentation of experience, the identity diffusion, the disturbed modes of perception and communication, and certain other characteristics of the acute reactive schizophrenic's structure are to a significant extent derived, by process of internalization, from characteristics of the family social organization" (p. 215). In some cases the role structure of the family is internalized by the patient as a primitive superego which directly determines behavior. The person's self is embedded in the superego; his identity is largely determined by its actions. A schizophrenic panic can then occur at some critical phase in development when the self attempts to separate itself from the primitive superego. The authors make the point that pseudomutuality is a phenomenon which may be observed generally in families, although it is especially intense and enduring in families in which there is a schizophrenic member. The acute schizophrenic episode represents a breakdown of pseudomutuality, an attempt to restore it, and an attempted individuation by the disturbed family member in which only partial individuation is attained.

Wynne (1961) more recently describes concepts of alignment and split in the families of schizophrenics. Alignment is defined as the perception that two or more family members are joined in a common bond and have positive feelings toward one another in carrying out the purpose of their bond. In split there is an experience of opposition between family members, with a negative emotional component involved. To a large degree, the alignment and split in families determine the emotional equilibrium. In the same paper, Wynne also describes a concept of pseudohostility as behavior in which there seems to be a split ". . . which may be exceedingly noisy and intense but remains limited to a surface level of experience and interaction . . . Pseudohostility serves to blur and obscure the impact, on the one hand, of anxiety-producing intimacy and affection and, on the other hand, of deepening hostility unfolding to destruction, acknowledged helplessness, and lasting separation" (p. 110).

A study by Ryckoff, Day, and Wynne (1959) describes a particular role pattern observed in families with a schizophrenic member in which family roles were oversimplified, rigid, and stereotyped. This inhibiting pattern prevents adequate identity formation and contributes to serious crises. A yet more recent study (Schaffer, Wynne, Day, Ryckoff, and Halperin, 1962) inquires into the interesting predicament that occurs when the value systems of the therapist and the family clash. The authors summarize the predicament as follows:

The psychiatrist, in his efforts to introduce the idea of relation and continuity, violates the culture of the family: In just the same way, the family's responses—the systematic destruction of meaning and the denial of authenticity—are experienced by the psychiatrist as acts of extreme violence. These exchanges—which have very little to do with conversation—both among the family and between them and the psychiatrists, are essentially characterized by the mutual failure or inability to understand, tolerate or confirm the other's experience (p. 44).

In 1956, Bateson, Jackson, Haley, and Weakland published a report in which they sought to formulate a comprehensive theory of schizophrenia. The paper presented broad outlines of a theory focusing on the aspect of communication, both verbal and nonverbal. The important concept of the double-bind was elaborated in this paper. The requirements of the double-bind situation are as follows: at least two persons are needed, including one who may be designated the "victim"; there must be a repetition of important themes or experience made to the victim; there must be negative injunctions; there must be conflicting levels of injunctions with threat of punishment for disobedience; and there must be further injunctions which prevent the victim from escaping the field of communication. The so-called "victim" comes to perceive his life as based on a certain number of key double-bind interactions with important personages, such as parents. More than two persons can be engaged in double-bind interaction; for example, with an offspring one parent may negate at a more abstract level a communication of the other.

Bateson *et al.* (1956) described the pathologic double-bind situation between the schizophrenic and his family as follows: a mother who is made anxious and hostile by the threat of too much closeness with her child and who responds to her hostility by assuming a too loving attitude toward the child; and the absence of a strong and insightful figure (for example, the father) who could support the child. The mother's great problem is control of her anxiety in connection with the child. She aims to do this by manipulating communication in order to produce the degree of emotional proximity she can tolerate. The child may come to be aware that her too loving attitude cloaks a basic hostility, but if he is to retain whatever love she can give he must not permit himself to communicate this knowledge to her. He recognizes that it is dangerous for him to interpret accurately her deeper feelings and thoughts. As the authors put it: "The child is punished for discriminating accurately what she is expressing, and he is punished for discriminating inaccurately—he is caught in a double-bind" (p. 258).

The pathologic double-bind produces a wide range of disturbing affect: helplessness, fear, exasperation, and rage, among others. These reactions in the child may be completely ignored by the mother. The father may be outraged by the mother's behavior toward the child, but he remains passive because of the peculiar relationship he has with his wife. The child's psychosis is a means of dealing with the double-bind situation. It has on the one hand the effect of disrupting the double-bind; yet on the other hand the patient often merely recreates the same double-bind situation or creates new ones which are even more pathologic.

Jackson (1957) is a strong exponent of the family treatment method. He has described a concept of family homeostasis, a hypothetical condition in which change in one family member effects changes in others in the family. In one case he cites, a husband called the psychiatrist to inform him that his wife, who had been undergoing psychotherapy for recurrent depression, was planning to commit suicide The psychiatrist replied that he thought the wife had actually shown improvement in her condition. The husband shot himself to death the day after the telephone call. Jackson's conclusion was that there was a pathologic homeostasis between the marital partners; the husband became self-destructive when the wife began to give up thoughts of self-destruction.

In another paper, Jackson (1961) discusses some of the advantages and disadvantages of family psychotherapy. One advantage is that use of the technique increases the chances of breaking the schizophrenic's communication "code." The therapist is present as the patient and family members attempt to qualify or disqualify their messages to each other, and so he can trace the process by which communication tends to move to a pathologic level. The chief disadvantage cited by Jackson is the danger that family psychotherapy will create severe family disharmony, with consequent outbursts of alcoholism, psychosomatic disorders, separation and divorce. In this paper, Jackson also mentions—and it is one of the first references to it—the problems inherent in the relationship between the members of the therapeutic team.

Haley (1959) has considered ways in which the three persons of the nuclear family can interact in the instance of families with a schizophrenic member. In these families he contends there is incongruence between what is said and what is intended. Statements are made, then qualified and contradicted. Haley suggests that, by denying himself rational communication, the schizophrenic actually governs the communication of others. By excluding normal social relationships, he forces a situation which requires that he be hospitalized. Haley concludes: "The more a person tries to avoid being governed or governing others, the more helpless he becomes and so governs others by forcing them to take care of him" (p. 372).

Weakland (1960) says the double-bind situation involves a pair of messages of different levels ". . . which are related but incongruent with each other" (p. 376), and he points out that such concepts as the double-bind can be adapted to three-party as well as two-party interactions. He refers to concepts developed by such workers as Lidz, Bowen, and Wynne as ones which can fall within the purview of the communication theory of Bateson and his co-workers. For example, Wynne's concept of pseudomutuality ". . . implies the existence of some messages claiming closeness while others indicate the reverse" (p. 382). Weakland refers to a finding of Stanton and Schwartz (1954) that patients who became pathologically excited were often the objects of staff disagreement and frequently quieted when the disagreement was resolved in a mutually satisfactory way. Weakland uses this finding as an example of the way in which contradictory communication to the patient may be involved in very complex group interactions.

On the basis of experience with individual and family treatment undertaken concurrently, Boszormenyi-Nagy (1962) has developed the concept of pathologic need complementarity. He became interested in how unconscious needs for possession in the parents shape the psychic structure of the child. The unconscious needs are transmitted to the child as rigid superego demands which the child accepts in a passive way. By accepting such demands, the child's dependent needs are gratified. In this situation, needs are reciprocally gratified; parents and child mutually feed each other's narcissistic demands. Repetition of this reciprocal need gratification becomes a preoccupation of the child, and he fails to achieve an identity which would make possible an existence independent of the family.

According to Boszormenyi-Nagy, pathologic need complementarity may have the value of overcoming feelings of loneliness, helplessness, or isolation. Parents who have been deprived of their own parents through loss or separation may seek unconsciously to recover the lost parent through a relationship with the child, especially if the marital partner fails to gratify this need. The child is then transformed into a parent-like figure. Boszormenyi-Nagy contrasts his concept of pathologic need complementarity with Wynne's pseudomutuality, stating that: "Whereas the concept of pseudomutuality connotes a 'sense of relation' which becomes a 'hollow and empty experience' . . . the concept of need complementarity stresses a regressive, but 'meaningful' . . . experience of relatedness between family members. The complementarity of deep needs among the various family members, along with the other factors, such as specific communication patterns, or internalization of the 'overall family role structure' . . . help to make up a 'homeostasis' . . ." (p. 14).

Boszormenyi-Nagy and Framo (1962) have recently coined the term "family transference" to account for the tendency of a hospital setting—staff, physical surroundings, other patients, and so on—to evoke a family-like atmosphere for some patients. The authors point out a correspondence between the hospital setting and family living because both are ". . . uniquely conducive toward the stimulation of relatively unrestrained expressions of hostility and of infantile forms of sexuality (physical handling, bodily exposure, sharing of physical intimacies, etc.) with a minimum of social consequences. Intensive temptations and taboos pervade both family and hospital living" (p. 3). In the hospital setting described by the authors, it was possible for the patients to discover relationships which substituted for or diluted pathologic relationships established within the family. The therapeutic milieu developed sibling-like relationships between patients, and there was a tendency to recreate the parent-child relationship with the staff. Transference and countertransference were observed in some of the personnel who needed guidance in overcoming resentment when a favored patient seemed to reject or withdraw from their attempts to give aid.

In a recent publication, Whitaker, Felder, Malone, and Warkentin (1962) spell out their basic commitment to family-oriented treatment: "It appears now that the most effective way to neutralize critically pathogenic relationships is to treat the whole family of the schizophrenic as a unit" (p. 157). Their approach is described in the book edited by Whitaker (1958a). Whitaker and Malone describe a process in the marriage of the parents of schizophrenic children similar to that described by Bowen and Lidz: namely, the emotional separation of the parents. In their clinical work they find confirmation in families of schizophrenics of a dominant mother and inadequate father. The parents attempt to gratify needs through the children rather than through each other. These writers have made interesting use of a therapeutic technique involving the use of more than one psychotherapist per patient. They use an intensive relationship therapy to which they have sometimes applied the word "experiential."

An outstanding practical development affecting work in family psychotherapy is publication of a journal edited by Jay Haley, *Family Process*. The journal emphasizes systematic research in the various aspects of family life, and in a recent issue Haley (1962a) reviewed the various approaches to the study and treatment of the family. Haley himself described the family as a homeostatic system in which change in one part produces a reaction in another part. Change can be effective if it occurs at a key point. Haley (1962b) has also presented some problems involved in design, sampling, and measurement in family therapy research. He has attempted to classify certain transactions occurring among family members and has devised a novel setting and method of measurement of family behavior. Family groups were observed by him for the number and types of coalitions that occurred.

The concept of symbiosis was reviewed in another article in *Family Process* by Towne, Messinger and Sampson (1962). Symbiotic involvements in the family are more complex than ordinarily considered: they always involve a third party who is essential for the maintenance of the system. Three symbiotic patterns are described: the merger, conversion, and oscillation.

In one of the few papers on theory of technique of family psychotherapy, Framo (1962) has examined different aspects of resistance, transference, and teamwork in the therapy structure. Family therapy conducted in the patient's home has been described by Friedman (1962). He believes this method gives the advantage of direct observation of the natural habitat of the family. Sonne, Speck, and Jungreis (1962) studied a particular form of resistance in families which they term the "absent-member maneuver." This maneuver is thought to be a way in which the family resists maturation and a way of defending against anxiety generated in the course of therapy. MacGregor (1962) reports on multiple impact therapy with 55 families with problem adolescents; in this type of therapy the family and other involved persons meet with the therapists for intensive sessions lasting two or three days.

In another article in *Family Process*, Zuk, Boszormenyi-Nagy, and Heiman (1963) present evidence for the existence of a complementary process affecting the laughter behavior in family psychotherapy sessions with three family members, one of whom is schizophrenic. At the point in the sessions when laughter typically occurred most frequently in the schizophrenic daughter, it occurred least frequently in the parents; at the point it was least frequent in the daughter, it was most frequent in the parents. In a follow-up investigation of the meaning of laughter, Zuk (1964) presents evidence to show how laughter may be used to disguise or qualify information; how it may be used to maintain an alliance among family members against outsiders; and how it may be used to discourage psychotherapists from pursuing certain lines of inquiry.

Titchener, D'Zmura, Golden, and Emerson (1963) make a useful contribution by defining two terms frequently applied to family systems: pattern and style. The authors state that, "By *patterns* we mean a sequence of actions involving two or more family members which is repetitive, has some degree of automaticity, and is employed as part of the adaptive function of the family system. . . . When we speak of *style* we are referring to the whole organization and fitting together of many patterns in a family adaptation" (p. 113).

In a review article, Meissner (1964) describes some strengths and limitations of predominant theoretical positions. He points out that communication theory does not provide for the "fact" of the psychotic break, nor does it explain differences between psychotic and prepsychotic communication. Role theory does not explain why one child in a family "inherits" the psychotic role while another does not. Meissner asks whether any transactional theory can adequately incorporate the complexity of events in the family system. He suggests, however, that the really significant variables may reside in a yet to be developed theory of a primitive emotional level of existence.

Interesting recent papers on techniques and theory of family psychotherapy have, to be sure, appeared in other pages than those of *Family Process*. Rosenbaum (1961) discusses patient-family similarities in schizophrenia. James Jackson (1962) describes how he has used family therapy to help overcome stalemates in individual psychotherapy. Carroll (1960) reports on his experience with families of disturbed children in conjoint family therapy. Reidy (1962), Goolishian (1962) and Cutter and Hallowitz (1962) also report their experiences with conjoint family therapy in work with disturbed children. Goolishian's report describes the "multiple impact" study and treatment of the family developed by the group with which he is associated.

Work on family processes has also been reported by European and other foreign investigators. Lyketsos (1959), Main (1958), Elles (1962), Howells (1961) and Schindler (1958) have contributed significant observations on family psychopathology. Rubinstein (1960) has suggested a concept of "schizogenia" which stresses that the pathologic process occurs in the "genus," the family, in contrast to the concept of schizophrenia which has signified that the locus of the illness is in the individual.

A number of workers in the past few years, while not focusing their attention directly on the problem of schizophrenia, have made contributions of value to the study of family pathology in mental illness. Among those with a primarily clinical background are: Nathan Ackerman, John Spiegel, John Bell, and Martin Grotjahn.

One of the prominent exponents of family treatment and diagnosis is Ackerman (1957, 1958, 1960) who has been working with family groups for some time, primarily with parents and disturbed children. His system of diagnostic appraisal stresses the participation of the family as a whole from the very first. He believes that by seeing the family together from the first interview he obtains a more accurate impression of dynamic problems than if he interviewed family members separately or obtained a history from another professional person. Ackerman's technique is to focus on what is of immediate distress to the family rather than problems that might be recalled from the past. He participates actively in both diagnostic and treatment processes, often taking the role of an older relative or counselor in treatment sessions.

More recently, Ackerman (1962) has pointed out essential differences between psychoanalysis and family psychotherapy. The psychoanalytic model is a one-person phenomenon, and although influenced by an external agent, the psychoanalyst, this phenomenon is essentially nonsocial in that persons and situations affecting the daily life of the patient are not brought into the foreground of the therapy. The family psychotherapy model is a two-person or more phenomenon and fully social. Events of both intrapsychic and interpersonal origin are jointly considered in this type of therapy.

Spiegel (1957), although not primarily concerned with the treatment process in itself, has shown an interest in problems of role transactions in families in which one member is mentally disturbed. He points out that the family is a small-scale system that is constantly shifting in its equilibrium. There is a high level of complementarity of roles in the family, decision-making takes place at a low level, events tend to occur in automatic fashion, and there is considerable spontaneity in family members interacting with each other. These are features which tend to characterize all families. There are particular sources of strain, however, that give rise to disequilibrium. One source is role conflict. In his paper, Spiegel describes various means by which equilibrium is re-established in the family. Role modification can be an outcome of a new equilibrium; if it is, then the new solution is absorbed into the normal family routine. Also, role conflict can be internalized by family members and produce interpersonal difficulties both within and outside the family. Role conflict situations naturally give rise to states of disequilibrium.

Bell (1961), one of the earliest workers in the family treatment method, has described in a recent monograph his family treatment method in instances of disturbed behavior in children. His view of the therapist is of one who helps parents impose gradual and reasonable restrictions on the child's behavior in the course of therapy. The therapist helps parents communicate to the child the need to talk about problems, and he prevents parents from unfair exercise of their authority in the treatment situation. The therapist refrains from himself competing with the parents for the child, but he supports the child's verbalization. The supportive character of the therapy that Bell espouses is evident in his remark that ". . . no matter how chaotic the family life, the treatment confirms that each of the parents and each of the children is an integral and meaningful part of the group at the center of life, the family" (p. 52).

Recently, Grotjahn (1960) has described a method for psychoanalytic treatment of families in which the family as a whole could be described as neurotic. He maintains that the major aim of family therapy is understanding and treatment of the complementary family neurosis, not the symptomatic neurosis of an individual member. Grotjahn apparently does not regularly see families in conjoint sessions but prefers to explore the family neurosis through his analysis of the primary patient and sometimes in concurrent psychotherapy in which he treats members of a family or married couples at the same time but separately.

A number of social scientists have made noteworthy contributions to the study of family pathology as a major factor in mental disturbance. Although in most cases they have not been engaged in the study of schizoprenia, their work deserves mention. Theories and methods evolving from their work have had a significant effect on individuals working more directly with family treatment of schizophrenia. Among these scientists, psychologists and sociologists alike, are: Otto Pollak (1956), John Clausen and Melvin Kohn (1959, 1960), Talcott Parsons and Robert Bales (1955), Marvin Opler (1956), Robert Hess and Gerald Handel (1959), Reuben Hill (1949), Erika Chance (1959), Jerome Myers (1959, with Bertram Roberts), Rhona and Robert Rapaport (1961), Joseph Eaton (1955, with R. J. Weil), Florence Kluckhohn (1954, with John Spiegel), A. B. Hollingshead (1958, with F. C. Redlich), and John and Elaine Cumming (1962). Several empirical studies of large-group organizations in mental hospitals by social scientists seem to have important implications potentially for the understanding of pathology in smaller family groups. Among these are studies by Dunham and Weinberg (1960), Goffman (1957) and Scheff (1961).

A number of prominent psychotherapists, while not working mainly with the technique of family treatment, have made significant contributions to the understanding of the deeper relationship aspects in family treatment. Among these are: Rosen (1953), Fairbairn (1954), Will (1958), Searles (1959), Hayward (1961), Laing (1960) and Guntrip (1960).

Discussion

A core concept of family psychotherapy is that the mental illness of a member is a symptom or aspect of a greater interlocking family pathology, and perhaps the outstanding contribution to date of family psychotherapy studies has been the elaboration of shared unconscious pathology in families.

In the studies, emphasis has shifted from the concept of the pathogenic parent to the pathogenic family relationship, usually encompassing at least the nuclear family group. Family psychotherapy has begun to reveal the effects on a person of cumulative pathology; by this is meant that among the possible causes of schizophrenia now is included a disturbed marital relationship in not only the parents but also the grandparents of the patient. This current position can be viewed at least in part as a result of a discovery that the pathologic mother-child symbiosis has some of its origin in a prior series of unsatisfactory marital relationships: that of the mother to her husband and that of the mother's mother to her husband. This three-generation concept seems an important contribution arising from the study of family pathology.

The concept of schizophrenic symptomatology has itself changed when viewed from the standpoint of family psychopathology. Thought and affect distortions in patients are related to the context of similar distortions operating subclinically in their families. Such distortions in the patient may clear up only to be followed by a flare-up of pathology in another family member who was previously asymptomatic. Family pathology is thus held to follow the principle of homeostasis.

The concept of the schizophrenic patient as a passive victim has been altered in the context of family therapy studies. The power of this person to control family destiny has been described. There is, at least to some extent, a willing compliance to fit into a pathologic family process. Certain rewards are described for the patient for playing the role of the sick family member. The patient may believe, consciously or unconsciously, that no other role in life could give him equal satisfaction.

The major concepts developed in the field (for example, pseudo-mutuality, double-bind, three-generation hypothesis, pathologic need complementarity) seem to follow what might be called a "principle of economy" in psychopathology; that is, they suggest that at some point the tensions generated in a pathologic family system are reduced by a projection of tension onto a particular family member. The ego of the individual member is overwhelmed, with resultant psychotic behavior which may take the schizophrenic form. However, the continuation of the pathologic family system, without essential change once the tension has been reduced by this means, is assured. To be sure, the individual family member is "sacrificed" in order to maintain the threatened family system. But, in a sense, an important source of power of the so-called "victim" resides in his having played the role of martyr to the family.

Techniques of family psychotherapy are still in a preliminary phase of development. Criteria and objectives have not been fully elaborated. The role of the therapist varies greatly. Midelfort, for example, advocates that the therapist behave like an auxiliary member of the family. It is important, in his opinion, that the therapist be of the same ethnic and religious origin as the family. Ackerman has suggested that the therapist assume the role of wise friend and counselor. Whitaker and other members of the Atlanta Psychiatric Clinic describe a role for the therapist in which he invites the patient into *his* fantasy life, thereby directing the flow of affect in greater degree than if the patient's fantasy life were focused on. The prescription of the role of the therapist surely depends heavily on conceptual orientation. As yet, the conceptual orientations are lacking in proven validity and completeness and this condition reflects itself in the great variety of roles that have been prescribed for the therapist.

Adequate techniques and methods for evaluating the transactions observed in family psychotherapy are needed. The one-to-one dyadic model was found inadequate and discarded as a means of assessing the transactions. More comprehensive models are now being applied which can describe and assess the complex processes observed, such as, for example, coalitions, schisms, alliances, splits, and various forms of mutuality and complementarity. As Framo (1962) has aptly pointed out, the study of family treatment is still at the stage of hypothesis formation. Adequate methods to describe very complex processes are being sought. Adequate control of error has not yet been established. But despite these and other problems common to the early phase of development of any enterprise, family psychotherapy has rewarded its early exponents by exploring hitherto untapped levels in psychopathology.

The next decade of work in family treatment should see a more searching analysis of methods and concepts. Hopefully, the next decade will also see a more unitary theoretical structure within which family psychotherapy may be pursued, along with a clearer articulation of techniques and their effects.

References

ABRAHAMS, J., AND VARON, E. (1953). *Maternal dependency and schizophrenia: mothers and daughters in a therapeutic group.* New York: Int. Univer. Press.

ACKERMAN, N. W. (1957). Interpersonal disturbances in the family: some unsolved problems in psychotherapy. *Psychiatry 19,* 68–74.

ACKERMAN, N. W. (1958). *Psychodynamics of family life.* New York: Basic Books.

ACKERMAN, N. W. (1960). Family-focused therapy of schizophrenia. In S. C. Scher and H. R. Davis (Eds.) *Out-patient treatment of schizophrenia.* New York: Grune & Stratton, pp. 156–173.

ACKERMAN, N. W. (1962). Family psychotherapy and psychoanalysis: the implications of difference. *Family Process 1,* 30–43.

BATESON, G., JACKSON, D. D., HALEY, J., AND WEAKLAND, J. H. (1956). Toward a theory of schizophrenia. *Behav. Sci. 1,* 251–264.

BAUER, I. L., AND GUREVITCH, S. (1952). Group therapy with parents of schizophrenic children. *Int. J. grp. Psychother. 2,* 344–357.

BELL, J. E. (1961). *Family group therapy.* Washington, D.C.: Public Health Monograph No. 64, Dept. of Health, Education and Welfare.

BOSZORMENYI-NAGY, I. (1962). The concept of schizophrenia from the perspective of family treatment. *Family Process 1,* 103–113.

BOSZORMENYI-NAGY, I., AND FRAMO, J. L. (1962). Family concept of hospital treatment of schizophrenia. In J. Masserman (Ed.) *Current psychiatric therapies,* vol. II. New York: Grune & Stratton, pp. 159–166.

BOWEN, M. (1959). Family relationships in schizophrenia. In A. Auerbach (Ed.) *Schizophrenia.* New York: Ronald, pp. 147–178.

BOWEN, M. (1960). A family concept of schizophrenia. In D. D. Jackson (Ed.) *Etiology of schizophrenia.* New York: Basic Books, pp. 346–372.

26 INTENSIVE FAMILY THERAPY

BRODEY, W. M. (1959). Some family operations and schizophrenia. *A.M.A. Arch. gen. Psychiat. 1*, 379–402.

BYCHOWSKI, G. (1956). Interaction between psychotic partners: II. schizophrenic partners. In V. W. Eisenstein (Ed.) *Neurotic interaction in marriage.* New York: Basic Books, pp. 135–147.

CARROLL, E. J. (1960). Treatment of the family as a unit. *Penna. Med. J. 63*, 57–62.

CHANCE, E. (1959). *Families in treatment.* New York: Basic Books.

CLAUSEN, J. A., AND KOHN, M. L. (1959). The relation of schizophrenia to the social structure of a small city. In B. Pasamanick (Ed.) *Epidemiology of mental disorder.* Washington, D.C.: AAAS, pp. 69–94.

CLAUSEN, J. A., AND KOHN, M. L. (1960). Social relations and schizophrenia: a research report and perspective. In D. D. Jackson (Ed.) *Etiology of schizophrenia.* New York: Basic Books, pp. 295–320.

CUMMING, J., AND CUMMING, E. (1962). *Ego and milieu; theory and practice of environmental therapy.* New York: Atherton Press.

CUTTER, A. V., AND HALLOWITZ, D. (1962). Different approaches to treatment of the child and the parents. *Amer. J. Orthopsychiat. 32*, 152–158.

DUNHAM, H. W., AND WEINBERG, S. K. (1960). *The culture of the state mental hospital.* Detroit: Wayne State Univer. Press.

EATON, J. W., AND WEIL, R. J. (1955). *Culture and mental disorder; a comparative study of the Hutterites and other populations.* Glencoe, Ill.: Free Press.

EISENSTEIN, V. W. (Ed.) (1956). *Neurotic interaction in marriage.* New York: Basic Books.

ELLES, G. (1962). The mute sad-eyed child: collateral analysis in a disturbed family. *Int. J. Psycho-Anal. 42*, 40–49.

ELLISON, E. A., AND HAMILTON, D. M. (1949). Hospital treatment of dementia praecox. *Amer. J. Psychiat. 106*, 454–461.

FAIRBAIRN, W. R. (1954). *An object-relations theory of personality.* New York: Basic Books.

FISHER, S., AND MENDELL, D. (1956). The communication of neurotic patterns over two and three generations. *Psychiatry 19*, 41–46.

FRAMO, J. L. (1962). Theory of the technique of family treatment of schizophrenia. *Family Process 1*, 119–131.

FRAZEE, H. E. (1953). Children who later become schizophrenics. *Smith College Stud. Soc. Wrk. 23*, 125–149.

FRIEDMAN, A. (1962). Family therapy as conducted in the home. *Family Process 1*, 132–140.

FROMM-REICHMANN, F. (1948). Notes on the development of schizophrenia by psychoanalytic psychotherapy. *Psychiatry 11*, 267–277.

GALVIN, J. (1956). Mothers of schizophrenics. *J. nerv. ment. Dis. 123*, 568–570.

GERARD, D. L., AND SIEGEL, J. (1950). The family background of schizophrenia. *Psychiat. Quart. 24*, 47–73.

GOFFMAN, E. (1957). On some convergences of sociology and psychiatry. *Psychiatry 20*, 199–203.

GOOLISHIAN, H. A. (1962). A brief psychotherapy program for disturbed adolescents. *Amer. J. Orthopsychiat. 32,* 142–148.

GROTJAHN, M. (1960). *Psychoanalysis and family neurosis.* New York: Norton.

GUNTRIP, H. (1960). Ego-weakness and the hard core of the problem of psychotherapy. *Brit. J. med. Psychol. 33,* 163–184.

HAJDU-GIMES, L. (1940). Contribution to the etiology of schizophrenia. *Psychoanal. Rev. 27,* 421–438.

HALEY, J. (1959). Family of the schizophrenic: a model system. *J. nerv. ment. Dis. 129,* 357–374.

HALEY, J. (1962a). Whither family therapy? *Family Process 1,* 69–100.

HALEY, J. (1962b). Family experiments: a new type of experimentation. *Family Process 1,* 265–293.

HALEY, J. (1963). *Strategies of psychotherapy.* New York: Grune & Stratton.

HANDLON, J. H., AND PARLOFF, M. B. (1962). Treatment of patient and family as a group: is it group therapy? *Int. J. grp. Psychother. 12,* 132–141.

HAYWARD, M. L. (1961). Psychotherapy based on the primary process. *Amer. J. Psychother. 15,* 419–430.

HESS, R. D., AND HANDEL, G. (1959). *Family worlds: a psychosocial approach to family life.* Chicago: Univer. Chicago Press.

HILL, L. B. (1955). *Psychotherapeutic intervention in schizophrenia.* Chicago: Univer. Chicago Press.

HILL, R. (1949). *Families under stress.* New York: Harper.

HOLLINGSHEAD, A. B., AND REDLICH, F. C. (1958). *Social class and mental illness; a community study.* New York: Wiley.

HOWELLS, J. G. (1961). From child to family psychiatry. In *Third world congress of psychiatry proceedings,* vol. I. Toronto: Univer. Toronto Press, pp. 472–475.

JACKSON, D. D. (1957). The question of family homeostasis. *Psychiat. Quart. Suppl. 31,* 79–90.

JACKSON, D. D. (1961). The monad, the dyad, and the family therapy of schizophrenics. In A. Burton (Ed.) *Psychotherapy of the psychoses.* New York: Basic Books, pp. 318–328.

JACKSON, D. D., AND SATIR, V. (1961). A review of psychiatric development in family diagnosis and family therapy. In N. W. Ackerman, F. Beatman, and S. N. Sherman (Eds.) *Exploring the base for family therapy.* New York: Fam. Serv. Ass. of Amer.

JACKSON, J. (1962). A family group therapy technique for a stalemate in individual treatment. *Int. J. grp. Psychother. 12,* 164–170.

JOHNSON, A. M., GRIFFIN, M. E., WATSON, E. J., AND BECKETT, P. G. S. (1956). Studies in schizophrenia at the Mayo Clinic. II: observations on ego function in schizophrenia. *Psychiatry 19,* 143–148.

JOHNSON, A. M., AND SZUREK, S. A. (1954). Etiology of anti-social behavior in delinquents and psychopaths. *J.A.M.A. 154,* 814–817.

JOSSELYN, I. M. (1953). The family as a psychological unit. *Soc. Casework 34,* 336–343.

KANNER, L. (1949). Problems of nosology and psychodynamics of early infantile autism. *Amer. J. Orthopsychiat. 19*, 416–426.

KASANIN, J., KNIGHT, E., AND SAGE, P. (1934). The parent-child relationships in schizophrenia. *J. nerv. ment. Dis. 79*, 249–263.

KIRBY, K., AND PRIESTMAN, S. (1957). Values of a daughter (schizophrenic) and mother therapy group. *Int. J. grp. Psychother. 7*, 281–288.

KLUCKHOHN, F., AND SPIEGEL, J. P. (1954). Integration and conflict in family behavior. Report No. 27. Grp. for Advancement of Psychiat.

KOHN, M., AND CLAUSEN, J. A. (1956). Parental authority behavior and schizophrenia. *Amer. J. Orthopsychiat. 26*, 297–313.

LAING, R. D. (1960). *The divided self: a study of sanity and madness.* Chicago: Quadrangle Books.

LEVY, D. (1943). *Maternal overprotection.* New York: Columbia Univer. Press.

LIDZ, R. W., AND LIDZ, T. (1949). The family environment of schizophrenic patients. *Amer. J. Psychiat. 106*, 332–345.

LIDZ, T., CORNELISON, A., FLECK, S., AND TERRY, D. (1957a). Intrafamilial environment of the schizophrenic patient. I: the father. *Psychiatry 20*, 329–342.

LIDZ, T., CORNELISON, A., FLECK, S., AND TERRY, D. (1957b). Intrafamilial environment of schizophrenic patients. II: marital schism and marital skew. *Amer. J. Psychiat. 114*, 241–248.

LIDZ, T., AND FLECK, S. (1960). Schizophrenia, human integration, and the role of the family. In D. D. Jackson (Ed.) *Etiology of schizophrenia.* New York: Basic Books, pp. 323–345.

LIMENTANI, D. (1956). Symbiotic identification in schizophrenia. *Psychiatry 19*, 231–236.

LYKETSOS, G. E. (1959). On the formation of mother-daughter symbiotic relationship patterns in schizophrenia. *Psychiatry 22*, 161–166.

MACGREGOR, R. (1962). Multiple impact psychotherapy with families. *Family Process 1*, 15–29.

MAHLER, M. S. (1952). On childhood psychosis and schizophrenia: autistic and symbiotic infantile psychosis. In R. S. Eissler, A. Freud, *et al.* (Eds.) *The psychoanalytic study of the child*, vol. VII. New York: Int. Univer. Press, pp. 286–305.

MAIN, T. F. (1958). Mothers with children in a psychiatric hospital. *Lancet 2*, 845–847.

MEISSNER, W. W. (1964). Thinking about the family; psychiatric aspects. *Family Process 3*, 1–40.

MENDELL, D., AND FISHER, S. A. (1958). A multi-generation approach to the treatment of psychopathology. *J. nerv. ment. Dis. 126*, 523–529.

MIDELFORT, C. F. (1957). *The family in psychotherapy.* New York: McGraw-Hill.

MITTELMAN, B. (1956). Analysis of reciprocal neurotic problems in family relationships. In V. E. Eisenstein (Ed.) *Neurotic interaction in marriage.* New York: Basic Books, pp. 81–100.

MORENO, J. L. (1954). Interpersonal therapy, group psychotherapy and the formation of the unconscious. *Grp. Psychother. 7*, 191–204.

MYERS, J. K., AND ROBERTS, B. H. (1959). *Family and class dynamics in mental illness.* New York: Wiley.

NEUBECK, G. (1954). Factors affecting group psychotherapy with married couples. *Marr. & Fam. Liv. 16*, 216–220.

OBERNDORF, C. P. (1938). Psychoanalysis of married couples. *Psychoanal. Rev. 25*, 453–475.

OPLER, M. K. (1956). *Culture, psychiatry and human values.* Springfield, Ill.: Thomas.

PARLOFF, M. B. (1961). The family in psychotherapy. *A.M.A. Arch. gen. Psychiat. 4*, 445–451.

PARSONS, T., AND BALES, R. F. (1955). *Family, socialization and interaction process.* Glencoe, Ill.: Free Press.

POLLAK, O. (1956). *Integrating sociological and psychological concepts: an exploration in child psychotherapy.* New York: Russell Sage Found.

RAPAPORT, R. V., AND RAPAPORT, R. N. (1961). Patients' families; assets and liabilities. In M. Greenblatt, D. J. Levinson, *et al.* (Eds.) *Mental patients in transition.* Springfield, Ill.: Thomas, pp. 208–217.

REICHARD, S., AND TILLMAN, C. (1950). Patterns of parent-child relationships in schizophrenia. *Psychiatry 13*, 247–257.

REIDY, J. J. (1962). An approach to family-centered treatment in a state institution. *Amer. J. Orthopsychiat. 32*, 133–142.

RICHARDSON, H. B. (1948). *Patients have families.* New York: Commonwealth Fund.

ROSEN, J. N. (1953). *Direct analysis: selected papers.* New York: Grune & Stratton.

ROSENBAUM, C. P. (1961). Patient-family similarities in schizophrenia. *A.M.A. Arch. gen. Psychiat. 5*, 120–126.

ROSENZWEIG, S., AND BRAY, D. (1943). Siblings' death in the anamnesis of schizophrenia. *A.M.A. Arch. Neurol. Psychiat. 41*, 71–92.

ROSS, W. D. (1948). Group psychotherapy with patients' relatives. *Amer. J. Psychiat. 104*, 623–626.

RUBINSTEIN, D. (1960). The family of the schizophrenic. Paper read at Second Cuban Congress of Neurol. and Psychiat., Havana, January.

RYCKOFF, I., DAY, J., AND WYNNE, L. C. (1959). Maintenance of stereotyped roles in the families of schizophrenics. *A.M.A. Arch. gen. Psychiat. 1*, 93–98.

SANUA, V. (1961). Family environment and schizophrenia. *Psychiatry 24*, 246–265.

SCHAFFER, L., WYNNE, L. C., DAY, J., RYCKOFF, I. M., AND HALPERIN, A. (1962). On the nature and sources of the psychiatrists' experience with the family of the schizophrenic. *Psychiatry 25*, 32–45.

SCHEFF, T. J. (1961). Control over policy by attendants in a state hospital. *J. Health Hum. Behav. 2*, 93–105.

SCHINDLER, R. (1958). Bifocal group therapy. In J. H. Masserman and J. L. Moreno (Eds.) *Progress in psychotherapy*, vol. III: *tech-*

niques of psychotherapy. New York: Grune & Stratton, pp. 176–186.

SEARLES, H. F. (1959). Integration and differentiation in schizophrenia: an overall view. *Brit. J. med. Psychol. 32,* 261–281.

SIVADON, P. (1957). Du milieu familial anormal au milieu familial pathogene. Paper read at World Fed. Ment. Health.

SONNE, J. C., SPECK, R. V., AND JUNGREIS, J. (1962). The absent-member maneuver as a resistance in family therapy of schizophrenia. *Family Process 1,* 44–62.

SPIEGEL, J. P. (1957). The resolution of role conflict within the family. *Psychiatry 20,* 1–16.

SPIEGEL, J. P., AND BELL, N. W. (1959). The family of the psychiatric patient. In S. Arieti (Ed.) *American handbook of psychiatry,* vol. I. New York: Basic Books, pp. 114–149.

STANTON, A. H., AND SCHWARTZ, M. S. (1954). *The mental hospital.* New York: Basic Books.

SULLIVAN, H. S. (1948). The meaning of anxiety in psychiatry and in life. *Psychiatry 11,* 1–13.

SZUREK, S. A., AND BERLIN, I. N. (1956). Elements of psychotherapeutics with the schizophrenic child and his parents. *Psychiatry 1,* 1–10.

THOMAS, B. C. (1955). Mother-daughter relationship and social behavior. Unpublished doctoral dissertation, Catholic Univer.

TIETZE, T. (1949). A study of mothers of schizophrenic patients. *Psychiatry 12,* 55–65.

TITCHENER, J. L., D'ZMURA, T., GOLDEN, M., AND EMERSON, R. (1963). Family transaction and derivation of individuality. *Family Process 2,* 95–120.

TOWNE, R. D., MESSINGER, S. L., AND SAMPSON, H. (1962). Schizophrenia and the marital family: accommodations to symbiosis. *Family Process 1,* 304–318.

WAHL, C. W. (1954). Some antecedent factors in family histories of 392 schizophrenics. *Amer. J. Psychiat. 110,* 668–676.

WAHL, C. W. (1956). Some antecedent factors in family histories of 568 male schizophrenics of the U.S. Navy. *Amer. J. Psychiat. 113,* 201–210.

WEAKLAND, J. H. (1960). The "double bind" hypothesis of schizophrenia and three-party interaction. In D. D. Jackson (Ed.) *Etiology of schizophrenia.* New York: Basic Books, pp. 373–388.

WHITAKER, C. A. (Ed.) (1958a). *Psychotherapy of chronic schizophrenic patients.* Boston: Little, Brown.

WHITAKER, C. A. (1958b). Psychotherapy with couples. *Amer. J. Psychother. 12,* 18–23.

WHITAKER, C. A., FELDER, R. E., MALONE, T. P., AND WARKENTIN, J. (1962). First stage techniques in the experiential psychotherapy of chronic schizophrenic patients. In J. Masserman (Ed.) *Current psychiatric therapies,* vol. II. New York: Grune & Stratton, pp. 147–158.

WILL, O. A. (1958). Psychotherapeutics and the schizophrenic reaction. *J. nerv. ment. Dis. 126,* 109–140.

WOLF, A. (1950). The psychoanalysis of groups. *Amer. J. Psychother.* *4*, 16–50.

WYNNE, L. C. (1961). The study of intrafamilial alignments and splits in exploratory family therapy. In N. W. Ackerman, F. Beatman, and S. N. Sherman (Eds.) *Exploring the base for family therapy.* New York: Fam. Serv. Ass. of Amer., pp. 95–115.

WYNNE, L. C., RYCKOFF, I. M., DAY, J., AND HIRSCH, S. I. (1958). Pseudo-mutuality in the family relations of schizophrenics. *Psychiatry 21*, 205–220.

ZUK, G. H., BOSZORMENYI-NAGY, I., AND HEIMAN, E. (1963). Some dynamics of laughter during family therapy. *Family Process 2*, 302–314.

ZUK, G. H. (1964). A further study of laughter in family therapy. *Family Process 3*, 77–89.

2

IVAN BOSZORMENYI-NAGY

A Theory of Relationships: Experience and Transaction

As individual psychotherapy has stimulated the emergence of a dynamic model of personality organization (Freud), conjoint family therapy presses for an adequate model of transactional dynamics. This is not to say that in studying the family level of social organization one can dispense with Freudian psychodynamics. It means that family relations represent a higher, more complex organizational level which requires a broadened theoretical outlook in order to explain the family's emergent interactional and transactional phenomena. That the construction of a transactional language is of great practical significance is immediately apparent to those psychotherapists and psychoanalysts who, having been trained in individual-oriented theories and techniques of psychotherapy, have subsequently been exposed to the experience and practice of conjoint family therapy. The group process or the psychology of groups, as has been often stated, cannot be composed of the additive properties of the component individuals, and the individual's motivation

I gratefully acknowledge the helpful comments and suggestions for this chapter made by Dr. James L. Framo.

will be greatly altered when subjected to group psychology. Conceivably, family psychiatry can become the foundation of a general understanding of the deeper dynamics of all social relations.

In the literature on individual therapy, the question of the patient's personality characteristics in relation to his capacity for relating or to his treatability has occupied considerable interest. Helene Deutsch (1942) described the usually unanalyzable "as if" personalities whose apparent easy relating capacity covers an essential inner lack of spontaneity, masked by a mimicry-like identification. Balint (1958) describes patients with a "basic fault" which disqualifies them from conventional psychoanalysis; these patients respond to interpretations as if they were personal approaches, and the analyst himself becomes exposed to a constant "danger" of subjective involvement. In general, the relational component of psychotherapy tends to gain importance in proportion to the patient's ego weakness. It is one of the hoped-for contributions of this chapter that it stresses the need for the creation of a relational or transactional theory of the psychopathology and treatment of the whole family.

In addition to the introduction of the transactional viewpoint, the family therapist needs further extensions of conceptual framework. He needs a language that can express the private experience of relational transactions. There also is a need for a genetic or developmental view of the long-range dynamics of family relationships. In summary, certain unconscious, long-range determinants of family relationships cannot be understood without the construction of a comprehensive, transactional and at the same time experiential language.

The fact that we are unaware or unconscious of the texture of transactional process laws does not necessarily make them mere derivatives of the unconscious instinct-defense configurations of component individual minds. Family therapy experience shows that if the therapist is not able to conceptualize on a supra-individual, transactional level of organization, he is liable to lose control of what turns out to be a congeries of parallelly conducted individual therapies.

The four sections of this chapter are concerned with four main theoretical concepts and their applications. First, a dialectical[1] theory of personality and relatedness is introduced in an attempt to integrate certain conceptually analogous outlooks of present-day psycho-

---

[1] "Dialectical," a term frequently used in Hegelian philosophy and sometimes invested with political meaning, is used here as meaning the dynamic principle of the creative encounter (synthesis) of something and its opposite (thesis and antithesis), particularly of Self and Not-Self.

analytic ego psychology and existential phenomenology. The second section deals with the relational world of the person as composed of a spectrum of alternate choices for self-delineation. Third, a theoretical model of the formation of relational systems is presented. The fourth section is devoted to the concept and manifestations of what is denoted as the phasic relational process.

Dialectical Theory of Personality and Relatedness: Analogies between Ego Psychology and Existential Phenomenology

The conventional theories of personality are elaborated from an individual-oriented, objective vantage point. Though the individual is considered as, historically, a product of transactions, he is often analyzed as if he were a closed dynamic entity or a predictable universe. Even though the ego is frequently viewed as resulting from a compromise between instincts and reality, the adult mind is ideally regarded as a system, determined by its own laws. Fenichel (1945) writes: "Character attitudes are compromises between instinctual impulses and forces of the ego that try to direct, organize, postpone, or block these impulses" (p. 470). Although the basic notion of such a structural dichotomy is certainly correct, the closed system quality of character is open to question. Ordinarily, impulse control is not determined entirely by innate and introjected intra-psychic factors but also by the nature of the current relational fit between the individual and others. While two persons may complement each other positively in one area, they may create a detrimental emotional (instinctual) feedback system in other areas. A precocious child may complement a childishly demanding parent, for example. Furthermore, control of one person's impulses is often achieved through the acting out of others who are unable to control the same impulses. In other words, the other ego may have to be considered a constitutive agent rather than a mere segment of an indifferent social reality. This is one reason for avoiding the labeling of any one member of a family as "sick."

The transactional view of social relations regards action organizations (systems) rather than persons as units. One or several persons may make up a system of actions, and any action, whether attributed to a person or to a system, implies a subject and an object. Translated into experiential language, the subject appears as Self, either a singular Self (I) or plural Self (We). Each real, or anticipated, transaction creates or contributes to a symbolic delineation of both entities: the one or the ones who act (subject) and the one or the ones who are acted upon (object). The structure of any transaction implies a figure-ground-like polarity of relating, and each transaction redefines personality boundaries. As long as one participates in mob violence, for instance, one's person is fused with the other mob members and all are collectively defined as subjects against the victim as object. A more covert plurality of the subject position is exemplified by the instance of a mother's unconscious assistance and vicarious participation in her daughter's impulsive acting out. One could say that the mother's own sexual role delineation is trans-acted via her daughter's behavior toward males. In other words, the motivational determinants of one person's actions may lie in another person's self-delineation needs.

The concept of *social reality* is often thought of as some impersonal force which requires adaptation on the part of the person, just as do changes of weather. Erikson (1962) stated: "We have studied man's 'inner world' with unprecedented devotion; yet we assign acutely decisive encounters, opportunities, and challenges to a nebulous 'outside reality' " (p. 457). Man depends on his social environment. Yet, a person can be enviably successful in terms of worldly pursuits and nevertheless unhappy. The unhappy person can move from job to job, from one marriage to another, and still feel that he has to keep changing his social reality until he finds the right environment, i.e., himself. It is as if his personality were a figure looking for a matching ground. Or, conversely, he may possess a matching ground but be unaware of this fact until the shock of losing someone, e.g., a sister or brother, makes him aware of a painful loss to his own Self, to his own meaning. Paradoxically, it may be a violently resented or hated Other whose loss leaves great emptiness and lack of purpose.

If anyone can constitute an important enough part of my person or Self to be needed so badly that his loss makes me feel as though I have lost a part of my Self, such Other has to be a constituent of my Selfhood. He may have been an extension of my Self because he was so alike or he may have been an antithetical Not-Self opposite to what I sensed as the symbolic content of my Self.

That the context or ground of the Self is a necessary constituent of Selfhood itself is beautifully expressed by Gabriel Marcel (1960): ". . . a human life has always its center outside itself; though it can be centered, certainly, on a very wide and diverse range of outside interests. It may be centered on a loved one, and with the disappearance of the loved one can be reduced to a sad caricature of itself; it may be centered on something trivial, a sport like hunting, a vice like gambling; it can be centered on some high activity, like research or creation. But each one of us can ask himself, as a character in one of my plays, 'What do I live by?' And this is not a matter of some final purpose to which a life may be directed

as of the mental fuel that keeps a life alight from day to day"
(p. 101).

ONTIC VS. FUNCTIONAL RELATEDNESS

The Self can be related to an Other by way of two major types
of ties: functional and ontic. *Functional* relatedness can be described
in terms of instrumental performances among "interacting" partners.
In a purely functional relatedness the partner can be exchanged
for another partner without a feeling of loss, provided the new
partner performs the function at least as well as the previous one.
If, for example, in the middle of the dinner, our waiter is replaced
by a more attentive fellow worker, there is no complaint of loss.
Ontic relatedness, on the other hand, is based on a fundamental
dependence on the tie with the Other. The adjective was coined
by Heidegger and is defined by Spiegelberg (1960) as "descriptive
of a structure inherent in Being itself" (p. 721). The ontic element
in a relationship makes the Other an essential counterpart of one's
Selfhood, irrespective of any particular interaction. In this type of
relationship, the functional or instrumental role performance of the
Other lessens in significance, and in the event of loss, the relationship
cannot be re-established with equal or even better substitutes. The
survival of the tie by means of internalization constitutes the phenomenon underlying the important Freudian notions of mourning.

The concept of ontic dependence is implicit in psychoanalytic
developmental theories. Fenichel (1945) writes: "The concept of
reality also creates the concept of ego. We are individuals inasmuch
as we feel ourselves separate and distinct from others" (p. 35).
The implication here is that the Self depends on others for its separateness. Fenichel does not seem to make a distinction between
ego and self, whereas Hartmann (1950) defines the meaning of
self as "one's own person in contradistinction to the object," and
ego as "a psychic system in contradistinction to other substructures
of personality" (p. 84).

It is impossible not to recognize the parallel between Freud's
"structural" insights and the view of the existential phenomenolo-
gists concerning the Self-Not-Self encounter character of the core
of our personal existence. This parallel becomes manifest as Freud
(1923) talks of the ego as the "precipitate of abandoned object-
cathexes" or of an "alteration in character" being able to "conserve"
object relations (p. 36). According to Freud's structural point of
view, the ego repeats external object relations on a new, intrapsychic
"scene of action" (Freud, 1921, p. 80). It is obvious that the roles
enacted in the ego's innermost relational drama duplicate the experiential modes of external object relationships: approval, hatred,

love, indifference, etc. Here lies one of Freud's most lasting contributions: he has extended the principle of the encounter-like quality of existence into the inner realms of the psyche. Whereas Buber (1958) so succinctly states the existential-phenomenological position regarding the essence of man as being delineated by his fellow man ("I become through my relation to the *Thou;* as I become *I*, I say *Thou*. All real living is meeting" [p.11]), Freud's ego psychology explicitly formulates a relational principle of intrapsychic structuring or existence. The direction of progress from here on points toward explicitly relational or transactional doctrines of the personality (Melanie Klein, Fairbairn)[2] and, ultimately, of persons in relationship. Fairbairn emphasizes the object-seeking rather than pleasure-seeking nature of his dynamic concepts (1952).

The notion that the person originates from the antithesis of Self and Object representatives or Self- and Other-based perceptual rudiments is not new. Findlay (1962) reminds us that Hegel, and before him Fichte in the late 18th century, conceived of the existence of the Self (ego) as being based on the antithetical (dialectical) "positing" of Others (non-ego).

It is a corollary of the dialectical principle that neither the person nor his drive components are to be conceived of as having a substance-like character. According to this view, a sadist may cling to a masochist (and vice versa) not primarily because he has a sadistic urge that needs to be discharged, while for all other purposes he could be thought of as free of relational needs, but because he first wants someone as his object and it happens that it is through a sadomasochistic complementarity that he can discharge an important aspect of his (and possibly his partner's) needs for being defined or delineated. Or, as another example, paranoid suspiciousness can be regarded as the patient's need for a "bad object" as a context, rather than as a form of discharge for any of his particular "intrapsychic" impulses.

Regardless of the form of discharge or the communication patterns used, the need for a certain type of Self-delineating relationship has its own, configurationally dynamic function. Likewise, in a lasting "good" relationship the configuration of the "dialogue" of trusting interactions has its own unconscious structuring, based on the mutuality of the participants' ontic needs for delineation by "good" objects.

The dialectical principle describes a dynamic force which determines the choice of relational objects on the basis of their antithetical and complementary properties. In order to implement a drive dis-

---

[2] For a summary see Guntrip (1961).

charge, I need someone (object) who is receptive in the particular drive area in which I need to be active, and vice versa. The resulting sense of relating helps both me and my object to gain in individuation. One can say that individuation is a dialectical process. Conversely, primary identification or fusion through acting out tends to reduce the extent of individuation. Extreme loss of individuation results in experiences of depersonalization.[3] According to dialectical dynamics, many instances of rigid projections and transferences are due to unconscious configurational requirements for individuation and for avoidance of the ever-present horror of depersonalization.

Individuation through the formation of subject-object boundaries probably precedes any other "psychological" motivation. Being the source of the experience of Selfhood, Self-Not-Self discrimination is a prerequisite of the pleasure principle. The compulsive repetition of neurotic or psychotic symptoms is aimed at Self-restitution as well as Object-restitution. From the dialectical point of view symptoms are aimed at the formation of ego boundaries through Self-Not-Self polarity. The hypochondriac substitutes "intrapsychic organ representations" for "intrapsychic object representations" (Fenichel, 1945, p. 261). The psychotic "needs" his hallucinated voices, as exemplified by a patient who admitted that he relied on his voices because "they are there" when he was alone. The common observation that paranoid psychotics experience great relief when they first formulate their suspiciousness and anxiety in the form of organized delusions supports our notion about the value of even a purely intrapsychic Self-Not-Self boundary. Furthermore, the apparent detachment or withdrawal of cathexis between marital partners is also often due to investment of Self-delineating intrapsychic object representations. The latter seem to constitute a more secure dialectical ground for the Self than even the closest of external relationships. Finally, external relationships are frequently overvalued because of projective distortions due to internal object relations.

The transactional core of the dialectical concept of personality becomes apparent when it is recognized that the experience of the Self as a symbolic unit depends on the selective availability of a matching Not-Self. The important concepts of autonomy, dependency, and fusion have to be re-evaluated in the light of the person being viewed as a complex of structured Self-Other situations. Is there any meaning in the concept of autonomy if some aspect of an Other has to participate in the very formation of the Self-ex-

---

[3] Feelings of passivity or of being influenced are characteristic experiences of depersonalized psychotics, and the so-called object-restitutive phenomena are obvious efforts at restoring a sense of subject-object relatedness.

perience? Where are the limits of health and pathology regarding identifications and vicarious action patterns then? Can successfully internalized relationships help the "mature" person to become really free of the need to depend on Others for basic Self-delineation? Is there a difference between projecting the "bad" Self and projecting the bad (object) context of the "good" Self? Is it necessary to identify with the Other with whom one is overinvolved? Ultimately, a theory of relationships will have to define the criteria of the Other as (a) constituent of the symbolic structure of the Self *experience* and (b) party to a *transactional* system.

The family therapist will tend to be equally interested in the relational or transactional aspects of any impulse discharge and in its possible intrapsychic ramifications. A daughter's vicarious acting out of her mother's repressed impulses is a good example here. Viewed in isolation, the prudish mother could be regarded as a person using the "intrapsychic" defense of "reactive character formation" against her overtly unacceptable impulses, and the overt transactional system of acting out seems to consist in this instance of the acting-out daughter and a man. Yet, identification between mother and daughter may make them joint subjects of an impulse, which is transacted toward the man as its object. Self-Other delineation takes on an implicity plural Self character here, based on the covert motivational fusion of mother and daughter. A dialectical or transactional orientation to psychopathology would tend to focus on the dynamic factors that prevented a Self-Other distinction between this mother and daughter, rather than on the intrapsychic motivational roots of the particular impulse responsible for the daughter's acting out.

The intrapsychic perspective of classical, individual-based, maturity-oriented individual theory and the relational orientation of family therapy are linked through two branches of contemporary "ego psychology": the theory of ego autonomy and internal relationship theory. The family therapist, explicitly or implicitly, functions on the assumption that it is futile to consider intrapsychic (e.g., ego vs. instincts) mastery except in the context of interpersonal autonomy. As Rapaport (1958) has stated: ". . . ego autonomy from the id and the ego autonomy from the environment mutually guarantee each other only within an optimal range. Maximization or minimization of either disrupts their balance" (p. 32). The possibility has to be seriously considered that if one family member's intrapsychic mastery is tenuous, he will fortify it at the expense of another member's autonomy. Many family therapists have accepted the applicability of the term homeostasis for that aspect of family functioning in which improvement in one member may lead to another member's taking the sick role. It is as though in certain families an autonomous role can exist only if it is balanced against a non-autonomous one on the part of another family member. The term autonomy, however, is fraught with various "objective" meanings that imply independent existence, and therefore the term tends to under-emphasize the transactional or relational element which is a *sine qua non* of the Self being viewed as experience. Internal object-relation theories of the personality, on the other hand, concern the formal properties of the unconsciously determined relational aspects of need and gratification dynamics.

Modes of Relating

There are many ways in which relationships can be categorized, among other things, according to their underlying instinctual and affective charges. From the point of view of the dialectical theory, however, a more precise, yet broad-based description of the structural characteristics of relationships is needed. Take love and hatred, for example, which are concepts with multiple meanings. Though con-tradictory on an affective level, both terms connote relatedness be-tween involved, more or less distinct individuals, though being in love is frequently conceived of as a merger between two partners. On the other hand, even though a capacity for love is a requirement of "healthy" or "mature" personalities, distinct selfhood is clearly a more desirable maturational ideal than love at the expense of merger or fusion with another. The complete dialectical assessment of relatedness, therefore, has to account for both the nature of in-volvement and the degree of the participants' Self-Other distinctness.

The first requirement of the dialectical relationship theory resem-bles the figure-ground principle of gestalt-theory. The Self is incon-ceivable without "having" some object, just as with the loss of the ground, the figure, too, is lost. A partial loss of ground of the Self is known to occur in cases of pathological mourning. Due to the familiarity (predictability) of his actions and reactions, the lost Other has become a segment of the transactional context of the mourner's Self as subject. In order that the Self be freed of this dependency on particular objects, it is required that early relation-ships be transformed into a structural relational context, involving intrapsychic Self- and Object-representations. From then on the in-ternalized relational set exerts a selective influence on the choice of new external relationships. Each internal Other or Object-repre-sentation is a derivative of composite memory traces from various past partners.

The transactional theory of the person implies that the experience of Selfhood depends on the existence and intactness of a *boundary*, formed through the polar division of the person's relational agents into two symbolic regions: a proximal region of Self-referent and a distal region of Not-Self-referent agents. Agents of the proximal region are all experienced as constituents of either a singular or a plural Selfhood (I or We), whereas the agents of the distal region make up the spectrum of Others or, generally, the World. The growth of the personality depends on continuous enlargement of both, Self- and Not-Self-referent regions. Buhler (1962, p. 22) quotes George Bach in saying, "I consider growth through 'identification with' a transitory process, while self-actualization through 'differentiation from' is a life-long mode of self-assertive living." The vicissitudes of a person's identification models and differentiation molds are inadequately represented in most current dynamic personality models.

The boundary that exists between Self-referent and Not-Self-referent agents of the person is essential in the development of the discrimination between identifications and relationships. The growing child can respond to its parent's actions with either identificatory imitation and fusion or reciprocal complementation and differentiation. The little girl identifies not only with mother's femininity but also with her coquetry vis-à-vis her father or males in general. In other words, the little girl learns the feminine role vicariously through both an identification model and the latter's complementary role or relational context. Thus, according to the dialectical principle, each Self-referent agent depends on a conscious or unconscious Not-Self-referent as its context. Certain aspects of our person are grounded in a reciprocal or complementary relationship to a whole family's—not just to one person's—mode of functioning. Significant introjected familial transactional networks may have to be symbolically transferred ("family transference," Boszormenyi-Nagy and Framo, 1962) to our current relational contexts. A hospitalized patient, for instance, tends to develop family transference toward the staff and the other patients.

The assumption that the person as a Self depends on a set of matching Not-Self-referents implies that he, in turn, has to be a Not-Self-referent for others. Part of our relationship with the others is based on our usefulness for their self-delineation. We are, by principle, excluded from experiencing ourselves as a Not-Self-referent or Self-delineating ground as we appear for others. As an example, no one can really experience his or her "sex appeal"; it can only be learned from the reactions and comments of others. A woman can sense her own feminine identity as a Self-referent but her sex appeal is a Not-Self referent to the masculine identity of her male admirer. Her identity as a woman of sex appeal is defined through her being an object for others. Although knowledge of our-selves as image for others can contribute to our social poise, it never becomes a constituent of the sensed Self. Pfuetze (1961), a student of G. H. Mead's theories, fails to give recognition to this distinction when he states: "The distinguishing characteristic of the Self is that it is its own object" (p. 101). In our view the Self can never become identical with its object or with itself as an object because the Self-Object encounters are dynamically antithetical.

Having defined the need for possessing a Self-delineating Other as a fundamental (ontic) need, we have to explore relatedness as to its phenomenological criteria. What are the characteristics of per-sons in relationship? How is it any different to be a subject as opposed to an object of relating? If person A makes a relational move, person B can do one of four things: (a) join the move (merger, primary identification), (b) counter it with a different move or striving, (c) become the object of A's move or striving, or (d) be indifferent to the move. These choices constitute four modes of ontic or existential attitudes of relatedness. The first three choices result in an interpersonal relationship regardless of whether the relationship is satisfactory emotionally. The fourth choice, indiffer-ence, may coincide with B's turning to his internal relational world as a response to A's move. Being an object, rather than subject, of a relationship is a question of *differential* of initiative or "strength." Whereas acceptance of being an object may (though does not have to) mean a captive relational role, merger always leads to at least partial and temporary extinction of the person as a discrete dynamic entity. The vicissitudes of these relational positions are reflected in the participants' ego boundaries (Federn, 1952).

From its own vantage point the Self can be viewed as a unitary or synthetic reference point for a multitude of matching sets of Not-Self- or Other-referents. The experiential stability and continu-ity of the sensed Self depends to a great extent on a flexible *inter-changeability* of its various composite object worlds. The integration of the Self- and Not-Self-referents constitutes a homeostatic system. The Self's Other-referents fall into four categories: (a) internal Sub-ject-Other (e.g., superego; persecuting, delusional object-representa-tions); (b) internal Object-Other (hated or desired parental imago; hallucinatory voice, loved because of its "availability"); (c) external Subject-Other (admirer; hater); (d) external Object-Other (beloved one; target of one's aggression). It is likely that internal (intra-psychic) Others, once acquired, are never lost again, though their manifest significance may lessen. In accordance with the unconscious homeostatic laws that govern object-interchangeability, the loss of one Not-Self-referent is bound to be replaced by an internally fitting substitute. Upon the "loss" by assassination of President Kennedy, a previously rather subdued, inactive, hospitalized patient became belligerent and threatened to kill several previous work associates for "robbing him of ten years of his life" during which period he was made to feel "like a nothing." It is possible that the profound loss of sense of Self, suffered as a result of the loss through the murder of a parental figure, contributed to the reactivation and subsequent projection of the bad internal counterparts of the persecuted Self as Subject. Possibly, the loss of this patient's sensed Selfhood was restored through his role assertion vis-à-vis an imaginary persecuting subject and persecuted object.

The search for Self-delineation can be manifested in unconsciously structured, symbolically meaningful actions, fantasies, and relational modes. Fantasies reflect identity configurations and other cognitive aspects of Self-delineation, whereas actions help define the Self through motivational integration and goal-elaboration. The various relational modes represent degrees of demarcation regarding Self-Other complementation. Relational modes are constituents of the participants' character traits. Furthermore, entire families or certain of their subgroups may also be characterized by a habitual relational mode. The more consistently a person's distinct Self-Other demarcation is, the better will he be protected against the anxiety of object loss and its accompanying fear of annihilation.

The classification of relation modes has to begin with *unrelatedness* as its baseline. Unrelatedness, as a quality of experience, can be found among people with comparatively good social functioning. Naturally, the extremes of unrelatedness as they occur in autistic infantile psychosis and chronic "deteriorated" schizophrenic pictures provide the clearest illustrations of lack of Self-Other demarcation or ego-dedifferentiation. As we go down the list of more and more effective relational modes, pathology retreats in favor of security and effective life functioning. The six relational modes are: (a) intrasubject boundary; (b) internal dialogue; (c) merger; (d) being the object; (e) being subject; (f) the dialogue.

Figure 1 depicts a hierarchic series of six relational modes, each defining the Self's boundaries in a specific fashion. Each circle segment represents a biological individual and each broken line represents an ego boundary formed through a dialectical (relational) contraposition of Self and Not-Self. The arrows represent the directional character of relational involvements, particularly the circumstance that from the "proximal" vantage point of the Self as a subject everything, even other Selves appear as (distal) objects. The first two relational modes do not involve a real Other; the third mode consists in a nondialectical, intersubjective merger; the fourth and fifth modes are unbalanced, one-sided, dialectical subject-object encounters; and the sixth mode, the dialogue, is characterized by mutuality. Seen from an interpersonal point of view, the first three modes are "nonrelational" and futile object-restitutive efforts, whereas the last three represent increasingly satisfying and stable

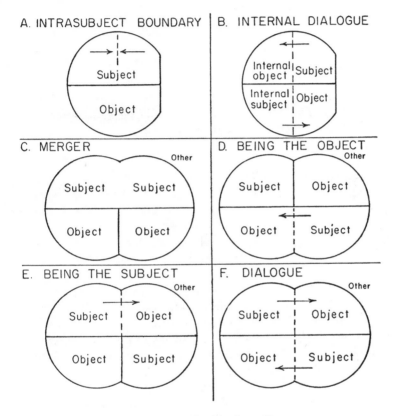

Fig. 1. Six relational modes.

"real" relationships. The diagram shows that the dialogue is more than the sum of two self-centered efforts, (d) and (e); it is an integrated feedback system of two whole persons.

INTRASUBJECT BOUNDARY

In a cognitive sense the person is capable of looking at himself from an introspective, observing vantage point. A frightening and disrupting splitting of the Self into subject and object parts can occur in early stages of psychotic depersonalization. Subsequently, self-vindicating and self-accusatory preoccupations may serve to alleviate the anxiety over imminent depersonalization, as illustrated in the following clinical example.

A patient described retrospectively a thought that seemed to have been her preoccupation during the initial phase of psychotic isolation: "I wanted to believe I was bad." The dialectical configuration of this statement obviously differs from notions concerning the ego' wanting to become an object to the id (Freud, 1923). In analyzing the statement: "I_1 WANTED [me_2 or another aspect of my Self] TO BELIEVE I_3 [me] WAS BAD," we notice that I_1 is the observing (synthetic) ego of the present, whereas me_2 and I_3 are mutually antithetical, past ego-structures, of which the first one is the subject and the latter the object of a belief. Concurrently, at least on an overt level, the past subject (me_2) becomes the object of the present subject (I_1). The act of assigning a bad role to I_3 makes it appear as though there were two agents interacting.

INTERNAL DIALOGUE

A fundamental corollary of Freud's structural theory is the construction of intrapsychic dynamics as if they were an *intrapsychic dialogue*. According to the dialectical construct, the Self depend on a transactional field, even in the absence of relations to external Others. In view of this internal subject-object polarity, it becomes critically important to distinguish between what gets introjected into the Self versus into the internal Other. Since the Self can be both subject and object of internal relationships, the designation "internal object" is less accurate for the present usage than "internal Other." The Freudian model of the ego seeking the love of the superego can be translated into the dialectical view of the Self being compelled to rely in its ontic dependence efforts upon a delineation which makes it an object to an internal subject (superego).[4]

As we have noted, Freud's structural theory supposes the existence of an intrapsychic relational world which serves as the storage of "learning" regarding transactional patterns of behavior and impulse discharge. We have designated structural sets of internal relational needs as *relational need templates*. In its development, a real (interpersonal) relationship passes through a period of adjustment, on the one hand, between each person's relational need templates and on the other hand, between internal and "real" demands. The in

---

[4] It must be noted that, as a rule, Freud's usage does not distinguish between Self-representation, ego, and mind: "Let us reflect that the ego now enters into relation of an object to the ego-ideal which has been developed out of it, and that all the interplay between an external object and the ego as a whole, with which our study of the neuroses has made us acquainted, may possibly be repeated upon this new scene of action within the ego" (1921, p. 103).

ternal relational need template (or its fitting object) may or may not be consciously represented in a person's mind. An example of a manifestly internal relational configuration occurs in the early phases of a paranoid hallucinatory or delusional condition. In the process of treatment or of other attempts at "real" relating, the internal accusations of a voice or imaginary person are likely to be projected upon real Others. From then on, any interpersonal relationship that falls under the shadow of the paranoid need template will be *selectively* perceived as fitting the criteria of the Other's internally presumed maliciousness and cruelty.

Projecting the inner need configuration onto a real relationship provides the paranoid person with the necessary sense of (false) validation of the particular type of malignant Not-Self which vindicates his own defective sense of Selfhood. Delusional transference is bound to be more rigid and "unchangeable" than neurotic transference because the former represents a major and indispensable dialectical framework for the Self's existence. In the more mature ego structure of the neurotic, on the other hand, transferring the internal dialogue to interpersonal relationships does not represent a vitally important means of major Self-delineation.

In an oversimplified way, Figure 2 illustrates the two principal implications of the person's being involved in an internal dialogue. In (a) the internalized subject-object relationship appears as a "dynamic counterweight" to external relationships. Internal relational attitudes can, in the mature person, blend with accurately perceived interpersonal relationship elements. The person can fall back on his internal relationships as a resource, and he does not have to feel reduced to a shapeless nonentity following the loss of valued external Others. The richer the spectrum of his internal relational attitudes, the more capable will the person be of coping with a great variety of external relationships.

Figure 2 represents that aspect of dyadic relationships which is characteristic of transference distortions and delusional projections. The Other is seen here through, as it were, the distorting glass of persistently cathected internal relationships. Here the Self, in addition to being deprived of the perception of itself as object-to-the-Other, cannot even establish any representation of the Other-as-his-object without having it contaminated by perceptions of the Self's own internal Other. Though the Self preserves its subject and object aspects respectively, the Other's address to the Self will be indistinguishable from the messages coming from the internal Subject Other (e.g., a censuring superego). By means of selectively perceiving the Other's messages only if they fit the internal Other, the Self manages to use the internal dialogue as a "buffer" for regulating the interpersonal dialogue. The more "pathology" the less is the person's capacity for truly perceiving people as they are or as they realistically behave toward him. The severely paranoid psychotic may withdraw into almost exclusive preoccupation with internal relationships. He may spend most of his wakeful time listening to and arguing with his "voices." Yet, as long as his world allows for a Self-Other boundary, he is saved from the horror of depersonalization.

An important and very fundamental mechanism of mixed internal-external relating is based on the projection of the split-off

A. DYAD AS DIALOGUE

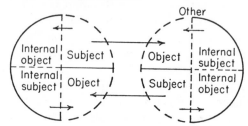

B. DYAD AS MUTUAL PROJECTION

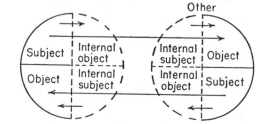

Fig. 2. The dyad and the internal dialogue.

bad aspects of an internalized parent. As a result of the projection, the external Other (e.g., the marital partner) is seen in a scapegoat-like "bad" role so that the remaining internal parental image can remain "good." Thus, a mutual "conversion game" begins. The Other is assigned the role of the "bad" parent who could and should improve but does not want to. Naturally, the assignment of the bad parent's role does not have to be explicit. In fact, the more cunningly the assignment is done ("double-bind") the more effectively caught the Other will be. The mutually scapegoating conversion pattern is decidedly a more complex configuration than the mere sum of two individuals' projections. It may even be part of a larger transactional system wherein a third person becomes the object for both participants' projection of an idealized or bad parental image.

Family members who relate to each other in a predominantly distortive, "narcissistic" (Brodey, 1961) manner are ordinarily considered unfit for individual psychotherapy or psychoanalysis because of their "weak ego structure." The experience of family therapy does not contradict this. It does propose, however, that there is an indication for therapeutic techniques which can explore the entire multiperson relational unit in interaction. With an opportunity to observe all the relevant relational feedback mechanisms, the treatment of transactional "pathology" becomes a less hopeless undertaking.

MERGER

Intersubjective merger or fusion is a nondialectical relational mode which lacks the polarity of subject-object demarcation in its transactions. Based on mechanisms of primary identification (Fenichel, 1945), projective identification (Klein, 1963), or vicarious participation, the relating person clings to the Other parasitically. This type of quasi-relating is often seen in psychopaths ("as if" personality; H. Deutsch, 1942) or in recovering psychotics. It is as if the parasitically dependent or symbiotic person were exempted from the necessity of being a person. People attached to one another in this engulfing manner appear to share each other's feelings and motivations, instead of mutually recognizing their disparate traits. They seem to lack those ego boundaries requisite for individuation; it is as though they hoped to participate in the Other's Self-Other demarcation processes.

The essence of merger is not an imitative effort. It is, rather, in the clinging, possessing attitude which, if successful, eliminates the need for even imitation. After the person has "merged" with the host, the latter's relationships are used to fill up the parasite's feeling of emptiness which stems from his lack of sense of Selfhood because of lack of relatedness. To use a Freudian phrase, one can state that in these persons the "castration complex extends into the ego" (Waelder, 1960, p. 210).

BEING THE OBJECT

Although, from the purely centrifugal view of the person, the various internal and external relationships appear to be interchangeable, the nature of dyadic relationships is complicated by the existence of two opposing, centrifugal and centripetal, relational attitudes. What is centrifugal from one partner's vantage point is centripetal from the Other's viewpoint. The relational world of the dyad, thus, is more complex than merely an encounter of two subjects' competing assertions. The structure of a relationship apportions subject and object positions to the relating partners, and as long as one remains "in relationship," the Other's needs become one's secondary needs through one's becoming an object to the Other's strivings and a ground for his assertiveness. Permitting the Other to make one his object without a chance for reciprocity in the dialogue can result in what Sartre (1956) calls an "internal hemorrhage" into one's world. Both Freud's and Sartre's relational orientations seem to stress the psychic economic value of one's capacity for making active use of others as objects of one's drives or projects, although even as subjects we may need an empathic identification with the Other's own centrifugality or assertion. Whereas Sartre's man would always consider an object-for-Other role as an ego-dystonic intrusion, Freud's structural concepts of the mind make allowance for an ego which has to "co-exist" with the superego that makes the ego an object of either its love or contempt. That mutual relatedness through an *alternation of subject and object roles is a vital structural* component of the personality is implied in Buber's theories of the dialogue (Friedman, 1960a, Pfuetze, 1961).

The Other's strong investment in assigning a particular object-significance to one may not only be conflictful but, if excessive and successful, detrimental to the development of one's own object-seeking, i.e., the autonomous, subject aspect of one's personality. This captive position is the destiny of the young child who is assigned a parental position by its parent. The child's molding into a parent-like role clashes with his need for developing a necessary dependence on adults. The child's prematurely developed, adult-like attributes fail to satisfy both his own needs for dependency and for supporting objects as a Not-Self context. Using the analogy of immunity, the more the child is exposed to the antigen (the parent's childishness), the more he acquires a complementing active immunity, i.e., altered state of responsiveness. The child turns parental, rather than dependent. In self-defense, the child learns to turn an actively hostile attitude toward the intrusive world, perhaps for a lifetime.

In extreme cases the child's self-image may become completely choked off because of his force-fed object role opposite the parent. One may wonder whether there is not a dynamic connection between the grandiose, unrealistic assertions of superhuman wisdom in a 17-year-old schizophrenic boy, on the one hand, and his mother's recollections of her having regarded the boy, even at age 1, as a miniature-sized but grown-up man. It is interesting in this regard that the personality description of the pre-psychotic (usually pre-adolescent) period of the future schizophrenic patient is frequently that of a "good," nondemanding, retiring (object-like?) child. The impression one gets from these descriptions is that there must have been an almost complete lack of aggressive expression in early childhood, perhaps based on the absence of the preverbal dialogue of playful romping between mother and baby. Being forced into a role of Not-Self for the parent, the child fails to develop its active, subject-like Self.

The psychotherapy of schizophrenic patients can provide interesting examples of transition from desperately inadequate to more satisfying modes of relating. A psychotic young woman who long had alternated between paranoid and assaultive states showed a gradual transition from unrelatedness to internal and finally to external subject-object dialogue. At first, she would be either nonverbal or rather incoherent in her rage attacks. Later on she began shouting fragmented phrases pertaining to some woman being a "whore" or a "bitch." At this stage it was impossible to find out whom she wes referring to: Self or Other? Then she told me about some voices that were telling her that she was a "whore." Finally, she *knew* for certain that *I* thought of her as a worthless, immoral person. Thus, she managed to become object first to an internal then to an external Other. At this time, it became possible to engage her in an actual dialogue through the externalization of her objectively "inappropriate" but internally meaningful relationship needs. Resolution of at least some aspects of this patient's deep ambivalences became possible and she started to re-invest her family relationships on a less psychotic level.

Being the object, as a relational mode, is related to the concept of "passive receptive mastery." The latter term, as the word "mastery" suggests, implies narcissistic gratification by means of becoming the object of one's own impulses. Fenichel (1945) writes: "The stage of primary narcissism, in which omnipotence was felt and "mastery" was no problem yet, is thus followed by a period of passive-receptive mastery in which difficulties are overcome by influencing powerful external objects to give what is needed" (p. 41). Fenichel's wording retains the term "object" for the partner who is being manipulated into active giving. The concept of secondary gain is a good example of such mastery. Yet the Self, while becoming the object of certain interactions, nevertheless remains the motivational source. Being the object in the true relational sense, on the other hand, connotes an action sequence which stems from the Other's motivations.

BEING THE SUBJECT

Although a striving for being the subject of actions opposite to Others as objects of actions is fundamental to the structure of motivation, a flexibility that permits an alternation between subject and object roles is needed. Without such flexibility we are barred from lasting, mutually gratifying relationships. A rigid insistence on the subject role is synonymous with the desire to make the world comply with all one's needs, and if two people in relationship do nothing but mutually strive to create the Other as an object, the two will be in the insoluble dilemma of trying to fit interpersonal relationships into intrapsychic ones.

The term *subject* connotes the centrifugal aspect of the Self which is contrasted with both the Other as Not-Self and the Self as Object-for-the-Other. Viewed in isolation from its object world, the subject is a mere abstraction. More concretely, the subject can be thought of as the agent of a set of strivings, bent on attaching objects to itself and grounding itself in them as context. It is appropriate to our viewpoint to speak of the Self's *affinity* for a fitting set of relational Others. The choice of the term affinity is meant to diminish emphasis on the motivational dichotomy of ego vs. instinct. Two people in relationship encounter each other's ego as well as instincts. Therefore, our configurational rather than quantitative theoretical framework de-emphasizes degree of *cathexis* by mental (instinctual) energies. Affinity is a configurationally determined, constitutive, and synthetic law of relationships. Unconscious components of relational affinity are to be sought in those implicit configurational laws which determine selective attraction and the sense of complementation between the entirety of two persons' *need templates*. Need templates, on the other hand, are largely unconscious amalgamations between inherited, phylogenetic patterns and past learning (imprinting) from formative encounters with significant Others.

The concept of affinity between two persons' relational need templates could be considered a simple renaming of wishful fantasies or derivatives of aim-inhibited impulses. These individual-based concepts, however, neglect the dynamically structuring properties of mutual subject-object complementations between persons. In order to illustrate the difference, let us take the examples of masturbation and heterosexual relationship. The element common to both is a tendency toward a complementary fitting of one's need templates with objects, as is consistent with the universal human (symbolic) striving for the "patterning" of every, even the most nebulous, impulse. We know that masturbation is usually associated with selective fantasy patterns, i.e., internal object configurations. Similarly, we know that, in man, the preparatory phase (foreplay phase) of sexual intercourse is heavily dependent on a wishful fitting of the object to the subject's internal need dispositions. Yet, if the dyadic relationship is to be at least comparatively constant, elements of the Other's wish configurations must become components of the configuration of one's own needs and this is what happens: the lover's affinity for his mate encompasses his being the object of the mate's impulses. In contrast, in masturbation the only feedback originates from fantasy creations.

Perhaps it is valid to compare the heterosexual situation, as an example of a dyadic relationship, to the acquisition of active immunity or allergy. In active immunity the organism, due to its exposure to an intrusive agent, acquires a tendency which, though external to its original "need dispositions," will from now on characterize its immunological responsiveness. By analogy, in relationship the partner's needs impinge on one as antigens or allergens, extraneous to one's needs. The masturbator or the daydreamer (delusional or otherwise) avoids being exposed as object to the, at least initially, ego-dystonic wishes of an Other. In the harmonious love relationship, on the other hand, pleasing the Other becomes part of one's own goal. Fitting oneself as object to the Other's needs can, however, take excessive "pathological" forms in which one pays the price of assuming a negative identity.

Of the many possible illustrations of how a valued negative identity stems from being the object, one can be mentioned because of its technical significance in the conduct of long-range, intensive conjoint family therapy. We have found that one of the most prevalent transactional systems between the parents of a schizophrenic patient is a pointless, endless bickering. Quite often the deeper structure of this transaction involves the wife's inability to face her own negative, critical attitudes toward or about her parents, along with the need for a simultaneous assignment of a "bad" object role to her husband. In those cases in which, usually after one or two years of therapy, the wife becomes able to explore her ambivalent feelings toward her parents, her tendency to transfer the parents' "badness" to the husband diminishes. One would expect a better marital relationship from there on, but, paradoxically, this phase seems to frighten the husband, apparently because he is used to the marital dialogue based on his "badness" role. In some of our cases the husband has made repeated efforts at incriminating himself in the shortcomings of the wife's parents. He seems to be in alliance with his wife's distortions in order to preserve his role and identity.

The concept of need template connotes more than the sum of the components of an instinctual tendency. Need templates are more inclusive than the sum of strivings within a zone or developmental stage of the Freud-Abraham scheme. Although the concept encompasses the Self's needs for a symbolic ground, the biological, instinctual origin of some of the components of the subject's need templates is self-evident. The core of the personality originates from the undifferentiated biological matrix of the mother-child unity. The process of differentiation between the rudiments of Self and Not-Self takes place in the earliest, preconceptual origins of mental life. The origin of subject-object polarity is linked to experiences of separation and reunion with parental figures. It is probably fair to assume that in man, as in primates (Harlow, 1962), the main affective response to the earliest separation experiences is jointly attached to both tactile-kinesthetic and oral-alimentary type of sensory organization. In Harlow's experiments baby monkeys were raised without their mothers. The mothers were substituted for with (a) soft "cloth mothers" and (b) metallic but feeding "wire mothers." After a given period of adaptation, threat stimuli were used to test which "mother" was used more often as a comforting object to cling to in times of stress. In its search for security, the threatened young monkey ran more often to the cloth mother than to the wire mother. As far as the dialectical concept of Self-Not-Self separation is concerned, this preference suggests the importance of the warm contact between the embryo and the uterine wall rather than the mouth-nipple antithesis as experiential sources and reference points of security obtained through object-availability.

That the concept of need templates ought to include a broader range of inherited behavioral patterns than does traditional psychoanalytic instinct theory is suggested, among other things, by data from ethologic observation. The trend of combining psychoanalytic with ethologic concepts (Rapaport, 1960b, Bowlby, 1960) substantially enriches the exploration of the preconceptual roots of infantile need templates. Bowlby (1960) cites Hermann and other workers of the Budapest school of psychoanalysis as the first to emphasize instinctual aspects other than orality in the child's early relation to his mother. According to these workers and the ethologists, clinging and following are primary instinctual needs in their own rights. Conceptualizations about the character-forming role of the flexibility and rigidity (fixation) of relational need templates obviously have to take into account the nature of a multitude of instinctual drives and their "derivatives," i.e., their interlocking with early "imprinted" experience or learning.

It has been demonstrated that the relationship patterns of a "territorial" animal change radically if it is moved from its territory (Lorenz, 1959, p. 181). On the other hand, other animals' secure functioning depends on a personal bond formed with a companion. Is this a preconceptual precursor of the Self-Not-Self dialogue of humans? Are the territory and the companion equivalents of trust-giving love objects? Lorenz states that, although two animals of almost any vertebrate species will fight each other if placed in the same cage, they will do so only if they feel at home in the locality. The dialectical structure of these relational patterns of animals is striking indeed. A familiar context in the animal's existence organizes the animal's intraspecies relational patterns as though the animal operated on the basis of the internalization of its relationship with its territory or with a fellow animal. Apparently, the animal becomes more assertive when it can rely on a habitual (internalized) Other, symbolized by the "personal" meaning of his environment. It seems as though the companion or territory were more than mere props which help form a self-delineating context. That even man does not live entirely in the sphere of human (or animal) encounters is proposed by Searles (1960).

In accordance with the assumed transactional nature of the core of personality, one can conceive of what are known as dependent oral drives as manifestations of intrapsychic relational configurations of a dyadic nature in which the one who demands in a dependent fashion assumes a filial position and the one toward whom the demand is directed assumes a parental position. Apparently, we never give up the unconscious wish to correct the parental or giving capacity of our parents. In adult life we may have sublimated this drive into serving humanity, into doing good. Humanity, God, and fate are idealized replacement objects; they are the wished-for, improved editions of our internally preserved parent-objects. As long, however, as the dependent demand is channeled into adult interpersonal relating, whoever is able to transform the Other into a parent wins the object-role assignment game. The newborn may win it through its helpless crying, the sick adult through his suffering, the demanding family member through his "unrealistic" perpetual bickering and guilt-arousing blame. The member who gets "hooked" into the dyadic position of a parental object seems to be the loser in the contest, as documented by observations of the endless efforts of family members to make someone else feel responsible for their inner disappointments, expecting the Other to repent and to reform thereafter.

Although the range of possible relational objects is wide, the complexity of man's need templates makes it rather unlikely that two individuals can find a matching reciprocity of needs and satisfactions (relational dialogue) without considerable adjustment efforts. The principle of the dialogue requires that any lasting relationship ought to be reciprocally satisfactory to both partner's self-delineation needs. The knowledge of reciprocation builds reward into one's consideration of the Other's needs.

THE DIALOGUE

The concept of the dialogue can serve as a bridge between the individual-based and transactional or system-based motivational theories. A purely individual-based motivational theory is, for instance, the instinct theory. According to the instinct theory the subject, searching for an object of his drives, is an open system. He will select one or several objects for his drives and he in turn may be selected by one or several Others as their object. The dialogue, on the other hand, is a closed system, based on the feedback between two subjects. One of the interlocutors has to be subject and the other an object in each of their transactions. This give-and-take builds up trust and anticipation as mutual rewards. Possession of the partner becomes a secondary motivational aim which is instrumental in assuming one's primary need gratifications within the structure of the dialogue. If one partner's trust in the give-and-take is insufficient, the danger of his wanting to exploit the Other as the object increases. Of the six relational modes shown in Figure 1, the dialogue is the only one that can assure mutual and therefore secure possession of a relationship.

Probably the greatest importance of the dialogue lies in its contribution to both partner's self-delineation rather than to their impulse discharge. The trusted relational partner offers a context or ground for the delineation of the Self, both as subject and object. Once a love partner has been chosen on the basis of an increasing relational complementation, sexual, aggressive, and dependent drive discharges can each take their turn within the context of the two persons having entered into close relationship. In describing Buber's concept of the dialogue, Friedman (1960b) states: "What really matters in genuine dialogue is my acceptance of the "otherness" of the other person, my willingness to listen to him and respond to his address. In monologue, in contrast. I only allow the other to exist as a content of my experience" (p. 27). "True confirmation means that one confirms one's partner as . . . an existing being even while one opposes him. I legitimize him over against me as the one with whom I have to do in real dialogue, and I may then trust him also to act towards me as a partner" (p. 86). What is referred to here as legitimization amounts primarily to helping the Other to be delineated as a subject opposite to oneself as an object of the Other's needs. Since offering oneself as an object to the Other amounts to "giving," the act of mutually trusting the Other is an important structural requisite of the dialogue. The trust, i.e., the anticipated reciprocation on the part of the Other, removes the emotional flavor of being used or taken advantage of. The atmosphere of trust changes the *economy* of "giving emotionally."

The fact that in the process of dialogue one is alternately subject and object has many, previously unexplored implications. The relative complexity of the "relational engagement," as compared with "object choice," stems from the fact that the former term encompasses "subject choice" as well. By this is meant that one assesses empathically the probable range of the partner's object-seeking drives, along with assessing him as a possible object for one's own drives. My choice of him as my object depends on my intuitive assessment of the ways in which he might turn to me as object of his needs. The complete human dialogue is therefore made up of the two (simultaneous or successive) opposite, part-relational processes. One school of thinking emphasizes the mutually exclusive nature of simultaneously being a subject and object toward the Other (Sartre, 1956). Whereas I don't consider the two components of relatedness as mutually exclusive, I believe that making the Other an object to one's needs is more gratifying than offering oneself as an object for the Other.[5]

Although an empathic perception of the Other's needs is an important requirement for the differentiation between Self and Other, it is the give and take, the alternation of subject and object roles, that makes the dialogue the foremost means of establishing a truly dynamic Self-Other demarcation. According to Buber, each relational move consists of two steps: "primal setting at a distance" and "entering into relation" (Friedman, 1960a, p. 80). By a reciprocal alternation of moves the dialogue becomes a safeguard against symbiotic merger. Mastery of the dialogue thus is a requisite of ego strength and autonomy. Failure to achieve the dialogue can be a source of social isolation and attendant relational "pathology."

Conversely, without autonomy on the part of the participants, we cannot speak of dialogue. Integration of conflicting attitudes through an exchange of points of view, which tends to increase rather than decrease the autonomy of the participants, implies a mutual respect for each other's growth. Mature love, rather than being a fusion as often stated, is a true dialogue in which each participant complements in succession the other's subject *and* object needs. This is the reason why playful boxing, for instance between father and son,

---

[5] It is difficult to illustrate the difference between the subject and object positions expected of the Other. In the course of paranoid delusion formation, for instance, the patient chooses to picture himself as object to imaginary persecuting, or tempting internal Others as subjects. The subject of a relationship provokes responses; the object responds.

turns out to be a friendly rather than mutually destructive encounter. One offers himself to the other's aggressive needs in exchange for gaining an object for his own needs for punching someone else.

Despite its crucial significance for the survival of the dialogue, empathy itself is not its chief constituent. Let us take Buber's example illustrating the importance of empathy: "A man caresses a woman, who lets herself be caressed. Then let us assume that he feels the contact from two sides—with the palm of his hand still, and also with the woman's skin" (1947, p. 29). The dialogic character of this situation is described by the first part of Buber's poetic formulation which contains the information that the object "responds," i.e., "lets herself be caressed." Without a true response the man's feeling the contact "with the woman's skin" would belong to "primary identification," i.e., an imaginary assumption of relatedness on his part, outside the woman's awareness.

Heterosexual "love" or encounter presents a possible example of a *simultaneously* reciprocal dialogue. Both man and woman need confirmation, which they give to one another by merely expressing their respective physiologic needs. The man's assertiveness in his role seems to make him automatically the object of the woman's assertiveness in her role and vice versa. But the test of the true dialogic maturity of the man-woman relationship comes at a time when the physiologic sexual urges are satisfied or absent. What is the nature of the total *personal* relationship then? No one wants to play the role of an object to the Other's needs permanently. To keep the Other in a unilateral object role, one has to pay for this state of affairs by means of wealth, physical beauty, social importance, or fame, or perhaps with notoriety. If sexual possession is the main attempt at solving man's ontic need for confirmation, sooner or later new demands arise for coping with the resulting disappointment. Entering into an intimately sensuous relationship, if it does not lead to total mature dialogic complementation, may cause one or both immature marital partners to regress, reviving their nonreciprocal needs for a parent, i.e., a captive supporting (anaclitic) object. Without resolving the ontological problem of mutual dependent needs, the marital partners are bound to land in an impasse even regarding their physiologic sexual need complementation. If they cannot develop a dialogic system, one or both may feel used by the other as a mere object for his own "selfish" needs. One or both can turn sexually nonfunctional through impotence, premature ejaculation, frigidity, etc., as an unconscious protest against being used as object by the other.

Considerations of the dialectical nature of relationships lead to the apparently paradoxical conclusion that the same process (dialogue) which guarantees the maintenance of the participants' distinct and autonomous Self-Other delineation constitutes a state of mutual dependence as well. Even the partner who has the active initiative or choice is dependent on the other partner as his object or ground. The one who is in the object position seems to have given up his active autonomy, yet the mere fact of his being a complement to the Other's assertion prevents him from a fusion with the Other, thereby confirming his distinct Selfhood. I believe that, just as the concept of internal relationships has to be incorporated into the thinking of existential phenomenology, the relational modes of being a Not-Self context or an object for the Other and the dialogue require further exploration in the context of psychoanalytic personality theories.

Relational Systems in Families

The concept of transactional systems is of great practical significance in the understanding and treatment of family difficulties. Since most family therapists have originally been trained in the field of individual psychotherapy or analysis, their theoretical framework is that of a dynamic relationship among an individual mind and its subsystems (id, ego, superego, conscious, unconscious, etc.). The practicing family therapist, however, is compelled to realize that the level on which pathology exists and therapy takes place is that of a system which is more than the sum total of pathologies of the individual members as discrete entities. It is appropriate to assign a higher level of system organization to the multipersonal totality of family transactions. Consequently, as in all cases of systems of varying complexity, the laws of lower level systems (e.g., hydrogen and oxygen) have to be jointly considered with the emerging new system laws appropriate to the higher order system (e.g., H_2O). The practical implication of this viewpoint is likely to produce a radical departure from the traditional individual-based nosologic orientations of psychiatry to one that is "system-based."

How can the concepts of the dialectical model be applied to the description of family health and pathology? The transactional character of the model postulates transpersonal or multi-individual units of subject-object discrimination, often masked by what appear to be individual-based motivations. In other words, a person, while saying *I*, may actually, and often unconsciously, mean *We*. Any actual or intended transaction can, of course, be conceived in terms of a subject-object relationship or boundary. One or more participants may make up either side of the relational boundary. For example, the boundary of intermember loyalty may shift quickly from a husband-wife vs. child to a mother-daughter vs. father configuration. The term boundary is not meant here to denote a rigid dividing line between two territories. It rather connotes the fact of a discontinuity, and of a dynamic, feedback-like relatedness between subject and object. The Self's delineation or meaning can be accentuated either by its antithetical contraposition to the object or by its fusion with a co-subject respectively. A subject-object contraposition is one of the basic requirements of the dialogue and the healthy family consists of a network of relationships of the dialogic rather than fusion type.

The essence of the scapegoating process is that someone is assigned an object role by the collusive action of several other members. The role is not necessarily "bad." We have seen family members caught in an idealized "good" position, having been assigned the task of improving the ostensibly hostile interrelationship of the parents. Neurotic parents can unconsciously utilize the peacemaker inclinations of their anxious children who, in their efforts to save their parents' marriage, offer themselves as responsible, parent-like transference objects. The child's go-between role may take the form of an angry censor or now one, now the other parent. Many times the go-between child may be the only channel for constructive communications in what appears to be a life-and-death battle between the parents.

Any family member who becomes caught in an object role in the network of relational systems is at a considerable disadvantage. He is at the whim of the Other's internal need templates, a motivational field which is basically inaccessible to his own needs. Perhaps his best countermove is to make the Others the relational objects of his needs and selectively to perceive only the ego-syntonic aspects of the transaction, but the result can be a mutually paranoid and defensive attitude on the part of both sides.

A symbiotic and increasingly nondialectic relational network can come into being if the Other's role becomes predictable. Gradually, A comes to know B's responses so well that A's address to B actually contains B's predictable response. The predictability of the member's responses transforms them not only into captive objects with respect to each other but into components of an *intersubjective continuum*. The latter term describes a state of fusion among members which eliminates one-to-one subject-object relatedness. The system may become threatening to individuality: if there is no Not-Self, there can be no Self-experience; if there is no masculinity, there is no femininity; if there is no clear-cut parental role, there is no satisfying child role. Eventually, each member becomes bound by the rules of the fused system. As they become objects to a *system of predicta-*

ble transactions, they lose their freedom of choice as individuals. As the subject-object dialogue becomes impossible, the transactional system obtains the character of "pseudo-mutuality" (Wynne, *et al.*, 1958). It is futile to look for the contours of the individual members' position in such a system. Each position is contingent on the state of the system as a whole. For the same reason, there are no real alliances in such families. The only lasting configuration is an intra-familial fusion opposite to extrafamilial Others. Usually it is this need for a trustable predictability rather than any secret that keeps the Other (e.g., therapist) outside the family; only relatively well-differentiated groups can maintain true secrets. Interestingly, the same tendency which keeps the amorphous family apart from the outsider, the intersubjective fusion, is the force that works toward an eventual, merger-like incorporation of the stranger also. The predictability of the family members' responses eventually tends to provoke predictable, cliché-like responses from the outsider (therapist), and whoever permits himself to be involved in a predictable response-feedback becomes fused himself with the intersubjective system. Such fusion per se is different from, but often preceded by a phase in which the outsider is vested with a "transference" object role.

The structure of a predictable response system, by serving as a basis of the members' self-delineation, becomes the structure of inter-member trust. Whereas the individuated give-and-take of the dialogue sustains trust through the participants engaging in evolving subject-object roles, intersubjective fusion can not tolerate any autonomous change on the part of its members who participate in a shared (plural) Self-experience.

The fused family can also be characterized by Buber's concept of the "primitive We" (Friedman, 1960a). An "amorphous" We experience can replace the individual members' Self-experiences whenever the multiperson system becomes a major channel of impulse discharge in the same manner as the ego is the organized agency of the individual's impulse management. But whereas the unity of a single organism provides a single point of reference, the unitary function of a family system depends on the *predictability* of the action patterns of all members. The system becomes a necessary channel for the members' gratifications. As long as all members are committed to the system, their sense of satisfaction is not threatened. At its extreme, such a system does not permit any individual choice. In less extreme instances, the system can permit some freedom on the part of the members, and the members' commitment to the system is insisted upon only in certain symbolically meaningful rituals, e.g., in spending Christmas, New Year's, or Thanksgiving Day together.

The transactional system characterized by an amorphous We represents more than intersubjective merger; experimentally it is an Us-Object as well as We-Subject system. Together, family members may react to outsiders with shared persecutory fantasies and paranoid tendencies. Termination or conjoint family therapy may be experienced by a family as a victorious expulsion of the "bad" intruder. If there is a marriage of one of the offspring, the pseudoindividuated young wife, for instance, may be retracted into the family system by guilt, just like a pseudopodium into the amoeba. The husband finds himself confronted with an entire system to which his wife seems to give greater allegiance than to her marriage.

Recent interaction-oriented theories of family behavior have produced the notion that certain patterns of transactions, e.g., "pseudomutuality" (Wynne, et al., 1958) or "double-bind" (Bateson, et al., 1956), directly interfere with the participants' autonomy. In the instance of double-bind, the formulation explicitly includes a binder and a victim. The victim is conceived of as prohibited from escaping from the field, both by the initial, ambiguous set of conflicting injunctions and by a tertiary negative injunction. The authors add: "However, it seems that in some cases the escape from the field is made impossible by certain devices which are not purely negative, e.g., capricious promises of love, and the like" (p. 254). The concept of being unable to escape from the "field" is very similar to what we call *captivity of object-role assignment*. In a more recent paper by the authors of the double-bind concept the dyadic context of binder and victim is de-emphasized, and the double-bind situation is described in terms of a person being "caught up in an ongoing system which produces conflicting definitions of the relationship and consequent subjective distress." (Bateson, et al., 1962, p. 157).

In our terms the captive aspect of the object-role assignment becomes apparent when the person who is "caught up" is, by definition, unable to act as a subject, i.e., to reciprocate according to his own needs by assigning object roles to others. For instance, he may be made to listen to or care about others without being able to make the others comply with his own needs. The captive of a relationship can be made to "give" without himself being given to. As an example, a young schizophrenic man ran over to me at the beginning of the first family treatment session, grabbed my throat in a menacing manner, and shouted: "I am depleted, emptied! I can't give any more." It turned out that he was indeed wedged in the family system through what seemed to be irreversible bonds. The mother immobilized the boy by making him feel guilty for any sign of autonomy, while the father offered a deceptive protectiveness as if it were a defense against the mother. The boy was forced to be a receptive channel to both parents, while at the same time they were impervious to his needs. The ostensibly (over) protective alliance of the parents isolated their child; he could not "get" from them.

The concept of captivity by object-role assignment implies that, regardless of the nature of the underlying specific (aggressive, libidinal, etc.) needs, the accomplished assignment secures the availability of an object to the captor(s). The "bind" is not of a communicational nature, not just a "conflicting definition of the relationship" (Bateson, *et al.*, 1962). Its essence is *possession* or merger, frequently exemplified by slips of the tongue: "My mother would not put my . . . I mean *her* arm around me." In this example, the child wishfully makes the mother's arm her own possession, an object of her needs. What Bateson and his co-workers have called inability to "escape from the field," more specifically should be called the inability to escape an assigned object role, which is co-determined by the captive member's unconscious collusion with the binding system.

Previously, we have described that basic trait of "symbiotic" or pathologically close family systems which, by elimination of both individual choice and unpredictability, transforms these relational networks into an intersubjective merger. The definition of a pathologically close family system does not rely on the number or quality of extrafamilial contacts. Rather, it is a function of the extent of intersubjective or transpersonal merger as opposed to autonomous initiative on the members' part.

The nature of part-object role assignments in symbiotic systems differs fundamentally from the dialogic role relationships of differentiated individuals. Moreover, the multiperson, *intersubjective sharing* quality makes these object-role assignments differ even from immature, partial object-role assignments on a one-to-one basis. In the example of the sadist and the masochist, the partial object role (e.g., the one who causes or takes suffering) is assigned by one person to another and, usually, vice versa. Their commitment to the relationship is at least numerically symmetrical. In the family system of intersubjective sharing, on the other hand, the expectations of the multiperson system assign roles, (e.g., scapegoat or parent) to individual members. The object-role assignment is done here with so much *collusive* sharing and rigid predictability that it precludes dialogic or subject-object contraposition. Further, since in these families no one is ever fully committed to relate to other members as a whole person, and no one is ever able to offer himself as one whole object to any other member's strivings, no reciprocal relationship can ever be formed. The resulting, deficient relational and emotional development becomes fixated by the fact that all members contribute unconsciously to the maintenance of the state of intersubjective sharing. Not only are the members' personalities the products of symbiotic systems but they have a vested interest in the system which diminishes the danger of separation and of consequent depersonalization experiences.

At its outset any relationship, even a mature or dialogic one, has to rely on two, basically nonreciprocal object assignments, one on each partner's part. The Other becomes attractive as a symbolic validation of or imaginary coincidence with an internally needed prototype (e.g. in the case of the girl: strong man, kind man, intelligent man, or, on a deeper level, "a man like I wished Daddy to be"). This stage of relating is not only *unidirectional* but *partial*. In a selective fashion, only that part of the Other is perceived which fits the criteria of the internal prototype. If the relationship remains fixated on this level, an autistic system (Chapter 3) develops. The prototype of such systems is the unhappy combination of a love-hungry baby with its deprived, parent-seeking young mother.

As the relationship evolves, a network of co-ordinated responses develops out of a congeries of individual, unilateral object-role assignment efforts. The uncertainty of the Other's responses diminishes; his reactions become more predictable. To the extent one perceives the Other's responses as confirmatory of one's object-seeking, role-assignment efforts, one begins to feel confirmed in self-assertion and trust. Concurrently, the I-experience takes on the characteristics of a We-experience. One could postulate that the nature and vicissitudes of the We-experiences characterize the family as a relational system. Ultimately, an entire family will be experienced as within the boundaries of a We. The purely autistic family system may lack a We-experience. Other types of family systems can be characterized by either an *amorphous* or a *differentiated* We experience on the part of their members. The amorphous We is mainly based on intersubjective fusion among all members; the differentiated We is characterized by distinct subject-object positions (dialogue) between members of healthier families.

The stress of being approached, and later penetrated, by strangers (e.g., therapists) may accentuate the family's tendency for intersubjective merger. As an example, let us observe a family at a typical family evaluation interview. They come into the interviewing room and sit down somewhat suspiciously, perhaps partly because of the microphone and the one-way mirror. In most cases it takes only a few minutes for the observer to identify each member's role in the presenting family system. One child will be somewhat boisterously hyperactive; one parent will tend to act as a controlling force; perhaps one member has the solemn look of an actor inwardly rehearsing his role prior to stepping on stage. To the extent that each role is not just incidental behavior but a meaningful, quasi-predictable expression of the family as a whole, each member has a partial, subject-like responsibility for the other's behavior. The first statements made by one member to the therapists are essentially made by the entire family. At this stage, one member speaks for even those members with whom he will later disagree most decidedly; he opens up the family dialogue opposite to the therapists who represent both intruders and potential parent-objects for the entire family. Members who later will turn out to be jealous contenders for the therapists' attention join each other now to test how far the therapists can be engaged in a quasi-parental role.

Experienced therapists will soon pick up signs of disregard for discrete individuality or *autonomous otherness* among family members. Members will finish each other's sentences or claim to express each other's innermost feelings, etc. They don't regard the Other's address as important; they don't allow the Other to be a subject opposite themselves as available objects. An example of this phenomenon is the "overprotective" parent who supersedes the autonomy of the child by being hungry or cold *for* the child. The symptoms of the designated "sick" member often seem to be complementary to family patterns of fusion and vicarious participation. A psychotic daughter who was designated as patient, first appeared bizarre as she tried to defend her promiscuity, but later she turned out to be merely a caricature of her "normal" father, who for many years had claimed the "right" to reject his marriage in both words and in token actions. The lack of father-daughter role complementation was apparently made up by unconscious, imitative duplication. In another family, in which the mother's main complaint pertained to her two sons' unwillingness to help her with the dirty dishes, both boys' psychotic symptomatology culminated in compulsively frequent taking of showers, with special attention to anal cleansing. A chronically psychotic woman habitually inflicted wounds on her own body and thus strived to enlist the sympathy of her six siblings who visited her in the hospital with great regularity. History revealed that this family's early "system" had initially centered around the sick mother whose martyr role had been ambivalently revered by her helplessly immobilized children. The designated psychotic daughter lived in a partial fusion with the deceased mother.

The amorphous family organization may take the form of an ostensibly well-functioning transactional system. Intersubjective sharing may deceptively appear as intensive relating. On closer observation, however, members of such families turn out to be incapable of genuinely reciprocal commitments to each other. They seem to selectively disregard messages and meanings that may be conducive to individuality and autonomous growth. A habitually bickering parental couple displayed a basically collusive design for holding their sixteen-year-old daughter in the assigned object role of a "giving" parent. In one of the family therapy sessions this girl attempted to discuss her interest in a boy friend whom she had been meeting in a library. The parents could not "hear" anything else but her refusal to be more responsible and giving toward the family. The two parents kept repeating that the girl read too much and that she neglected the family in favor of the library. Both parents limited their involvement with their daughter to their transference demands on her, refusing thereby to become available as parent objects to the girl's needs.

No family system is entirely amorphous or entirely differentiated. Often the test comes in the form of losing a member. Although even mature, individuated families resist the painful act of separation, their resistance is different, at least in degree, from the desperate defense displayed by the amorphous system against any attempt at individuation, let alone separation. Members of a differentiated family system have to cope with object loss and mourning, but members of an amorphous family system have to fight the felt self-disintegrative threat inherent in the separation of any member. They do not seem to be able to partake of that type of growth of the ego which is said to proceed via abandoned object relationships (Freud, 1923) because of the intersubjective fusion, rather than subject-object demarcation quality of their relatedness.

It is consistent with our transactional point of view to assume that the relinquishment of any object tie is possible only if the person has sufficient inner resources for a remodeling of the crucial (dialectical) delineation of his Self through the substitution of other, either external or internal subject-object antitheses. Since each family member constitutes a participant ground (object) for the subject aspect of all other members, any one member's departure will be resisted by the members of any, even "healthy" family system. True separation always implies a subjective feeling of loss, or, symbolically, of death. Acquisition of relationships or involvement, on the other hand, beginning with the act of nursing, symbolizes the principle of life. The family's shared relational stagnation, while helping to ward off the pain of object relinquishment, amounts to an obstacle to vital relational growth on each member's part.

IS THERE A COLLECTIVE PLEASURE PRINCIPLE?

If two or more people join forces in helping each other to avoid the pain of emotional growth, their escape from reality amounts to a shared venture, as though their regressive mental economy was guided by a *collective pleasure principle*. The economic gain for the participants, however, is only partly related to "receptive dependence and the necessity for immediate discharge" (Fenichel, 1945, p. 42). No one member is able to enjoy immediate impulse discharge as an individual, nor is he a mere passive, dependent participant of the system; the maintenance of the system requires co-ordinated role-playing among members, which demands, in turn, that the individual be constantly "tuned in" to the pertinent actions of the others, instead of being "in conflict with the whole world, with the macrocosm as well as with the microcosm" (Freud, 1929, p. 27). Viewed in its complex interactional context, the behavior of the participants of an amorphous dynamic system is only partly unreal. The participants are not given to isolated, autistic daydreaming to the exclusion of all social reality. Their "pathological complementarities" (Boszormenyi-Nagy, 1962) amount to partial, implicit, but *de facto social validation* through sharing of a psychic economic gain. The symbiotic goal of the amorphous system is usually unconscious in the members, but the forces that maintain the system over the years must act on a preconscious or conscious level of ontic, self-delineating, and self-confirmatory gain.

The presumed ego weakness shared by the nonautonomous members of the amorphous system which penalizes separation and allows postponement of mourning is not always manifested in the participants' proclivity for immediate impulse gratification. Rather, their state of interminably prolonged "absence of grief" (H. Deutsch, 1937) is based on a complex structuralization which requires great investment and delay for its maintenance. The system represents an unconscious contract among the participants. Adherence to the contract is supposed to protect the participants against the possibility of the threat of disastrous object losses. At times the system is manifested in an apparent lack of attachment among members. The symbiotic state itself is based not only on the denial of the loss of original love objects but also on a denial of the attendant failure in accomplishing a progressively integrated, reciprocal Self-delineation among the participants. The gain, on the other hand, is not pleasure of discharge but security through "not rocking the boat." The repetition of rituals which maintain these stagnant family systems lies, so to speak, beyond a group pleasure principle.

Turning now to the question of implementation of object-role assignments within amorphous family systems, we have to admit the great limitations of our knowledge in view of the wealth of man's relational strategies. In any case, covert assignments of object roles make up the texture of relational systems. I plan to describe some of the empirically observed manifestations (schemes) of pathological family systems in a later section. But first an attempt will be made here to enumerate two transactional dimensions along which object assignments are often made by family members: goodness vs. badness and relational differential.

ASSIGNMENT OF THE ROLES OF GOODNESS
AND BADNESS

Few of the families in our treatment center have stayed free of an almost compulsive assignment of good and bad roles for any prolonged period of time. It seems that at times of stress, or perhaps after a given time of self-imposed restraint, the system of family interactions simply must include a certain amount of scapegoating of certain members along with a complementary idealization of others (assignment of Devil and Angel roles). Quite frequently, the only expression of tensions in the parental marriage occurs in the form of the parents' joint censure of a psychotic offspring's misbehavior. At other times the intolerable tensions developing between a mother and her adolescent daughter are expressed in an explicit scapegoating of the father, not entirely without his willing compliance. Although the assignment of good and bad roles to certain members may be regarded as attempts at a system-based, complementary self-delineation, these relational patterns serve the members' basic needs for impulse discharge as well. To the extent, however, that external relationships become mere impersonations of familially shared fantasies, a genuinely reciprocal dialogue among participants, as whole persons in their own right, becomes impossible. The complete predictability of the sequence of all transactions robs the members of any choice or true initiative. Scapegoating, for example, deprives the scapegoat of both, either clarifying himself, or hitting back in a reciprocal, appropriately aggressive, yet acceptable and accepted manner.

The family therapist must be cautious about accepting intrafamilial interactions at face value. Although their disparaging manifestations may appear to be undesirable, they may fulfill important intrapsychic need constellations. Intrapsychic "relatedness" to values of goodness and badness is an important factor of relational choice. Feelings of guilt, for example, can be attributed to an *internal transaction* with one's internal critic: the superego. The superego, as an imago or intrapsychic object representation, is a natural heir to the self-delineating role of originally external relational objects: the parents. Consequently, the perpetuation of one's own sense of guilt may be regarded as a relational aim; it provides a ground or "mental fuel" through the painful internal transaction itself. What from the ego's conscious viewpoint is unpleasurable may thus be maintained in the interest of unconscious configurational needs for Self-Other discrimination.

Various kinds of real, external relationships can be examined from the above point of view. Patterns of apparent hatred are maintained with what may seem to be reciprocity between members. Can hateful relationships be truly reciprocal or is their persistence due to an interlacing of autistic needs in two members, each relating to his own bad internal objects? It is an empirical fact that one of the characteristics of families of schizophrenics is the production of countless variations on the theme of finding a culprit for the unhappiness of now one, now another member. We have come to regard this chronic bickering in family therapy sessions as one of the manifestations of an underlying symbiotic inseparability and, paradoxically, as a main channel for the expression of belonging among family members. In this regard our view is related to that aspect of Wynne's (1961) concept of "pseudo-hostility" which serves to "blur and obscure the impact . . . of anxiety-producing intimacy and affection" (p. 110). If we assume—on well-supported clinical grounds —that family members are navigating between the Scylla of primary identification (merger) and the Charybdis of lonely unrelatedness, both leading to a loss of Selfhood, it is understandable that, in spite of its "badness," an atmosphere of constant discord may prove to be conducive to an optimal definition of the members' ego boundaries. This view is consistent with Erikson's (1959) position concerning the apparent advantage of some forms of negative identity choice over the dread of lack of identity.

Though self-delineation with the help of "bad" relationships may be preferable to unrelatedness, it is also true that society does not usually reward those whose suspicious and hostile attitudes become diffusely generalized. Such attitudes entail another danger of annihilation: an overflow of destructive or hostile propensities. Thus, it is easy to empathize with the relief of the patient who in an intermission between two paranoid phases reported to her therapist: "When I feel good toward you, the entire world seems to be good too." The agony of a world of hatred is illustrated by another schizophrenic patient's statement made in an individual therapy session during an acutely disturbed psychotic phase: "I hate my whole family, I guess . . . I hate everybody in here . . . You can't get revenge on people because they don't feel they are doing something wrong . . . I wish I'd have been able to go to my mother when I was little and tell her: Mother, these people are hurting me . . . they hate me . . . you hate me . . . that would have hurt her so bad . . . I don't think my mother cared . . . When you hate everybody you are afraid you are going to die . . . I can't confide in anyone . . . That's the way I know how to get close to people: by hurting them!" It is obvious that this patient is concerned about the social implications of the "bad" relational choices, dictated by her relational need-templates, based on negative identity choice.

One of the important applications of the assignment of the role of a "bad" object is the phenomenon described as "scapegoating." Scapegoating is an age-old practice, designed for the magical riddance of evil. It requires the existence of a group, the members of which feel threatened by some implication of evil (plague, sin, etc.) and who agree to use an Other (goat, slave, prisoner, etc.) to impersonate evil, which is ultimately to be gotten rid of through destruction of the scapegoat. Scapegoating, thus, requires at least three participants. Though one person can attempt to project badness upon another, ordinarily he cannot exert a social sanction alone; he needs a third one who will validate his notions of the "bad" identity of the scapegoat. Furthermore, a person can become scapegoated by a collusion between his critical superego and an outside Other.

The assumption that scapegoating situations have a minimally triadic structure has important implications for certain malignant interactions in families of the schizophrenic. As one becomes more familiar with the interaction patterns of these families, one is likely to discover mechanisms which appear to be aimed at possessive control through the threat of inducing psychotic disintegration. A patient, after having spent years in a "chronic" psychotic state, began to show definite signs of improved social functioning. This state of affairs produced, or at least coincided with, a diffuse variety of anxiety in the other members. In one family session, for no apparent reason, the mother burst out, "Susan, you may have improved with the help of these doctors, but I know that deep down you will always harbor the same old resentments toward me that you used to have before." This communication produced in the easily discouraged patient a feeling of helpless rage, as well as leading to the collapse of her efforts at improved behavior. The scapegoating implicit in this type of situation relies on the parent's "alliance" with maliciously critical internal objects within the patient. The validation of the destructive superego's verdict by the parent, who is genetically related to the superego, can amount to an ineludible bind based on the simultaneous operation of guilt and anger.

There seems to be an interrelation among "mental illness," assigned object-role, and the need for self-delineation. Acting-out or self-paralyzing psychotic behavior may represent aspects of a captive object role assigned by the family system. It is possible, for instance, that whenever in the father-mother-daughter relational triangle the parents are assigned the pattern of "good" interrelatedness, a concomitant assignment of the "bad" role to a child manifests itself in the child's acting-out behavior. Conversely, an unconditionally forgiving and protective attitude on the mother's part toward the child as a "good" object often complements a bad object assignment to the husband. Having been assigned a good object role, the family member would tend to repress and unconsciously direct against the Self all aggressive tendencies, curtailing his autonomy seriously thereby. The person may experience a disintegrative threat to his existence as a result. In this light, it is worth exploring the role of the "good sibling" opposite the bad, acting-out one. Jerman Rose has observed the rather regular occurrence of a "good," somewhat effeminate brother in the families of sexually acting-out adolescent girls (1963).

There are many forms which the assignment of bad roles within family systems can take: a young child may be accused of having an innately bad character, two children may be ascribed the role of being incorrigibly hostile and destructive to each other, the marriage of the parents may habitually be referred to as "bad," or one parent's genetic make-up may be blamed as defective. In any case, collusive good or bad object-role assignments are important components of intersubjective patterns and are indicative of deficient person-delineations.

The splitting of relational objects into good and bad ones corresponds to the type of organizational pattern described by a group of British psychoanalytic authors (summarized by Guntrip, 1961) as characteristic of endopsychic relational structures. Melanie Klein calls the earliest psychic developmental phase the paranoid position, characterized by splitting of fantasied good and bad aspects of both mother-objects and ego. Fairbairn (1952), who originally conceived only of exciting and rejecting bad internal objects, later admitted the existence of both good and bad internal objects opposite to what he called the "central" ego. The split (good and bad) object-relational model itself is reminiscent of the configuration of the classical formulations of the oedipus phase in which identification (merger?) with the "aggressor" parent of the same sex coexists with a sexually tinged "good" relating to the other parent. The powerful, triangular, person-delineating configuration may never be fully given up as a model of deeper relationships, and it results in a variety of later triangles which some marriages seem to need in order to exist. The involvement of the future schizophrenic child in the parental marriage appears to be analogous to the triangular involvement of a grandparent, paramour, or other third party, as evidenced in several of the families we have observed by the fact that the onset of a schizophrenic process in the offspring occurred shortly after the death of a grandparent who had been deeply involved in the nuclear family.

The ultimate motivational determination of the need for assigning the dichotomous roles of goodness and badness to others can be conceptualized in such alternate frames of reference as good and bad archetypes, life vs. death instincts, or love vs. aggression. From the point of view of dialectical theory, a lastingly negative or ambivalent relating can be interpreted as a mutually needed, though not consciously desired, figure-ground complementation of each other, rather than merely an interpersonal channel for the discharge of innate aggressive impulses. It is probably correct to assume that the dialectical model of the person postulates a need for at least an occasional *simultaneous bilateral identity delineation,* i.e., one toward both good and bad objects. The latter assumption amounts to a transactional, ego-structural theory of ambivalence.

THE RELATIONAL DIFFERENTIAL AS ASSIGNED ROLE

Long-term observation in therapy can reveal layers of relational gains that are not immediately connected with the content aspect of symptoms. An important relational (secondary) gain is implicit in the concept of *regression*: the regressed adult restores the child-adult differential between himself and the others. In this sense, its net effect is the same as that of any transference-shaped relationship. The often-described instantaneous transference of the psychotic is one facet of the same relational gain, of which another facet is the childishly regressed symptomatology. Obviously, the weakness of a certain internal relational equilibrium is dynamically responsible for this aspect of psychopathology.

To be dependent on an Other is ordinarily conceived of as a subordinate, weaker relational position opposite to a stronger Other. A newborn child, found on a sidewalk, would depend absolutely for survival on the passerby. Viewed from the vantage point of biological contingency, the situation defines the infant as the weak, subordinate partner of the relationship. However, in the context of the value systems of society as they are internalized in the average member of the human race, it is the infant who, through its hold on the passerby's superego, makes the passerby a captive object of its needs. The infant can instinctively capitalize on the ontic needs of the passerby, who, in turn, needs to have himself defined as a decent person even though his own functional needs would cause him to prefer freedom from responsibility. The weak one wins through passive mastery, i.e., through having assigned the superior (parental) position to the stronger one.

Many intrafamilial struggles appear to be aimed at assigning the superior position to another member. It is known that one of the most effective ways of disciplining a child is through the inducement of guilt feelings. Manipulation of the Other's feelings of responsibility and guilt is one of the most powerful means by which to influence people's decisions without the guilt-assigner having to play an authority role. Passive mastery amounts, in effect, to a very *active* object-role assignment. Many types of pathological behavior can be regarded as essentially aimed at the secondary gain of assigning the superior side of a relational (dependency) differential to others. Being labeled as sick or drunk, for instance, accords one a socially tolerated state of lowered responsibility, while assigning to the healthy or sober one an implicit burden of higher responsibility. We have seen infantile, "psychotic" regression and psychosomatic sickness alternate between mother and son, as unconsciously performed maneuvers, aimed at care and attention from the rest of the members. The delinquent who acts out invokes a protective, controlling response on the part of society.

More subtle means of assigning a superior role-differential is needed if the assigning person is in a position of intrinsically higher authority. This is the case with the "parentification" of children by there parents. Martyr-like devotion, sickness, or excessive material giving can all amount to powerful binding of the child through his superego, i.e., his internal value orientation. Paradoxically, withholding of emotional "giving" to the child can in itself lead to a captive object-role assignment, probably through more complex means. The child's frustration and emotional hunger may tie him to the parent, even though the latter represents a questionable "giving" resource. Incestuous involvement between parent and child can lead to complicated binds of captivity, from which the child cannot extricate himself without outside help. Joint infantile regression of both parents (e.g., endless pointless bickering, continuous threats of separation and murder) are powerful means of binding the child in a responsible, essentially parent-like role. We have seen "good" children erupt in furor in the course of family therapy at the point when they can finally face their accumulated and long-suppressed anger over having to be a go-between for irresponsibly quarreling parents.

The Phasic Relational Process

The concept of process connotes an ordered temporal sequence. In this section both the family members' *transactional or group "behavior"* and their subjective, experiential, *intrapsychic develop-*

ment will need to be explored as organized sequences of events. The term process is used, further, in the sense of a "series of actions or operations definitely conducing to an end" (Webster's New Collegiate Dictionary, 1949) rather than as the antonym of "personal" or "experiential," as used, for example, by Guntrip (1961). In fact, a true psychological personality theory has to develop process constructs of both impersonally observable aspects of interactional behavior and the vicissitudes of private Self-Other experiences.

From the point of view of observable group behavior, the family's long-range life process can be compared to that of a biological organism. The biological common denominator of human and even subhuman family processes is the procreative cycle: mating, birth, child-rearing, maturation, mating, etc. Within the long-range, generational cycle there exist brief, functional relatedness cycles. The mother, for instance, engages in a complex of feeding relationships with each newborn, followed by consecutive phases of gradual weaning and increasing autonomy. The Freud-Abraham scheme of instinctual development and Erikson's epigenetic phases of psychosocial development can be considered as important examples of a psychodynamic process theory of relationships. Erikson's theory integrates familial with extrafamilial relational processes into a broader conceptual framework.

Whereas the sequence of behavioral development in families constitutes the subject of psychosocial "ecology," the role of relationships in Self-delineation experiences is the subject matter of dialectical personality theory. The concern of this section is with the relational (dynamic) roots of the *development* of Self-experience ("ego-feeling," Federn, 1952). This experiential focus is related to, but more personal and "anthropomorphic" than, Erikson's (1959) premise based on "the mutual complementation of ego synthesis and social organization" (p. 26). If we assume that one's discrete Self-experience depends on the vicissitudes of one's Self-Other encounters, the intrapsychic and interpersonal relational realms assume interconnected causal significance. The internalized relational patterns will, to a certain extent, predetermine the external relational preferences and the fate and level of involvements. External relationships, on the other hand, can contribute to the content and quality of what evolve as building stones of the endopsychic structure of Self and Other representations. Common clinical illustrations of the above are the "projection" of superego attitudes upon external relationships, on the one hand, and the incorporation of the attitudes of significant, quasi-parental others into one's superego configuration, on the other.

The specific goal of the present section is the construction of an inclusive framework for the sequence of phases of both social interaction as observable behavior and Self-Other delineation as inner experience. Since our focus is chiefly concerned with subjective experience as a dynamic source, our orientation for ordering process phases has to be based on an experiential-phenomenological conceptual framework. The key dimension of the experiential-phenomenological framework is the Self-Other demarcation, rather than the synthetic, organizing, adaptive, and executive ego function. What the proposed phasic theory implies, then, is that there is an interrelation between the styles of interactional or transactional (group) *behavior* and modes of self-experiences of individual members. At the same time, for instance, when, from the observer's vantage point, members alternate between uninvolvement and close involvement, the members themselves feel that they fluctuate between *singular* ("I") and *plural* ("We") *modes of self-experience*. To the extent that any experiential event is organized around the plural Self as a basis for Self-Other delineation, various Others may share in the We-experience. However, my subjective structuring of my Self-Other boundary might not coincide with the ways other members' subjective experience causes them to structure the Self-Other boundaries of the We-group from their vantage point. Each new developmental phase of the family's relational process is marked by a new alignment of transactional patterns and modes of Self-Other delineation.

A simple enumeration of the important stages of personality development from birth to maturity could provide a model for the experiential side of the relational group process. Mother and newborn infant start interacting ostensibly from a baseline of complete unrelatedness. It is true, on the other hand, that there have been certain anticipatory sets which, to some degree, determine their subsequent relating: the infant possesses an inborn instinctual apparatus, and the mother brings her conscious and unconscious wishes, idiosyncratic sensitivities, etc., into the relationship. She is related to previous, internalized Others and she will turn some of her past relational expectations toward her child as a transference object. Thus, in its early phase, the mother-child relationship can be called *autistic*. The early phase of lack of relatedness or exclusive transference relating is soon replaced by a sense of symbiotic fusion. The dynamically most crucial moments of this affiliation can be characterized as an "amorphous We" experience. As the infant grows, gradually a Self-Other (ego-object) differentiation takes place, based on both participants' ability to distinguish between what the Self wants and what the Other wants. Along with the recession of the amorphous We experience, an internalization of the Other takes place, and this phase can be called that of *individuation*. One can also say that at this stage the private experience of relatedness takes the form of a "differentiated We" with an increasing distinctness of I-Thou relationships between singular Selves and Others. It must be added, though, that the relationship usually remains, at least to a degree, interspersed with amorphous, symbiotic We experiences. The We experience can only be given up if it is replaced by the establishment of discrete, singular, Self-Other boundaries in the intrapsychic world of the participants. Since relinquishment of old ties is a requisite for new relationships, the individuation phase prepares the ground for the *separation* stage. It is implicit in this latter, mourning-like stage that, in order to complete it, the member, has to be able to internalize not only his partner's contribution to his amorphous We experience but his own antithetical, Other-aspect as well. In the separation stage the relinquishment has to be actual, not just structural; the individuated member has to become capable of physical separation. It is obvious that this stage cannot be successfully resolved without the accomplishment of the individuation phase. After separation, or concurrently with it, *reinvolvement* in a new relationship (e.g. courtship, marriage, etc.) can follow. Thus the cycle of relational process is completed and a new cycle starts with a new nuclear family and new offspring.

In terms of object-role assignment, the relational process can be characterized as consisting of consecutive *phases of increasing integration of internal and external relational perceptions and attitudes.* In this sense the autistic phase is mainly characterized by anticipatory, internally determined object-role assignments, with a minimum of empathic perception of the Other's needs. The affiliative or symbiotic stage is characterized by a confusing clash of the respective object-role assignment efforts, along with a gradually increasing awareness of the Other's subjective needs. In fact, certain partial need-object complementations may appear to the participants here as mutually ego-syntonic, although the relationship as a whole has not yet been delineated. Instead of being a dialogue, the relatedness takes the form of either an avoidance of differences or of desperate attempts at convincing the Other of one's own point of view. At the stage of individuation the improving dialogue between the partners introduces a synthetic alignment of inner expectations with a more adequate understanding of the Other and consecutive object-availability to the Other on the Self's part. Reciprocity or mutuality is based here on a clear distinction and acceptance of differences rather than on avoidance of conflict. The alternation of compatible subject-object complementations constitutes the dialogue of two individuated persons. With the increase of the members' capacity for personal commitment, anxiety due to amorphousness and lack of delineation tends to diminish. In families, one of the signs of this development is the narrowing of the spectrum of topics that are taboo for discussion.

As the "dialogue of needs" becomes established, it becomes one of the greatest sources of relational security and trust. Its accomplishment permits the posing of real demands, i.e., of transiently nonreciprocal kinds of object-role assignments, in the knowledge that the Other will subsequently feel free to demand the same in turn. In a way, the mutually rewarding quality of the dialogue extends the freedom of need expressions. Postponement of complementarity or mutuality becomes increasingly possible as a result of anticipated future give-and-take. The structure of the dialogue is not based on a constant complementation of needs. Instead, it is a contract for the free exchange of both partners' noncomplementary need assertions, based on their reliance on the over-all mutuality of each other's object availability. The experiential structure of the dialogue of needs is then something like this: "I know that you know that I shall put up with your demanding; therefore I am turning to you with my demand."

A simplified schematic representation of the phasic relational law is given in Figure 3. This schematic drawing attempts to represent the unity of the transactional, behavioral, and experiential-personal aspects of the phasic process. It ostensibly is a scheme for changes in the global aspect of relating, although the phasic relational law is applicable to the—much more frequent—part-relational, e.g., oral, anal, or genital, involvements. Since the scheme depicts the ideal timetable of maturation, it does not account for relational stagnations.

Phase A signifies the autistic stage in which a parent-child relationship is merely anticipated. The dotted lines in the parents' circles indicate the object-seeking internal relational attitudes (remnants of past relationships) of each parent turned expectantly toward a prospective (recovered) love object. Another relational expectation of the parents has been partly fulfilled by the marital relationship, as is indicated by the overlap of their two circles.

In Phase B expectation has been replaced by real relationship, and the impact of the affiliative forces weakens person delineations (boundaries). The extent of intermember conjunction achieved here predisposes each participant to inner experiences of interpersonal merger or fusion with symbiotically vicarious, fused patterns of action.

Phase C indicates a beginning relational distance along with the formation of tentative ego boundaries. More significantly, however, it signifies the first appearance of internal relationships in the child.

The nature of the relationships with internal objects will determine the success of the individuation phase as a preparation for the next phase. The beginning of a satisfactory resolution of the oedipus complex and consecutive superego formation are illustrative of this phase.

Phase D represents the painful phase of actual relinquishment of family ties, which at the same time is the gateway to emotional

TRANSACTIONAL PATTERNS		INTRAPSYCHIC EXPERIENCE
	A. EMBRYONIC LIFE EARLY INFANCY	A. AUTISM (PARENTS WITH INTERNAL RELATIONAL EXPECTATIONS)
	B. AFFILIATION CONJUNCTION SYMBIOSIS	B. BASIC TRUST, MERGER
	C. INDIVIDUATION AUTONOMY	C. SENSE OF DISTINCT SELFHOOD (EGO BOUNDARY FORMATION)
	D. SEPARATION DISJUNCTION	D. GRIEF
	E. REINVOLVEMENT ENGAGEMENT MARRIAGE	E. LOVE, TRUST, MERGER

Fig. 3. P = Parent; C = Child; E.O. = Extrafamilial Other.

freedom and fulfillment on a mature level. The proof of successful accomplishment of the separation phase lies in subsequent reinvolvement with genuine commitment. Many of the abrupt separation moves of adolescents serve, however, only to highlight the lack of accomplishment of levels C or B and to recreate the supremacy of phase B as a family goal.

In Phase E the child has grown "mature" and, as a discrete individual, he is ready for re-involvements with peers. His well-delineated internal relationships enable him, the young adult, to seek complementary type relationships (dialogue) without the concomitant threat of arousing a need either for fusion with or for "transference distortion" of the partner as if the latter were a desperately longed-for parental love object.

The five phases of the scheme represent partial goals of the cyclic maturational process, and each shift (from A to B, B to C, etc.) represents a dynamic change, a relational realignment. Transition from one phase to another is comparable to the "work" of mourning whereby the capacity for absorbing losses represents a maturational goal.

AFFILIATION OR SYMBIOTIC PHASE

Affiliative motivations can be based on the participants' internal (transference) needs for assigning to each other the roles of representatives of internalized objects. These needs are bound to elicit mutually disappointing expectations and demands. An atmosphere of frustration and desparate seeking of object possession is characteristic of the "orally" demanding, symbiotic type of families. It is as though the members have reached the extent of closeness necessary for posing demands for relational availability without having achieved the level of reciprocal give-and-take or dialogue of needs. The aim of the struggle is to make the other member "care," i.e., become a willing ground to one's wished-for self-delineation.

Frequently, apparent complementarities between the expectations of parent and child can amount to counterautonomous, symbiotic binds. A mother revealed that the more annoyingly hostile and demanding her daughter used to get, the more self-sacrificing and self-controlled would she herself become, because, as she stated, her daughter wanted her to be that way. The daughter, on the other hand, felt that she had to behave in uncontrolled fashion in order to help her mother express anger. More subtle gratifications among family members may take the form of less overt complementarity. A mother may ostensibly disapprove of her daughter's self-destructive sexual behavior yet participate in the behavior pattern through unconscious identification and sharing. Such "superego lacunae" (Johnson, 1949) may lead to powerful symbiotic bonds which contribute to self-experiences based on an "amorphous We."

The phase of affiliation manifests itself in both overt and covert interactions among family members. The conjunctive nature of these interactions may be cloaked by ostensibly disjunctive overt behavioral attitudes. Manifestations of affiliative, symbiotic needs may be found in: (1) observable behavior (e.g., a young wife *leaves* her "impossible" husband and children and *rejoins* her mother, concealing from herself her unconscious wish for union with mother); (2) content of thoughts (a patient reports that she has to consult a fantasied, introjected mother before making any decision); (3) gross disorders of thinking (hearing mother's "voice" all the time); (4) quality of subjective experience ("Everybody reminds me of my mother" or "I don't feel like a person" or "I go to pieces when she is around"). Formal and content characteristics of dreams and projective test material may also provide evidence of a psychological state pervaded by affiliative motivations.

Unconscious possessive needs can be classified according to levels of increasing specificity. There can be a (a) global need for having someone as captive object for closure through relatedness. Most typically, the demand is concealed "between the lines," not admitted overtly. A corollary to this need is an unconscious expectation that the family member, e.g., a child, will fail in his growth effort if the effort is seen to lead to eventual separation. The fiancé of one of our patients received a warning letter from the girl's mother, bluntly advising the young man against marriage and adding that raising her daughter had been to the mother like "putting money in the bank." Another level of need is (b) to have the object need satisfied in the most gratifying manner, that is, through having the Other adjust constantly and unilaterally to one's needs for a specific, complementing object or "resource" person. Applied to the parent-child relationship, the unconscious dynamic of the parent's object-restitutive needs can be expected to shape the child's emotional growth. The child who is selected for this role is usually the one who has shown the most capacity for empathizing with the parent's needs. At other times, the constitutionally most defenseless child may fall most easily into such a nonautonomous role. The whole system of the various members' mutual disregard for each other's autonomous personality needs, combined with the demand that the other members provide the expected person-complementing ground, can be related to the phenomenon of "pseudomutuality" (Wynne, et al., 1958). A third level is (c) to have the captive object offer positive and loving object and subject attitudes. If the libidinal expectations of the child remain bound to the parents, the emptiness of the parental marriage is rendered more tolerable. In one of the families we treated, the father preferred his daughter to his wife, both as an intelligent companion and as an accepting audience for his ambitious social and political aspirations. The mother, on the other hand, expected her daughter to be like she had always wished her own mother to be: warmly loving and ready to correct her at all times. A curious oscillation between "good" and "bad" companion roles was expected of another young schizophrenic girl by her mother. Every summer, while the other, preferred daughter was out of town, the patient was expected to become nonpsychotic and a warm companion for her mother, a role to which she conformed eagerly. With the advent of autumn and the return of the other daughter, the patient slipped back into a psychotic role and went into "deep freeze" in the hospital until the following summer.

INDIVIDUATION PHASE

Individuation is the second phase of the relational process; it represents progress beyond the accomplishment of affiliation or symbiosis. The individuated offspring can relate heterosexually or as a parent, provided there exists a capacity for an active and spontaneous induction of a reciprocal process (dialogue). The phase of individuation, however, applies to the family system as a whole. Although the next two phases, separation and new involvements, lead beyond the system of the family of origin, individuation is a shared phase of development. Individuation, in other words, can occur only in a group which allows it. It is pointless, for instance, to expect that a child take steps toward genuine individuation before he has absorbed a sufficient quantity of truly giving involvement from his parents. More precisely, the child cannot incorporate the model of trust and self-reliance if the parents have been unable to act genuinely parental. Only if the parents have given true recognition to the child's growth needs and arrived at a trusting reciprocity, will the child's personal existence become authentically autonomous.

Many examples of parental incapacity or ambivalence relative to helping the offspring to individuate can be given from family therapy experience. Parents who seem to agree to disagree and never reach resolution of any issue or disagreement perpetuate an atmosphere in which the child's need for a firm orienting point becomes badly frustrated. It seems as though parent and child were contending for a maximally irresponsible position so that someone, the organizations of the larger community, e.g., police or court, eventually will have to step in as quasi parents. The captive child is at the mercy of an abruptly alternating role: he is either expected to act as a mature judge between two childishly fighting adults or is enticed into agreeing with one parent against the other. In either event, the child has no trust-inspiring parent to listen to his own problems and needs. One family changed radically in therapy when the quiet, "good" daughter burst out in anger, "You two parents are always fighting like chickens when you should act like responsible grown-ups . . . my own feelings are completely left out."

Further, it is not only external relationships within the family that may oppose the autonomous strivings of the offspring. Certain internalized motivational (value) systems, described under "counterautonomous superego structure" (Boszormenyi-Nagy, 1962), act as internal hindrance to even thinking of oneself as moving toward eventual autonomy. The child becomes imbued with the conviction that he is obligated to "straighten out" his parents and that individuation on his part would amount to treason.

The adolescent or young adult offspring's turning from affiliation to individuation can present the parents' maturity with a severe test. This is particularly true if the parents need the child as a transference object for their vitally important, unconscious internal dialogue with their own parents. The parents' inability to complete mourning may make clutching to the offspring the most important goal of their unconscious motivations. We have seen parents offering to trade their marriage relationship for a protracted close involvement with the psychotic offspring. The parent's underlying possessive motivation may be disguised by a rationalized readiness for any necessary sacrifice to help the child get well. The desperately longing parents usually are blind to the fact that they overburden the child with their dependent demands. These parent-child relationships tend to provoke mutually frustrating, unilateral, and defensively autistic attitudes in both parties.

SEPARATION PHASE

Separation of the offspring is a most important "healthy" goal of the nuclear family. Separation as a physical process connotes a clearly disjunctive move on the part of one member and, implicitly, on the part of all. As an emotional process, separation is the expression of a crucial developmental phase of the entire family. Insofar as family members represent a most important segment of each others' dialectical personality ground, relinquishing the Other as a partner to the dialogue means a painful loss to every member's subject-object configuration. Individuation, a prerequisite for separation, has already meant a partial end to amorphous, symbiotic family togetherness. The separation of one member not only affects the separating member's one-to-one relationships with every other member, but it sets off a chain reaction of compensatory relational changes among the other members of the family system. The outcome of the compensatory rearrangements depends on the maturity of the family as a whole, in addition to the maturity of the members as individuals. More specifically, to the extent that members can absorb each other's "exposed" need templates, they can adjust to relinquishing a member. Conversely, the loss of a sibling, for instance, by marriage or death, can "precipitate" psychosis in one of the other children, or even parent, who had been previously compensated.

Separation is an extremely complex process and its successful accomplishment requires prior satisfactory achievement of the goals of affiliation and individuation. Only after having achieved close, trusting, and reciprocal relationships with members of the family and having internalized these relationships will the offspring be able to sever the familial ties and replace them with extrafamilial attachments. Separation is often preceded by a realignment of the offspring's intrafamilial relationships, e.g., the shifting of the adolescent girl's closeness from mother to father or to a brother.

Various complex family forces may counteract a member's moves toward separation even in the "normal" family. A certain child may come to represent symbolically an unconscious family concept or a fantasy of loyal "togetherness." We have seen families in which one of the daughters has been "selected" for the role of staying with the mother after the other children are married. The moral pressure for the acceptance of this caretaking role may come in the form of an unquestioned expectation from the siblings, parents, friends, or religious advisers. It is as though one sibling were selected to repay to the mother the obligation of all the children. The unspoken family agreement will "confirm" this daughter's personal identity needs only on condition that she performs the assigned caretaker role and thereby appeases the other members' guilt.

REINVOLVEMENT PHASE

The emerging extrafamilial relationships normally call for more active subject roles and more generously accepting object-other roles on the young adult's part. He should be able to express his—more mature—wishes to his new love object and to respond to the—not always mature—wishes of the partner. Schizophrenic and severely neurotic young adults discover painfully that friends, colleagues, marital partners, and, to a great extent, their own children tend to reject their clinging, parasitic attitudes. The demands of new close relationships and the responsibilities of reciprocal commitment naturally arouse anxiety in the young adult. The nature of these anxieties is often blurred by a guilt-laden nostalgia for the parents or for the symbiotic state of the past. One is apt to feel guilty about having received more from one's parents than one could ever repay, perhaps, paradoxically, the more so the less one has acquired in trust and security from one's parents.

Concluding Remarks

Questions of the "pathology" of intrafamilial relating are inevitably connected with the issue of family "health." In our view the question of family health and illness has to be separated from considerations of health of individual members. The concept of the dialogue may help to define the transactional structure of healthy family relations. The give-and-take of the true dialogue presupposes a high level of trust among family members. One can maintain a lasting receptiveness to the Other's needs only if one can trust that the Other will reciprocate. The alternation of subject-object roles among participants is a safeguard against intersubjective fusion or undifferentiated, symbiotic, amorphous relating. Presence or absence of an atmosphere of trust can characterize the entire relational system, not just individual members. The "pathology" of a system is more than the sum total of the pathologies of individuals.

The transactional concepts of health or pathology, growth or stagnation have to rely on notions of trust, i.e., a "temporal" predictability of reciprocal transactions. If the predictable reciprocation leads to Self-confirmation in the participants, the resulting mutual "possession" assumes the pattern of a dialogue. Improving capacity in the family for the dialogue is both a most important goal and in itself a good prognostic sign. If the predictability of consecutive transactions is not conducive to improved Self-confirmation in the members, the pattern of collusive, intersubjective fusion is bound to increase. Since without a minimum of subject-object or dialogic Self-delineation the members' basic security is threatened, even "negative" relational patterns have to be regarded as preferable to amorphous fusion. In order to "help" the family through the stages of inducing dialogue and challenging stagnant, nonreciprocal systems of interaction, the therapist himself has to go through the phases of a "therapeutic" relational growth process. His strength to change others issues from his own freedom to change continuously and become progressively more himself through give-and-take.

References

BALINT, M. (1958). Three areas of the mind; theoretical considerations. *Int. J. Psycho-Anal. 39*, 328–340.

BATESON, G., JACKSON, D. D., HALEY, J., AND WEAKLAND, J. H. (1956). Toward a theory of schizophrenia. *Behav. Sci. 1*, 251–264.

BATESON, G., JACKSON, D. D., HALEY, J., AND WEAKLAND, J. H. (1962). A note on the double bind. *Family Process 2*, 154–161.

BOSZORMENYI-NAGY, I. (1962). Concept of schizophrenia from the perspective of family treatment. *Family Process 1*, 103–113.

BOSZORMENYI-NAGY, I. AND FRAMO, J. L. (1962). Family concept of hospital treatment of schizophrenia. In J. H. Masserman, (Ed.) *Current psychiatric therapies*, vol. 2. New York: Grune & Stratton, pp. 159–166.

BOWLBY, J. (1960). Ethology and the development of object relationships. *Int. J. Psycho-Anal. 41*, 313–317.

BRODEY, W. M. (1961). Image, object, and narcissistic relationships. *Amer. J. Orthopsychiat. 31*, 69–73.

BUBER, M. (1947). *Between man and man.* Translated by R. G. Smith. Boston: Beacon Paperback, 1955.

BUBER, M. (1958). *I and thou.* New York: Scribner's.

BUHLER, CH. (1962). *Values in psychotherapy.* Glencoe: Free press.

DEUTSCH, H. (1937). Absence of grief. *Psychoanal. Quart. 6*, 12–22.

DEUTSCH, H. (1942). Some forms of emotional disturbance and their relationship to schizophrenia. *Psychoanal. Quart. 11*, 301–321.

ERIKSON, E. H. (1959). Problem of ego identity. In G. S. Klein, (Ed.) *Psychological issues,* Vol. I, no. 1. New York: Int. Univer. Press.

ERIKSON, E. H. (1962). Reality and actuality. *J. Amer. Psychoanal. Ass. 10*, 451–474.

FAIRBAIRN, W. R. D. (1952). *Psychoanalytic studies of the personality.* London: Tavistock.

FEDERN, P. (1952). *Ego psychology and the psychoses.* New York: Basic Books.

FENICHEL, O. (1945). *Psychoanalytic theory of neurosis.* New York: Norton.

FINDLAY, J. N. (1962). *Hegel: A re-examination.* New York: Collier Books.

FREUD, S. (1951), originally published 1921). *Group psychology and the analysis of the ego.* New York: Liveright.

FREUD, S. (1961, originally published 1923). *The ego and the id* in Standard Ed., vol. 19, London: Hogarth Press.

FREUD, S. (1957, originally published 1929). *Civilization and its discontents.* London: Hogarth Press.

FREUD, S. (1949, originally published 1938). *An outline of psychoanalysis.* New York: Norton.

FRIEDMAN, M. S. (1960a). *Martin Buber: The life of dialogue.* New York: Harper Torchbooks.

FRIEDMAN, M. S. (1960b). Dialogue and the "essential we." The bases of values in the philosophy of Martin Buber. *Amer. J. Psychoanal. 20*, 26–34.

GUNTRIP, H. (1961). *Personality structure and human interaction.* New York: Int. Univer. Press.

HARLOW, H. F. (1962). Development of affection in primates. In E. L. Bliss (Ed.) *Roots of Behavior.* New York: Hoeber.

HARTMANN, H. (1950). Comments on the psychoanalytic theory of the ego. In *Psychoanalytic study of the child,* vol. 5, New York: Int. Univer. Press.

JOHNSON, A. (1949). Sanctions for superego lacunae of adolescents. In K. Eissler (Ed.) *Searchlights on delinquency: New psychoanalytic studies.* New York: Int. Univer. Press, pp. 225–245.

KLEIN, M. (1963). *Our adult world.* New York: Basic Books.

86 INTENSIVE FAMILY THERAPY

LORENZ, K. (1959). Role of aggression in group formation. In B. Schaffner (Ed.) *Group processes.* Transactions of the 4th Conference, Oct. 13–16, 1957. New York: Macy, pp. 181–252.

MARCEL, G. (1960). *The mystery of being, vol. I, Reflection and mystery.* Chicago: Gateway.

PFUETZE, P. (1961). *Self, society, existence. Human nature and dialogue in the thought of George Herbert Mead and Martin Buber.* New York: Harper Torchbooks.

RAPAPORT, D. (1958). Theory of ego autonomy: A generalization. *Bull. Menninger Clin. 22,* 13–35.

RAPAPORT, D. (1960a). Structure of psychoanalytic theory. In *Psychological Issues,* vol. II, no. 2, monograph 6.

RAPAPORT, D. (1960b). Psychoanalysis as a developmental psychology. In B. Kaplan and S. Wapner, (Eds.) *Perspectives in Psychological Theory; Essays in Honor of Heinz Werner.* New York: Int. Univer. Press, pp. 209–256.

ROSE, J. (1963). Workshop on family therapy. Annual meeting of the American Orthopsychiatric Association, Washington, D.C., March.

SARTRE, J. P. (1956). *Being and nothingness. Essay on phenomenological ontology.* Translated by H. E. Barnes. New York: Philosophical Library.

SEARLES, H. F. (1960). *The nonhuman environment in normal development and in schizophrenia.* New York: Int. Univer. Press.

SPIEGELBERG, H. (1960). *The phenomenological movement. A historical introduction,* 2 volumes. The Hague: Martinus Nijhoff.

WAELDER, R. (1960). *Basic theory of psychoanalysis.* New York: Int. Univer. Press.

WYNNE, L. C. (1961). Study in intrafamilial alignments and splits in exploratory family therapy. In N. W. Ackerman, et al. (Ed.) *Exploring the base for family therapy.* New York: Fam. Serv. Ass. of Amer., pp. 95–115.

WYNNE, L. C., RYCKOFF, I. M., DAY, J., AND HIRSCH, S. (1958). Pseudomutuality in the family relations of schizophrenics. *Psychiatry 21,* 205–220.

3

IVAN BOSZORMENYI-NAGY

Intensive Family Therapy as Process

Intensive family therapy differs from all other mental health approaches in its application of principles and techniques derived from
dynamic individual psychotherapy and, to a lesser extent than might
be supposed, from group therapy, to helping all family members
through direct observation and modification of their interactions.
Although family therapy offers some of the deepest and clearest
insights into intimate relationships, its practitioner finds himself confronted with problems on a unique multipersonal system level of
organization which involves the members' existence in a far more
global fashion than group therapy.

Psychiatric health and illness obtain new definition in family
therapy. The symptomatology of the presenting or "designated" pa-

The author wishes to acknowledge with gratitude the assistance of the Commonwealth of Pennsylvania and the Administrative Officers of the Eastern Pennsylvania Psychiatric Institute, including the Board of Trustees, Medical
Advisory Board, and Medical Directors Dr. John E. Davis and Dr. William A.
Phillips. They have provided a stable environment with academic freedom
which has enabled the author to establish and carry out a project of inquiry
into an unchartered frontier of psychiatric treatment.

tient is revealed to be only one manifestation of a protean, multi-person conflict. There exists in the family situation an individual *and* collective struggle in which the conflicting goals are autonomous identity on the one hand and security through symbiotic fusion on the other.

On a conscious level, both individuation and self-effacing submission to family loyalty are socially rewarded values. Each value is connected with a wide range of unconscious motivations in each family member. The clash of these motivations is frequently not revealed until the family relationships are exposed to conjoint family therapy sessions, since much of what is expected of a particular member and what he actually does in compliance is latent and perceived by other members with distortions. Various families show a wide range of responses to the suggestion that they explore the value of conjoint therapy. On one end of the continuum are families which clearly reject the suggestion of shared exploration of what they believe to be strictly one member's problem. At the other end we find families in which it is not possible for the members to be isolated for exploration on an individual basis. Frequently, though often unconsciously, they interpret the opportunity for conjoint exploration of problems as a sanction of their deep wishes for never-ending symbiotic togetherness.

The key to the understanding of "family pathology" and of specialized family therapeutic techniques is in the integration of individual and family system dynamics. In this regard the chapter serves a dual purpose: (1) the description of a case in order to illustrate some of the process involved in conjoint family therapy, and (2) the application of some of the concepts outlined in Chapter 2 for the identification of certain dimensions of multipersonal system dynamics.

In the successive sections of this chapter some thoughts on the relationship between individual- and system-based concepts of pathology shall be described, with extracts of a case history of family therapy, the questions of goals and rationale, and the problems of therapy and therapists.

Setting

The basis for observations and thoughts in this chapter originated from the author's six years of experience with intensive family therapy in the roles of therapist and administrator of a research therapeutic project at the Eastern Pennsylvania Psychiatric Institute.[1] Additional family therapy experience originated from five

---

[1] Members: Margaret Dealy, M.D., James L. Framo, Ph.D., Geraldine Lincoln,

years of association as part-time therapist with the U.S. Public Health Service project, "Family Treatment of Schizophrenia in the Home," at the Philadelphia Psychiatric Center (Project Director, Dr. Alfred S. Friedman). Teaching and supervision at EPPI, sharing of experiences and discussions with colleagues on both projects, and additional experience with family therapy in private psychiatric practice have all helped to shape the concepts presented in this chapter.

The Eastern Pennsylvania Psychiatric Institute Family Therapy Project grew out of a long-range psychotherapy project organized by the author in 1957. The project first focused on the exploration of the limits of intensive psychotherapy of schizophrenia from a relationship point of view. The latter orientation resulted from various sources: the author's many years of professional contacts with an early proponent of family psychiatry, Kalman Gyarfas of Budapest and later of the University of Illinois; another influence came from the author's affiliation (1956–1957) with the Department of Psychiatry of the New York State University in Syracuse, where, under the inspiring leadership of Marc H. Hollender, the significance of Fairbairn's object relationship theory was constructively explored by such penetrating thinkers as Thomas Szasz. The thought that the organizing factor of the ego is made up of patterns of relationships was consistent with the phenomenologic existential components in the author's psychiatric theoretical orientation.

Thus, the project started out with a design aimed at the exploration of the potentials of a psychoanalytically based but strongly relationally inclined psychotherapeutic approach with schizophrenics. The organization of a long-range therapeutic project in a state research institution seemed to have many advantages. The research setting provided an opportunity to select personnel and to give more than average staff attention to the patients. These circumstances were prerequisites for testing our assumption that certain psychotic conflicts can be "worked through" provided the appropriate relationship dimensions are in the focus of dynamic exploration and there is a sufficiently supportive and safe therapeutic environment. Our interest in intensive psychotherapy was maintained for over five years of long-term treatment of over seventy psychotic women.

A visit from Dr. Maxwell Jones in 1958 was another important influence upon the early development of the project. The spontane-

M.A., Leon R. Robinson, M.D., David Rubinstein, M.D., Oscar R. Weiner, M.D., Gerald H. Zuk, Ph.D. Previous Staff Members: Thomas Downs, M.D., Eddis Holden, M.S.W., Elaine Jones, M.D., S. G. Koepp, M.S.W., Jane Keenle, M.D., Elsa Katz, M.D., Kenneth M. Milgram, M.D., Laura Odian, M.D., Jerry Osterweil, Ph.D., Barry J. Schwartz, M.D.

ous informality of his approach to intra-staff and staff-patient relationships stimulated a reorientation of our concepts. It was at this juncture of intensive psychotherapy on the one hand and therapeutic community on the other that our project began to give more attention to family relationships and, toward the end of 1958, to family therapy.

The decision to begin family therapy was reached after the author's attendance at the American Academy of Psychoanalysis meeting on family therapy in San Francisco in 1958. It became increasingly clear to us that the working through of psychotic relational conflicts is bound to be much more meaningful in the context of the person's original primary relationships. The significance of the artificial or transference relationships (Boszormenyi-Nagy and Framo, 1961, 1962) in the therapeutic community receded, therefore, into a second choice position, provided we were able to involve the patient's family of origin in treatment.

As a first development, we established multiple family therapy meetings in June of 1958. In this program one or two therapists met weekly with a group composed of in-patient schizophrenics, their parents, and the nursing staff. The climate of these meetings has contributed to a gradual change in our clinical orientation in which treatment of single families became the prevalent approach. However, more recently, the need for amplifying the effect of family therapy led to the establishment of our Family Group Program with its day and evening shifts, each consisting of multiple family therapy sessions and of family activity programs.

We started treating single families in the second half of 1958. The designated patient (at that time a hospitalized schizophrenic female) and her parents were seen in weekly sessions by two therapists, one of whom was the patient's individual therapist. For the next five years our experience was based on concurrent individual and family therapy of young schizophrenic females. The patients came from a variety of socio-economic backgrounds and were often classified as "hard core" or "chronic" cases who had been given up by their former therapists as candidates for successful psychotherapy. Even if we discount our initial enthusiasm, the early response of our patients was most encouraging. Not only did most patients appear symptomatically relieved soon after the beginning of family sessions, but we began to see an unfolding of an increasingly meaningful though extremely complex multipersonal dimension of motivations. As we began to recognize the resistance forces operating in one family member toward change in another member, we gradually came to a new appreciation of the psychotic or otherwise malfunctioning individual's responsibility for the maintenance of his pathology. We also learned about the ways in which the apparent victim, the designated psychotic, was also contributing to the maintenance of "pathology" in the other members of the family. In short, the multipersonal "system" concept of deep motivation gradually emerged as a logically inevitable point of view. However, this emerging ideology began to require changes in administrative design.

The full realization of the significance of the family system concept first made the value of hospitalization appear questionable. We have discovered that many of our designated psychotics who were referred for hospitalization did better in out-patient family therapy. At the same time we stopped hospitalizing designated patients, we began to accept a great variety of other psychiatric cases besides schizophrenics. Family therapy proved to be a valuable approach to a broad spectrum of neurotic and character disorders as well. Altogether, some 50 families have been treated by the project staff in intensive, often long-term (up to four years) therapy; another 50 families have been seen for evaluation and/or short-term supportive therapy.

The transition from a mainly individual therapy to an almost exclusively family therapy orientation was gradual. As new therapists joined the project, each had to readjust his technical and value orientations through adopting a role that he first resisted emotionally and which he eventually came to adopt almost to the exclusion of other psychotherapeutic approaches. Most of the therapists have been psychiatrists who joined the project after completion of their psychiatric training. Others are psychologists with varying degrees of psychotherapeutic experience. In certain cases the project itself provided additional training and supervision in psychotherapy. We believe that a knowledge of the theories and practice of individual psychotherapy is an absolute prerequisite for the intensive family therapist. We have found no difficulty having well-trained professionals in psychiatry, psychology, and social work collaborate in interchangeable therapeutic roles. However, we question the wisdom of suggesting unmarried therapists for this work, with due respect to exceptional cases.

The emerging importance of therapy team relationships depends upon the "intensive" aspect of our approach to family therapy as well as other factors such as our prior interest and experience in the psychotherapy of "difficult" (psychotic, psychopathic, etc.) patients, our long-term commitment, our deep uncovering therapy goals, and our specialized experience in the simultaneous, dual (individual and family) therapy vantage points. On the other hand, in a number of cases we have offered a supportive type of shorter treatment to families because of the special nature of their problem or the limitations of their potential for deeper change. The dual teamwork method of therapy probably represents an even greater challenge to the beginner than the shift from treating individual patients to treating families. Observation of the work of each team through the one-way mirror by the rest of the eight therapists results in a complex process of mutual consultative and quasi-supervisory relationships which has developed within the project. This group process determines the ways in which therapists select each other as co-therapists for the evaluation and treatment of new families. The complex dynamics of therapist team relationships are reported in greater detail elsewhere in this volume and by Rubinstein and Weiner (1964).

As a rule, families are seen for approximately one hour once a week in a room which permits circular seating in comfortable chairs. We have found this seating best permits visual contact among all participants. The room is equipped with a microphone and a one-way mirror. At the time of the evaluation session the family members are asked to sign an application for family therapy and a release form giving permission for observation of sessions by professionals and possible publication of observations in professional journals, with the provision that their identities will be disguised. Soon after the acceptance of a family an appropriate fee is set according to a sliding scale.

Individual- vs. System-based Concepts of Pathology

If pathology is defined as the "science of diseases," can we speak of a pathology of the whole family? And, even if family pathology is a meaningful concept, the question remains: in what way is it more than the sum total of the diseases of the individual members? Without claiming to give definitive answers to these fundamental questions, an attempt shall be made to delineate several of the key distinctions between individual and family pathology.

From the point of view of phenomenology, the family members' individual pathology can be regarded as consisting of repetitious patterns of acting out. In its traditional sense, neurotic acting out consists in "purposive behavior, appropriate to an older situation in a new situation, which symbolically represents it" (English and English, 1958, p. 8). An inappropriate "nagging" attitude on a wife's part, for instance, may derive from the fact that as a child she got attention through persistent angry crying. But such an individual-based model of motivation will obviously fail to explain adequately the complex patterns of husband-wife interaction.

In order to fully explore the "appropriateness" of any individual's actions, the individual member's place within his relational feedback systems must be assessed. Usually it is difficult to distinguish pure individually based motivation from the social reinforcement effects reverberating among the various other members or within the whole family system. The marriage relationship system of the nagging wife, for instance, may comprise unconscious reinforcement messages on the part of the husband whose deep needs call for parental influence in the form of reprimand. Family therapy offers an opportunity to explore both the appropriateness of the individual members' contributions to their relational system and the system's appropriateness to the deep needs of the members. The question may then arise as to whether or not the recurrent actions (acting-out) of closely relating persons can truly be inappropriate.

The implications of the concept of acting out for the family's transactional "system" raise interesting nosological issues. The relative stability and utility for reality adaptiveness of some of the repetitive acting out behaviors is reminiscent of what in individual psychiatry is termed character trait rather than symptom. Acting out characters, however, are not necessarily identical with impulsive characters, as summarized in a report on a psychoanalytic panel on "acting out and its relation to impulse disorders" (Kanzer, 1957b). It is interesting to note that members of this panel found it necessary to introduce a relational framework into their basically individual-oriented explorations of the acting-out character. Greenson, for instance, pointed out the tendency of the acting-out patients to confuse identifications with object relationships. Frosch stressed the role of engulfment by the mother of the prospective actor-out, leading to weakly developed delay patterns. Adelaide Johnson described the superego defects of the acting-out child as mirroring those in his parents. Kanzer (1957a) stated about the actor-out that "the external behavior of a patient may leave us undecided as to whether we are dealing with sublimation, acting out, or symptom. This is all the more true since the decisive actions often take place outside the analytic situation and the patient's subsequent report may offer only an inadequate description." Later he adds that a "regressive need for immediate object possession is probably more primary than the motor activity which serves it" (p. 667). For our purposes it is important that acting out, as it is referred to in the foregoing statements, be considered at the borderline between intrapsychic and relational determination.

It is at the point of sensitivity to object loss that the implicitly collusive nature of the family members' acting out "defenses" becomes apparent. If, for instance, we conceive of two "object-hungry" family members as parts of a feedback system, the similarity and dovetailing of their impulse-defense-anxiety organizations makes it inconsequential (from the point of view of the symbiotic system) which of the two partners would threaten the other with engulfment, separation, or emancipation. Is it then more relevant to regard the situation as a relationship between two discrete "as if" characters (H. Deutsch, 1937), or rather to explore how an exceptionally vulnerable interpersonal fit may accentuate the partners' respective "ego-gaps"? The first of the two approaches is the traditional individual-based one and the second is the system-based, relational approach.

Viewed in its totality as a multi-person system, family pathology does not exclusively consist in a congeries of motor discharges, sublimations, projections, and displacements of individuals. It is rather an *interlocking pattern* of primary-process-like object conservative maneuvers. The nature of the primitive interrelatedness among members of a pathological family system is such that it prevents the necessary individuation which could lead to autonomous personality development and eventual separation. The system provides a field of immediate discharge for several members' fantasies through patterns of transaction or repetitive acting-out. In this atmosphere of shared primary process every member can assign an unconsciously wished-for parental role to another member. Role identities, passively assumed in the service of the family system, are bound to be unrealistic. The member who is being assigned a parental role is reduced to the state of "being an object" (Chapter 2), in conflict with his own autonomous growth aspirations. Any member who participates in assigning a fantasied (transference) parent role to another member is simultaneously exempted from the task of genuine growth through individuation; he puts off the painful process which leads to boundary formation opposite the lost parental objects of his own past.

The foregoing assumptions are of great practical importance for the family therapist. He will have to be guided by some hypothetical formula concerning the unconscious dynamics of the pathology that he intends to influence. An unconsciously maintained fantasy of the possession of actually lost loved ones can manifest itself in acting out through a distortion of present family relationships. In other words, the repeatedly acted out inter-member transference helps the family members to avoid the recognition of real losses. The symbolic meaning of the repetitious action patterns can be decoded in terms of an unfulfilled childhood wish, for instance a wish to be embraced, fed, or corrected. The unconscious fantasy through which the parent assigns his own parents' role to his children may result in bizarre, inappropriate actions. The connection between acting-out patterns and their underlying needs, e.g., the one for the assignment of parental roles, may be completely unconscious. Such regressive fantasies of the parents may result in demands for premature responsibility on the part of the children, who may comply with the parents' wish through precocious development. Feelings of hatred and wish for revenge originally connected with a parental introject can be acted out toward the child in unconscious transference, as illustrated by the tragic cases of severe child beatings and murder. Perhaps the worst cause of unconscious hatred toward one's parent is the feeling of rejection generated by early loss of one or both parents through death, desertion, or prolonged separation.

The deferment of the completion of mourning of lost relationships may lead to a de-differentiation of subject and object. As a measure of object conservation, a part of the Self may remain fused with the imaginary representation of the lost object. Such imaginary fusion may be reinforced by symbolically meaningful actions toward the member who is unconsciously viewed as a representative of the lost object. If the other member's transference needs for perceptual distortion and symbolic actions complement those of the first one, a mutual investment develops in the shared interactional system. Since, however, the one member is not truly an object of the other's strivings, neither becomes truly delineated as a subject of the relationship. In an atmosphere where this type of defense against loss is mutually practiced by several or all family members, the differentiation and the ordinary "constant task of testing" (Brody and Mahoney, 1964, p. 58) of subject-object boundaries is prohibited. The resulting state of fusion can be aptly called "undifferentiated ego mass" with Bowen (ch. 5).

The fantasy or inner formula through which a "pathological" action pattern is maintained is specific; each individual member has his own "relational need template" (Boszormenyi-Nagy, ch. 2). One may involve the other through childish helplessness or assign the parental role through objectionable acts that require correcting on the other's part. It is erroneous to assume that the context of conjoint family therapy is unsuitable for deep exploration of the individual members' fantasies. The experienced family therapist will find a key, for instance, in the many "slips of the tongue," which reveal the conflicting aspects of relationships as well as the members' confusion between relationships and identifications. Naturally one can expect an increasing number of slips as the acting out patterns begin to fail to "work" as defenses. For an optimal exploration of the intrapsychic and interactional dimensions the family's relationship with the therapist as well as the inter-member transference relationships have to be such that *spontaneous free play* can be given to the repetitious acting-out patterns, just as a capacity for free associating is fundamental to psychoanalysis.

The experienced and genuinely family-oriented therapist will develop a third ear for each member's unconscious object-assignment designs as well as for each partner's unconscious compliance with the other's narcissistic needs. Conflicts of an overtly dyadic nature frequently involve three or more members.

The father of a sexually delinquent girl was consciously enraged by the "craziness" of his wife because she did not allow him to punish the girl upon returning from her late night adventures because she believed that he would physically cripple the girl, even though he had never beaten his children severely. Yet, even though the father laughed at his wife's "crazy" assumptions, he also complied with them by making repeated threats to "beat the life out of the girl" if he had to deal with her. Possibly he was not aware of how his comments helped his wife in preventing him from the aggressively and perhaps sexually stimulating nightly encounters with his grown daughter. The wife, on the other hand, while stating to the therapists that she thought of killing herself for shame, paradoxically stated that if her "bad" daughter were jailed she would miss her even more than her other ideally behaving daughter. She even added that perhaps she might behave in the same way if she were her "bad" daughter's age. It soon became obvious that her nonverbal messages to her daughter were chiefly those of approval and appreciation, amounting to a condoning of her "bad" behavior. In summary, despite their complaints in this seemingly conflicting situation, the three members actually complied with each other's subtle cues and masked expectations.

It is important to examine whether neurotic compliance with the other's acting out constitutes a reciprocity. In terms of our list of modes of relating (ch. 2), even though the two sets of unconscious action patterns (being the subject and being the object) are complementary, they do not have to constitute a dialogic relationship. The relational complementation of two members' collusive, narcissistically regressive attitudes do not lead to mutual encouragement of growth and emotional maturation. These complementarities are collusive since they may contribute to an endless postponement of growth and resolution of mourning on the part of all participants. In the climate of projections and narcissistic distortions no one is forced to give up the objects of his past, no one has to individuate.

The Therapeutic Contract

Protection of the patient's interests and privacy has been implicit in the traditional "medical contract" for help. This tradition has guaranteed privacy to the patient even where members of his family are concerned, except for conditions of grave and incurable diseases or mental illness. The conventional psychoanalytic contract emphasizes the privacy of the patient-doctor relationship, characteristically to the exclusion of the family members. On the other hand, the very privacy of the individual therapeutic or analytic relationship may prevent direct therapeutic exploration of the pathological social *interaction* patterns. The patient may become trapped in the privacy offered to him. He alone carries the "blame" for dyadic or triadic relational pathology while, of course, being offered help in becoming a more autonomous and integrated individual. In the individual-responsibility-oriented framework of psychoanalysis the patient's references to family members' contributions to his "pathology" are usually discouraged and designated as resistance to thorough self-exploration. Admittedly, however, not all patients are capable of working according to such requirements. Consequently, the indications for family therapy as either an exclusive approach or an addition to individual therapy should be examined.

Family therapy traverses the boundaries of the cultural stereotype of psychotherapy as it requires all family members to open up long-aching personal wounds in an atmosphere of mutually, though reluctantly, rescinded privacy. Furthermore, the conjoint therapeutic approach touches on an ethical issue, assuming, at least hypothetically, that consciously well-meaning family members are contributing causally to the overt psychiatric illness of other members. Consequently, the decision to undertake exploration of the family's problems requires the mobilization of considerable motivation on the family's part. Ideally, it should require the strength of wanting to change collectively, just as a motivation for change as an individual is the basis of therapeutic progress in individual therapy. Initially at least, family members are usually motivated solely on the basis of "helping the patient," i.e., changing the other one, and obtaining professional advice on how to handle the sick one. Even if certain members were genuinely motivated for change, others might, at least temporarily, benefit from the status quo. Non-symptomatic members of the family may be shielded from the recognition or even the consequences of arrested or distorted family growth by continued concentration on the overt "illness" in another member. Pseudomotivations for family therapy are often based on the desire to expose but not change *another* member's illness or attitudes.

The variability of motivations of individual family members is not the only complicating factor of the family therapy "contract." If, as has frequently been the case in our project, family therapy is *conducted parallel* with individual therapy, the relationship between the two approaches needs clarification. Can the same therapist wear two hats: that of an individual and of a family therapist? Every new member of our project staff has initially gone through a period of questioning the compatibility of the two roles. A further question arises regarding the distribution of roles within the treatment team. Does the presence of two differently involved therapists necessarily create a conscious or unconscious competitive intra-team struggle? Time has proven that these concerns have a relative validity only and that the advantages of the team approach eventually outweigh its drawbacks, provided the personalities of the two therapists are at all compatible. It is as though the process of growth in the given team relationship is interlocked with the family's growth process.

Another problem inherent in the "contract" for family therapy lies in the novel quality of family therapy as a treatment approach. The role of the psychiatrist or individual psychotherapist has become relatively well defined as part of the contemporary cultural scene; he seldom has to begin his work by justifying his approach and the aims of his procedure. The same is not true of the family therapist. Whether he likes it or not, families force him to "sell" his method as a valid treatment approach. The family therapist often is as undefended toward conventional attitudes and clichés of social prejudice as were the early pioneers of psychoanalysis.

Case Description[2]

The family selected for the illustration of the process of intensive conjoint family therapy has shown a deep and meaningful positive change during family therapy. Yet it is difficult to formulate and convey the interlacing of individual- and system-based points of view of dynamics of change. Because of a lack of relevant uniform conceptual foundations, this would be true even among therapists who have direct experience with intensive family therapy. For the description of individual therapeutic change I have used the conceptual framework of psychoanalytically based dynamic theory, and I have attempted to describe changes in family process on the basis of theoretical constructs of Chapter 2 and of constructs established in the literature on family therapy.

The S. family was referred to the Family Therapy Project for the treatment of Mary, age 16, who was first hospitalized for a

[2] The author gratefully acknowledges the value of numerous discussions with Oscar R. Weiner, M.D., concerning the clarification of Mary's clinical concepts throughout the entire course of the treatment of this family.

month for a condition diagnosed as schizo-affective psychosis. Her history was that of a precociously intelligent girl who was not considered a serious behavior problem until high school age. There was some concern about a fall in her early childhood and about her having been molested by a nine-year-old cousin when she was five. She was described as always physically healthy and as being physically mature at age eleven or twelve. She dressed neatly and was attractive. Before her admission to our unit as a voluntary patient she had been hospitalized three times. Mary's difficulties apparently began in the early part of 1960 when her concentration in school appeared to be impaired and her report cards became badly affected. According to the parents' account, she displayed numerous signs of rebelliousness and disrespectful behavior and ultimately she was hospitalized for "adolescent disturbance" in March of 1961. She was discharged at the end of the same month. In the summer of 1961 Mrs. S. became concerned about the possibility of Mary being sexually involved with several young men. At about the same time Mary ran away to New York, ostensibly to solidify her parents' marriage, which she thought was on the verge of breaking up. In October of 1961 she began to show hyperactivity and somewhat bizarre behavior at home and was admitted to a private psychiatric hospital unit. She was discharged in a month after having received intensive tranquillizing therapy. However, Mary's school and home difficulties soon returned, and in January of 1962 she was re-hospitalized with symptoms of insomnia, hyperactivity, and what appears to have been marginally delusional ideation. Shortly thereafter the family was interviewed to explore their motivation for family therapy, and Mary was transferred to the project.

The family consists of the two parents and two children, Mary, now 18, and Frankie, 16. The father is a "blue collar" worker, the mother has a clerical job. They live in their own home and seem to have social contacts with neighbors and members of Mrs. S.'s extended family. Except for Frank, the members of the family are quick to verbalize and they possess a vocabulary and a reasoning capacity which exceeds their overall educational level. Despite their capacity for debate and argument, it has been impossible to obtain from any family member a consistent description of the essence of their difficulties. It has been clear from the beginning that elements of Mary's condition and those of the parents' own life problems are inseparably interlaced in any descriptive account of the family's "problem." There has been no denial of the fact that the parents' marital relationship is far from satisfactory. Viewed from the therapy experience, the entire family is involved in the pathological process even though Mary is the only member who, as an individual, has fulfilled conventional criteria of being symptomatically ill. Retrospectively, it appears that her illness must have provided the family with a lightning-rod-like function through which she may have averted other much more catastrophic forms of pathology on the part of the other members.

Both parents were children of immigrant parents. Mrs. S.'s parents came from Lithuania. Mrs. S. lost her father when she was between 11 and 13; she stated repeatedly that she did not remember the time of her father's death and that her memories of him were extremely scarce. She was the youngest of four siblings in a family dominated by the mother. After the death of her father, the family moved to the country. Her mother did not insist on her finishing high school. She went to work early but stayed with her mother until her marriage in her late twenties. Mrs. S. is a tall, attractively dressed, intelligent woman with a quick grasp of issues.

Mr. S. was born in a family of Latin origin. He has two older brothers and a younger sister. He lost both of his parents when he was nine years old, his mother through death and his father through abandonment. He was raised in succession by a foster family, his elder brother, and an institution for boys. His account of his teens is full of bitter disappointments and hardships. He implied that he narrowly escaped a delinquent path of development. He went into the service shortly after he married. Mary was born while Mr. S. was in the service. Upon his return, he felt greatly disappointed by the fact that neither his 2-year-old daughter nor his mother-in-law seemed to be warmly accepting of him. In the ensuing disputes he was practically thrown out by his brother-in-law and he lived in separation and comparative poverty for about a year.

The details of the early phase of the parents' marriage were never stated in complete clarity, but it is reasonable to assume that their relationship was heavily marked by transference distortions. Mr. S. may have relived some of his boyhood separation experiences through the conflict with his wife's family, and Mrs. S. may have married her husband out of an unconscious urge to recover the lost father object. The marital relationship pattern at the time of admission was that of two extremely regressed, infantile partners, both struggling for justification through vindication of their rights for a parent.

The initial description of Frankie was that of a "well sibling" who had been no emotional problem to the family. He was quiet, obedient, and shy, managing in school as an average student. He gave the impression of a subdued member with very little emotional "life space" amidst the other three demanding members. In one of the first sessions that he attended, his only response to Mr. S.'s loud bullying was a helpless, painful, silent flowing of tears. Later he was kept out of the family sessions by the parents for over a year. He remains the least understood but possibly also the least engulfed member of the family system.

History of Mary's behavior revealed that she seemed to have turned from over-closeness to overtly hostile defensiveness regarding her mother. Concurrently, she appeared to be displaying some seductively tinged closeness toward her obviously affection-starved father. At the time of the admission Mary viewed her situation as intolerably stressful on account of the rivalrous demands of her parents. She felt that she was "in the middle" and that she had to "referee" between her parents who allegedly kept arguing over her love as though they were rivalrous "lovers." Direct observation of family behavior seemed to validate Mary's allegations. Instances of over-involvement and over-stimulation in the parent-child relationships were usually followed by mutually frustrating demands in the marital relationship. The verbal battles tended to deteriorate to uncontrolled rage and revengeful hatred on everybody's part. There was certainly a clear indication for separating Mary from the home environment.

The assumption that Mary was overstimulated by her parents is evident from the first family session, as shown by the following excerpt:

MRS. S. (to Mary): Why this change? Have we done anything to make that happen? Have I done anything?

MARY: Yes.

MRS. S.: Well, tell me what, Mary!

MARY: Fondling, petting, kissing on the lips.

MRS. S.: I thought that's what you wanted.

MR. S.: Didn't you want that?

MARY: No.

MR. S.: That's what you said. That's what you complained of. You didn't get enough love.

MARY: Did you have to kiss me on the lips?

MR. S.: Well, now . . .

MARY: Everytime I want to kiss you on the cheek, you want it on the lips! Not sincere enough . . . throw my arms around you . . .

MR. S.: I never questioned you which way you should kiss your . . .

MRS. S.: Mary, you're contradicting yourself. You've always said that you never get enough of loving.

The initial phase of treatment consisted of a combination of individual psychotherapy for Mary with weekly family therapy sessions which, in the beginning, ordinarily did not include Frankie. The reasons for not including Frankie at this stage were manifold. Not only was he detached and unproductive during sessions but there was hardly enough room for accommodating the talking needs of the three other extremely active members during the hour. In retrospect, however, the therapists felt that they should have insisted on this overly silent boy's presence from the beginning nevertheless.

Mary early formed an intensive relationship with her individual therapist who was one of the family therapists. Though she obtained obvious support from this relationship, she also tended to use the therapy for making her parents jealous. The parents initially utilized the family sessions for blaming their allegedly disloyal daughter and, subsequently, for their endless, angry bickering. After the first family session the family therapy was interrupted for two weeks because Mary was behaving in an acutely psychotic manner, wherein she talked under great pressure, became assaultive, predicted a hydrogen bomb explosion, saw herself as God or the Virgin Mary, and claimed that she was able to talk in any language. Following this short-lived psychotic episode, the family therapy was resumed and has been continued on a once-a-week basis with only one short interruption. At the time of this writing the therapy was in its thirtieth month.

It would be important, though very difficult, to describe the non-verbal aspects of the interactional structuring of the family sessions as they continued throughout the first one-and-a-half years of therapy. At times it seemed as though there was a contest among Mary and her parents, asserting themselves in the most regressed, childish ways. Simultaneous shouting at top voice, table pounding, and refusal to listen to one another made most of the sessions appear chaotic and devoid of any meaning. Seen through the one-way mirror, the apparent helplessness of the two therapists in their attempts at making sense gave observing colleagues an impression of poorest prognosis. Against the overwhelming intensity of this unceasing, meaningless bickering, the therapists could only consult each other in order to find some meaning. The therapists' statements or interpretations appeared to be repelled by the parents' rigid resistiveness. Mary's ostensible early alliance with the therapists, which at times made her appear to be a volunteer assistant family therapist, turned out to be a mere intellectual exercise, possibly designed to inflame the parents' jealous possessiveness. Despite all apparent bad prognostic indications initially, however, this family has changed perhaps the most meaningfully among two or three dozen families.

The process of therapy has produced an enormous amount of clinical material which can be conveniently studied on the tapes of the more than 100 family sessions. No exhaustive clinical analysis has been attempted in this chapter. The clinical material, in its deeper aspects mostly based on Mrs. S.'s revealed dynamics, is extracted from the total material for the purpose of illustrating concepts of multi-person, system dynamics. The complexity of even one member's dynamic oscillations can be overwhelming. It is even more unlikely that the totality of all four members' pathology could be satisfactorily explained by a single formulation. Nevertheless, it has been possible to delineate a typical modality of the recurrent, shared acting-out patterns and to postulate an underlying consistent dynamic formulation. It has also become possible to relate the acting-out pattern and the underlying hypothesis to a camouflage in the form of a "family myth," which becomes exposed as therapy progresses and the acting-out patterns begin to fade.

The *family myth* can be discerned from an interview between the two parents and Mary's individual therapist on the day after her admission.

THERAPIST: What brought the illness on?
MRS. S.: She [Mary] feels that her father does not care for her as much as he should and that the arguments we would have would be over her . . . and that it was brought to her attention that probably there wouldn't be half as much arguments if it wasn't on account of her.
THERAPIST: In what way?
MRS. S.: Well, if the father would reprimand her on something that he shouldn't have, there would be an argument over it. For one thing, I think my husband had been too strict with her in the very beginning from the time she was . . . well, I'd say 10 or 11 years old.

Ostensibly, the mother is here (and in many subsequent sessions) concerned about her husband's strictness and lack of care toward Mary as a contributing cause of her daughter's mental illness. But a closer observation of her sentences gives a rather clear indication of the intricacy of object-role assignments and identity confusions which constituted one of the main dimensions of the family's pathology. Mrs. S.'s first statement concerns Mr. S.'s alleged lack of "care" for Mary. We recall that Mrs. S. said her own father regularly spent evenings out of the home, an alleged cause for her amnesia about her father. In the second part of the same sentence Mrs. S. indicates that rather than not caring, she and her husband are overconcerned and that their arguments are over Mary. In fact, as therapy progresses, the emphasis shifts to Mr. S.'s inclination for reprimanding his daughter too willingly, rather than neglecting her. Specifically, he is being blamed for unreasonable strictness ever since Mary was eleven. We don't know why Mrs. S. refers to this period as "the very beginning." We only know that Mrs. S. lost her own father at about the same age. It is interesting in this regard that Mrs. S. complained about a lack of physical affection between Mr. S. and Mary and that Mary's physical development as a girl began at about the same age. Although material from later sessions will somewhat validate the assumption that Mrs. S. was inclined to confuse her own identity both with her mother's and Mary's, in the preceding excerpt the only hint in this direction is her use of the expression, "the father," instead of "Mary's father," or "my husband." In fact, throughout the majority of instances Mrs. S. kept referring to her husband as "the father."

Naturally, if the logic implied in the above statements is correct, Mrs. S. might indeed feel jealous rather than protective of Mary, though her jealousy has never been verbalized. On the other hand, if Mary is a passive victim of her father's strictness, it appears strangely inconsistent for Mrs. S. to have "brought it to her [Mary's] attention that probably there wouldn't be half as much arguments if it wasn't on account of her." This statement puts the blame explicitly on Mary. If she were a passive victim of her father's unjust harshness, why point it out to her that she is the cause of her parents' arguments, especially if the arguments concern Mr. S.'s strictness? It is possible that the strangely inconsistent, primary process-like logic of Mary's implication is based on transference of Mrs. S.'s feelings that were originally directed at her own mother, seen unadmittedly in the role of an intrigant. It is conceivable that the hidden ingredient of Mrs. S.'s logic is based on a repressed memory of competition with her mother for her passive father.

Actual observation of the family's interactions made the therapists increasingly convinced that Mr. S. was not nearly as much in control of his wife and daughter as he was controlled by them. Although the "myth" pictured Mr. S. as an unjustly punitive father, the truth seemed to be that usually he was manipulated by his wife into assuming the punitive role. Thereupon, with a sudden switch, she would attack him for being a harshly "reprimanding" father. The inconsistency of Mrs. S.'s behavior was matched by Mr. S.'s paradoxical willingness to repeatedly fall into a role for which he was soon to be repudiated in an equally "reprimanding" fashion. Finally, it was puzzling to observe why Mary was a willing tool for her mother's "game."

The first few months of family therapy revealed that one main "symptom" of the family pathology consisted in an oft-repeated triadic transactional pattern which involved the two parents and usually Mary or, occasionally, Frank. The transactional *pattern* involved four phases:

1. Mrs. S. lures or forces Mr. S. into reprimanding Mary (or Frank).
2. Once Mr. S.'s anger has been "worked up" to a high enough intensity, Mrs. S. turns against Mr. S. and accuses him of unreasonable harshness.
3. Mrs. S. then manages to direct Mr. S.'s reprimanding parental concern upon herself; a loud bickering develops between the two parents while the child fades out of focus.
4. Mrs. S. repudiates her husband's paternal behavior shortly after she brought it on.

In one of the early sessions a typical example of this four-phase pattern develops with Mary as the object. In Phase 1 Mrs. S. accuses Mary of several "faults," particularly of deliberately embarrassing and thoughtless behavior toward the last weekend's guests. The next five minutes of tape is filled with an outpouring of rather ineffective, repetitious, and mildly critical statements from Mr. S. toward Mary. At one point he asks Mary why she has to "pretend." At this moment Phase 2 begins, as Mrs. S. gives Mary a cue, uttered softly, in an intriguing tone of voice: "See? That's it." Instantaneously, Mary begins to cry. While Mr. S. talks considerately to Mary and offers her a paper tissue, Mrs. S. encourages her to speak up and tell why she is hurt, why she is crying. Mary explodes with great anger in her voice, attacking her father for having used the word "pretending." The rapidly evolving Phase 3 finds an angrily defensive father shifting the argument from Mary to his wife. The following excerpt is characteristic of the fully developed Phase 3:

MRS. S.: You always nag the other person.
MR. S.: I don't nag you, you're always . . . like I said before, there is never a time that you express something . . .
MRS. S.: Don't you nag your children?
MR. S.: I don't nag my children, I try to correct my children . . .
MRS. S.: Well, that's . . . to call it correcting . . .
(Both speak at the same time.)
MR. S.: I think I am correcting them. If I think they do something wrong and I feel as though they should be chastised because they'd done something wrong, I think that's correcting.
MRS. S.: Do they *ever* do anything right?

The latter question leads into Phase 4. Mrs. S. now repudiates her husband for being an unreasonable, irresponsible nagger, only a few minutes after he started out to reprimand Mary upon his wife's instigation.

It seems from our long-term observation that the issue of Mary's "illness" has also been utilized in the manner of this four-phasic dynamic sequence. Generally, Mr. S. tended to be doubtful about Mary's being ill, and his daughter's illness was often used against him as a club by his wife. For example, while Mary was in the hospital, her illness was used by Mrs. S. as an excuse for her disinclination for sexual intimacy. Almost every manifestation of control or discipline on the part of Mr. S. was interpreted by his wife as inconsiderateness toward his sick daughter. Another mechanism, used for the perpetuation of father-daughter conflict, has been Mrs. S.'s habit of discussing plans with Mary separately, to have Mary later confront her father with fully arranged situations (e.g., attendance at a party, etc.). The belated request for permission has tended to produce an inflexible, annoyed attitude on Mr. S.'s part.

Another instance of essentially the same four-phasic sequence involved Frankie. The two parents and Frankie went to a picnic with another family. Frankie and another boy of sixteen rented a row-boat to paddle up the creek. They were told to return by 5 p.m. but were more than half an hour late. Phase 1 began to evolve when Mr. S. became tired of reassuring his increasingly hysterical wife who thought that the boys might have drowned. When the boys showed up at 5:40, Mr. S. grabbed Frankie and beat him in front of the other picnicking families, telling him that he should not have upset his mother. Phase 2 developed quickly thereafter as Mrs. S. started to attack her husband for what she thought was an unreasonable harshness toward Frankie. In the subsequent Phase 3 the arguing parents overlooked Frankie completely and their ensuing, week-long bickering left Mr. S. with a newly reinforced label of the feelingless, brutal father (Phase 4).

The phasic acting out sequence suggests an implicit dynamic hypothesis, to be tested during the course of the family therapy. The hypothesis is based on three fundamental assumptions: (1) that a dependent, parent-seeking (object-restorative) motivation is one of the main dynamics of the acting-out family members; (2) that a wish for being reprimanded is a main need-template or channel for this dynamic in this couple; and (3) that the members involved in the triadic acting out scheme are—at least unconsciously—motivated to accept the "object" roles required by the rules of the pattern. With these premises in mind we can assume that a reassuring, dependent gratification of symbolically "having a parent" derives from first assigning the implied parent role to a third member and then assuming the role as object of the implied "parent's" reprimanding or chastisement. In other words, one's regressively wished-for identification with the child-self of the past is optimally provided when reenacted opposite to a willingly "correcting" parent. The hypothesized unconscious goal of possessing a long-wished-for chastising parental object is the exact opposite of the stated family myth. Although ostensibly the family myth condemns the father's "reprimanding" harshness, parental censure is deeply wished for as a regressive way of part-object relating. It seems that Mrs. S. reacted to Mr. S.'s readiness to reprimand Mary as though her daughter were overindulged with the same parent-daughter relationship that Mrs. S. had missed since early childhood. Therefore, for Mrs. S. to "latch on" to the role of the reprimanded object amounts to competing with her daughter for a dependent gratification. Then, as she repudiates her husband scoldingly, Mr. S. in turn obtains his share of gratification through being corrected for a fault. Thus, he too wins in competition with his daughter for his wife's parental attention. Finally, Mary is pushed into the role of an implicitly arbitrating third party, also a parent-like object role.

The clinical validation of our dynamic hypothesis became possible through the family's growing freedom for repeated acting out of the pathological patterns and through slips of the tongue and similar manifestations of unconscious determination. Frequently it appeared that in their behavior at home the family members were having a comparatively "normal" interaction and that they only assumed the roles of the four-phasic "plot" for helping its therapeutic exploration during the therapy session. This pattern is characteristic of families capable of therapeutic change, since the freedom for a spontaneous enactment of "pathology" is as important a requirement of intensive family therapy as the capacity for free associating is for psychoanalysis. Slips of the tongue usually occurred in the heat of these "reenactments" and they reflected the unconscious or dimly conscious texture of the members' wishes for assigning to each other the wished for transference identities.

Consistent with the wish for regaining their lost parental objects, the parents' slips frequently assigned a parental role to each other, as illustrated by Mr. S.'s slips (italicized) in the following excerpt from the first family session:

Mr. S.: My daughter, when she was growing up . . . I mean, she is a child, you treat a child as a child, like I've said before. But she believes that when her mother tells her to do something that there was a great . . . uh . . . uh . . . obstacle for her to do it and that she shouldn't do it because she . . . I was supposed to do it, I was her father, but I was supposed to do it, she was supposed to do nothing. In other words, when I didn't go along and wash the windows like my *mother* . . . like my wife would say, *Dad* . . . Frank, why don't you wash the windows? My daughter . . . if I would suggest to her and say "Well, Mary don't you think you should help your mother?" Which I believe was the correct thing to do because actually my wife went to work for her benefit, her [Mary's] brother's benefit and my benefit.

The two slips in the latter quote have interesting structural properties. In the first one Mr. S. unconsciously assigns the mother role to his wife, whereas in the second one he makes the parentifying slip *for* his wife, as though he were uncovering the unconscious motivations of both.

Many other slips could be collected to illustrate the parents' tendency to perceive themselves, in wishful fantasy, as being the child of the other parent. In one session the father makes the slip that his wife did not want to take the "two sons," i.e., himself and his son, to the ballgame. In another session his slip designates his wife and daughter as his "two daughters." In another slip the father reprimands his wife and his two children collectively ("the three of yous") for not acknowledging bad deeds: "They can't come and tell me: 'Dad, I've done it.'" Mrs. S. has made occasional slips calling her husband "Dad" and she almost consistently kept referring to him as "the" father.

There are many, at times subtle, hints and evidences to the assumption that being reprimanded or slapped can mean receiving love from a symbolically recovered parental figure. It is interesting in this regard to compare the tapes from two sessions. The first session contains an angry argument between the parents concerning how many times Mr. S. may have slapped Mary. First, Mrs. S.'s voice sounds sarcastic as she challenges her husband: "You slapped her *how many times?* Only *once?*" However, on closer listening to this recording, it becomes apparent that Mary is not too concerned about having been slapped and that Mrs. S.'s tone of voice sounds envious, perhaps because Mary has received what inadmittedly Mrs. S. has for so long desired for herself. The actual validation of Mrs. S.'s wish to be "chastised" comes from another family session, nineteen months later. By this time Mrs. S. has been undergoing a long, painful process of re-evaluating her attitudes toward her parental imagos. The "badness" of her father's memory is about to dissipate and her childhood amnesia begins to evaporate. She has recalled the story of one of her childhood misdeeds and she adds in a nostalgic tone of voice: "I remember getting a licking from my father, which was *only* once." This explicit shift in Mrs. S.'s evaluation of the value of paternal "strictness" signifies an important aspect of her gradual therapeutic change.

Throughout the first one-and-a-half years of therapy, however, the main struggle seemed to center around desperate attempts on both parents' part to assign parent-like object roles to each other, to Mary and, eventually in the transference, to the therapists. The parents made every attempt to frustrate Mary's emancipation. They ridiculed the only friendship she was capable of forming with another female patient of her age. They sabotaged Mary's return to public school, and if it were not for the therapist's intervention, this highly intelligent girl might have lost a semester of outstandingly performed school work. For over a year and a half it was practically impossible to obtain the parents' cooperation in any meaningful discussion of their background or of their possessive moves toward Mary. However, on a few occasions Mrs. S. was able to recognize her regressive tendency for confusing relationships with identifications as far as Mary was concerned.

An interesting incident took place during the months while Mary was still hospitalized, spending only weekends at home. Mary complained that when her mother had sent her out to buy some cake, she was humiliated for her lack of judgment in front of the guests because she had bought an insufficient quantity. Mother and daughter became highly excited while discussing this incident. Initially, Mrs. S. defended her position while Mary kept accusing her of inconsiderateness and humiliating treatment. However, Mary denied the suggestion that her mother wanted to humiliate her on purpose. Mrs. S. began to cry then and said that she believed Mary must have felt purposely humiliated. Thereupon she produced memories of her own childhood, recalling how she used to go out of her way to please her mother and how her mother would still be dissatisfied. At this point Mr. S. and Mary jointly recalled occasions on which Mrs. S. criticized various gifts received from Mary. Without denying the incidents, Mrs. S. then connected her own behavior toward Mary with her mother's attitude toward herself.

MRS. S.: . . . when I think of it now, it's just what my mother used to do to me . . . and . . . I am reversing the same thing onto her [Mary] where I shouldn't . . .

MR. S.: That's right.

MRS. S.: Because I used to do the shopping for my mother, I used to buy the meat for her. Every time I would bring it she'd say it [?] should smell it whether it was fresh or why didn't you get me this . . . The same . . . if I think of it, the same situation.

MARY: Problems of the parents.

MRS. S.: I used to get so mad that it [?] thinks she is ungrateful that I went out and bought it for her and she turns around and picks on it. But I never held it against her. I just took it as it came. I mean I just took her for what she was . . . I felt that's how she was and what am I going to do about it. The same thing if I went out and bought her a dress as a gift she'd say 'well, this does not fit me right,' and 'it does not look right' and 'I'd rather have another one' or something like that, and now that this meeting came out here today, I realize that that's just what my mother had done to me that I am doing to her.

It is quite obvious that in the preceding excerpt as well as on many other occasions Mrs. S.'s fluid ego boundaries shifted back and forth between (a) identification with Mary as her childish self, (b) herself being either Mary's extension or (c) her own mother. The sum total of transferences, misidentifications, reversals, and fusions amounted to a de-individualization of the family with an implicit weakening of all members' discrete ego-boundaries. Such ego fusion or regression to an "ego-mass" (Bowen, ch. 5) was reflected in the grammatical distortions of the preceding excerpt as Mrs. S. replaced the personal pronouns "she" and "I" with an impersonal, thing-like condensation, "it." Further, the first "it" refers to herself whereas the second one to her mother. The "it" represents a literally fused ego mass, consisting of Mrs. S. and her mother.

This aspect of the family's pathology was also expressed in certain typical verbal configurations, besides slips of the tongue. Such unconsciously determined distortions are known to express deeper motivations which intrude into and alter overtly conflict-free and appropriate perceptions and statements of relationships. For example, as a result of their incompletely resolved early object losses, the various members' primary process thinking may reveal an imaginary fusion of the Self with a Parental Other, a reversal of the generational differential, or other distorted perceptions of relationships and identities. Although Mr. S.'s slips often implied that he unconsciously accepted a parent-like position opposite to his wife, to his daughter he frequently made statements like: "I am not a parent," "I never was a parent." A playful but pain-inflicting arbitrariness of the parent-child differential was revealed in the following puzzling statements to Mary: "As long as I am your father," "Let us assume I am your father," as though Mr. S. hesitated to grant to his daughter that which had been denied him: the prolonged possession of a father.

Some of Mrs. S.'s slips gave the impression of an unconscious fusion between the images of Self and Parental Other. Two of these suggest important considerations in connection with the fact that both Mr. and Mrs. S. lost one of their parents at an early age. In a session dating from the beginning of the second year of family treatment, Mrs. S. made the following slip: "*I died when my fa* . . . I mean my father died when I was eleven years old." Another slip, implying perhaps the imaginary fusion of her husband's person with her own merged self, occurred at the beginning of the third year, at which time the therapeutic situation was undergoing a significant change. By the end of the second year Mrs. S. seemed less inclined to reproject her internalized bad parental imagos onto her husband. She had become depressed and had spent considerable effort re-exploring her forgotten childhood memories and feelings toward her parents. Mr. S. was very obviously annoyed by his wife's change which he made every effort to sabotage, despite his conscious cooperativeness. In one session he reprimanded his wife for criticizing her parents, saying: "A parent is a parent. You should respect them rather than blame them." At this point Mrs. S. burst out in anger: "Oh, Frank! How old were you *when you died* . . . when *they* died?" This slip not only seemed to fuse Mr. S. with his father, but perhaps also with the hated aspects of Mrs. S.'s own parental imagos. Furthermore, a fusion between Mrs. S.'s own father and Mr. S.'s father was implied by the word "they" in the last sentence. Her mother and father-in-law actually did not die until years after she and her husband attained adulthood, although Mr. S.'s father disappeared at the time when his mother died.

These slips expressed not only a shared but also a fundamental dimension of the two parents' developmental stagnation as shown by one of Mrs. S.'s dreams, reported in a session during the thirtieth month of family therapy. She dreamed that her husband finally decided to visit his mother's grave, and in her dream Mrs. S. felt very happy about it. It is noteworthy that it was at this same session that her husband first became able to talk about how lonely and deserted he had felt after having lost his parents. At one point he offered the spontaneous statement: "Maybe I did not want to live when my mother died and my father went away." It seemed to be a meaningful coincidence that on the subsequent week Mr. S. first reported, with great liveliness and pride, an act of unusual social activity on his part. In a delighted account, he told of inviting a group of his friends for a card game, potato chips, and cold drinks.

It is logical to assume that Mrs. S.'s dream was even more relevant to her own psychic stagnation or "death." It was revealed that she had not visited her mother's grave either. Apparently the content of the dream was not the only connecting link between Mr. and Mrs. S.'s childhood experiences. Mrs. S. also volunteered the following statement in describing her dream: "I couldn't be closer to my husband than in this dream."

As family therapy progressed, the parents became the main "patients." They seemed to be relieved of their guilt as Mary's psychotic symptoms subsided, and they could give themselves over to acting out their long-frustrated dreams and wishes utilizing the reassurance of professional support. The therapists functioned as a shield against real destruction, and therefore the parents could turn their hungry demands to each other and to Mary with increasing freedom. Even though these childish demands continued to force Mary into a parent-like position, by allying herself with the therapists she could withstand the pressure much easier. On the whole, Mary's behavior progressed from initial helplessness to mobilization of her defenses against enormous demands. In the first phase of therapy she appeared to be in flight both from her parents' demands and her own overstimulated adolescent instinctuality. Although we have no factual report on overt incest, Mary's comments in the first family interview regarding petting, kissing on the lips, etc., seem to have validated the assumption that she perceived her parents' approaches as sexual. Later on Mary reported that she acquired the habit of locking the bathroom while washing and getting dressed so that her mother could not watch her. The demands on Mary for becoming a parent to her parents were more subtle and masked, often disguised as childish bickering between the parents. At other times they were hinted at through slips of the tongue. Toward the end of the second month of treatment, one meeting was started by Mrs. S. as she turned to Mary with what amounts to a classic slip of the tongue:

MRS. S.: Come on, Mary, *give*. What do you have to complain about?
THERAPIST: Did you say "give"?
MARY: That's something to say, isn't it?
MRS. S.: Pardon me?
THERAPIST: Did you say, come on, Mary, give?
MRS. S.: No. I did? What did I say?
THERAPIST: Give.
MRS. S.: I said, come on, Mary, give? Gee, I must be saying things that I didn't know I was saying.
MR. S.: That's possible.
MRS. S.: I said, come on, Mary, start.

The subsequent ten minutes of tape recording contain an argument between Mr. S. and his daughter. He states that he has not slapped Mary more than five times altogether, most frequently for "back talking and disrespect for your mother and me." However, Mary argues that once she was slapped for merely talking with her mother about Mr. S. who was on the porch. As the heat of the argument abates, Mr. S.'s logic, his deep, parent-seeking needs come to the surface:

"All I can remember, like I said I do remember, *five times* is all I can remember slapping you and what I should've done was slapped you more across your backside. Maybe you wouldn't have been as bad as you are in different ways. Mary, you didn't think that you were treated wrongly the way you say. After all you just don't continually think that, like you say you've family problems. You won't say what family problems are. *I don't think that you have any concern about what your mother and I do.* That's between us."

The last two sentences imply deeply felt accusations on the part of both parents; by not caring, Mary becomes the scapegoat for her parents' childhood deprivations. It appears that this father who lost his parents before age ten is struggling with the shadows of his own deprived past: how can a parent give more than he or she has received from his or her own parents? This is one of the key conflicts of many a family's growth and development.

A few minutes later in the same session Mr. S.'s unconscious needs break through in the form of two slips of the tongue:

"All right. Now let me *answer* . . . let me ask you this question. How about when the child is in front of company and is very outspoken? What is the parent supposed to do at that time? How can they correct the child when the child is trying to *correct* the parent . . . trying to embarrass the parent in front of company?"

As the argument turns into bickering between Mr. and Mrs. S., the angrily defensive father reveals some fragments of insight:

"Why should the children feel: Well, here we've done something wrong and yet the father is being ridiculed and being chastised for something we did? Why should he . . . be . . . so why *shouldn't* there be this confusion all the time between child and parent?"

These slips suggest Mr. S.'s unconscious investment in a fantasied reversal of the parent-child role differential.

The excerpts quoted above illustrate also the *collusiveness* between the two parents' deep motivations, revealed too by their unconscious slips. Further, the tape is full of instances of "double-binding" on the parents' part and their jamming of Mary's utterances. The parents' hold on Mary amounts to a tight symbiotic inseparability. Perhaps this inseparability is best illustrated by a spontaneous statement which the father made in a family session: "Why do you doctors seem to question that I want my children to grow up? If you had a tree, wouldn't it be stupid for you not to want it to grow?" (approximate quote). The metaphor of the tree may symbolize a kind of growth which does not alter a person's state of captivity, i.e., a tree may grow but never walk away.

In the face of the parents' overt possessiveness, it was a doubly welcome sight to see Mary change from psychotic to rebellious teenager. Although she went through the motions of adolescent infatuation with a girlfriend, it is questionable that she ever formed any, even comparatively meaningful, peer relationships. It seemed that she sought friendships chiefly to aggravate the parents' jealous attachment to her. There was evidence that Mary tended to utilize the therapy relationships for similar gains.

Mary's relationship with her father seemed to fluctuate between long periods of arguing and shorter phases of warm closeness. They shared a lively interest in some sports and television programs. It seemed, however, that Mrs. S. would interpret any emotional closeness between Mary and her father as a dangerously hostile relationship and immediately intervene with what she consciously believed was a protective concern.

A great change occurred in the dynamics of the whole family treatment process toward the sixteenth month, at which time the therapeutic design was changed by the termination of individual therapy sessions. The reasons for this important decision were manifold. It became evident that individual therapy had exhausted its potential in "building Mary up" for participation in the family process. The very fact of a continued labelling of Mary as "patient" would have served the family's resistance against change. It became increasingly clear that other family members were covertly "present" in Mary's individual interviews. The extent of fusion between Mary's and Mrs. S.'s personalities made it inappropriate to deal with Mary's motivations as though they were separable from her mother's neurotic gains. Further, the therapist was constantly manipulated around the limits of his commitment to individual-based confidentiality, while Mary was able to use the interviews for both influencing family interaction and resisting exploration of family issues in family therapy sessions. Also, the parents began to utilize the dual therapeutic approach by trying to split the therapeutic team and create competition between the therapists. The therapists began to sense that their teamwork needed consolidation by increasing the focus on family interactions and eliminating the divisive influence of individual psychotherapy with its confidential nature.

Rejection in the individual therapy relationship may have caused an acute sense of loss in Mary, which she then tended to cope with by "acting out." She started to behave in an overtly bizarre and sick way. Telephone calls began to pour in at her therapist's office and even on his private phone, often during the night. Emergency services of hospitals called, and it was apparent that the family was playing with the "danger" of Mary being admitted to the reception ward of a state hospital. Yet the therapists remained adamant in refusing to readmit Mary to the project ward or even to deal with the problem outside the family therapy sessions. The family first responded by again refusing to bring Frankie to the sessions and finally by stopping family treatment for several weeks. Despite the family's lack of cooperation, the therapists did not terminate therapy. They expected the family to return with improved motivations for change and in a few weeks they did.

Shortly after the resumption of the family sessions, Mary disappeared. Later the family found out that she went to New York and was staying with an unknown family. During the three weeks of her absence the family underwent significant changes. The family therapy meetings were continued and Mrs. S., who was now suffering from an acute sense of loss, permitted herself a more overt expression of feelings than ever before. She rejected consolation through closeness with Mr. S. and Frankie. In response to this refusal, on one of the very rare occasions of direct expression of his feelings, Frankie remarked to his mother: "You are making a saint out of Mary." It was obvious that Mrs. S. was struggling with her ambivalence toward a lost, valued object, most likely her introjected mother in fusion with Mary. In a session, held one week after Mary had run away, Mrs. S. stated: "When she left Friday night, I said I wished she was dead, because then at least my worries would be over."

Later, after her return, Mary confessed that despite all her ostensible attempts to make her leave appear definitive, she was constantly hoping that her parents would come after her and force her to return. Nevertheless the period of this physical separation marked the beginning of a process of realignments in the family's network of relationships. The symbiotic closeness loosened up somewhat, perhaps because the family had survived their most painful separation to date.

By this time some of the patterns that had characterized the family sessions for over twenty months disappeared irreversibly. Mary changed from a provocative, rebellious, and somewhat exhibitionistic adolescent to a reticent rather subdued girl who expected her parents to give and be rewarded by her growth. She became interested in finishing high school and expected the parents to help her in planning toward the future. The most significant change occurred in Mrs. S.'s behavior. It seemed that she lost her motivation for continuing the pattern of constant rebukes between herself and her husband. Even when he tried to induce her to argue and fight, she tended to resist. Instead, Mrs. S. was now going through a period of depression and re-examination of her internal relationships, chiefly with regard to her mother. Her previously revealed unconscious wishes for fusion with her mother must have lost their defensive utility. She seemed to have acquired a new, more autonomous identity: a sad, deserted child-self. Most importantly, she ceased to implicate her husband projectively in what now became designated as the "faults" of her parents. In a session in the twenty-sixth month of treatment, there was an example of a new, reversed struggle between a Mrs. S., now bent on examining her feelings about her parents and a Mr. S., going out of his way in trying to become again the willing villain for Mrs. S.'s long-hated projections.

MRS. S.: I realize it now . . . that my parents weren't bad but they also did . . . uh . . . didn't know how to be a parent. Which they did to the best of their ability and as I think of it now I just wonder how . . . all of us grew up the way we did . . .

MR. S.: You don't have to explain it to me . . . (softly) I can't change it.

MRS. S.: You can't change it, Frank . . . I had good parents but they weren't actually parents as parents should be.

MR. S.: What do you call that a parent should be then?

MRS. S.: Have a concern what the children do or where they go and teach them right from wrong . . .

MR. S.: Well, I think I've been trying to do that all along with my children.

MRS. S.: You *have*. I don't say you haven't.

MR. S.: How come you never allowed it?

MRS. S.: Because of the fact the way I was raised . . . I thought that was the right way. Have faith and trust in your children, let them go . . . don't . . . uh . . . in other words be anxious as to where they go and know where they go, what they do, and forbid them to do this or that or that's wrong or that's right. You just feel that if you have enough faith you trust them to do the right thing but that isn't so.

MR. S.: You don't forbid any . . . you don't forbid anybody to do anything . . . they got to use their own common sense as they are supposed to do.

MRS. S.: You see you are doing just like my mother and father.

MR. S.: I am not doing like your mother and father.

In the last excerpt Mrs. S. seems to have given up the original myth completely. Rather, she now sounds accusatory toward her parents and guilty toward her children because of her previously permissive parental attitude. Moreover, when toward the end of the excerpt Mr. S. tries on the role (or caricature?) of the tolerant or liberal parent, Mrs. S. angrily attacks him, this time not for being harsh but, on the contrary, for preaching *laissez faire*, the very attitude she has attributed to her own parents. It would be interesting to understand the reasons why Mr. S. has also reversed his position. Previously, he used to repeat over and over: "I think that children should be corrected." It seems that his gain from continuing the "system" of husband-wife bickering is more valuable to him than maintaining his often stated strict position. It can be assumed that although Mr. S.'s dependent needs find satisfaction through "correction" implicit in the pattern of bickering, Mrs. S. appears less and less inclined to engage in these previously all-pervasive verbal battles.

In a recent family meeting the reporting of one of her night-marish dreams illustrates the important internal changes in Mrs. S.'s relational orientation. The dream was about her mother who kept moaning incessantly, in a "horrible voice like a man." After awakening, Mrs. S. continued to hear this guilt-provoking moaning, and she had to reassure herself several times that she could not really hear her mother's voice since her mother had been dead for years. Mrs. S. recalled that she actually used to be bothered by her mother's moaning while taking care of her in her sickbed during her last year of life. While describing these memories, Mrs. S.'s attitude to her mother changed from that of a defensive, guilt-ridden persecuted *object* into that of an assertive, freely critical *subject*. She stated that her mother had the habit of giving people the impression of more suffering than what she was probably experiencing. In contrast, Mrs. S. herself would not impose on others; she did not moan even while having labor pains. Gradually, she came to the conclusion that her mother used to control her through guilt. Apparently, helped by her reliance on the therapists, Mrs. S. succeeded in turning her passive relationship to her persecuting imagos into an active one.

At this point we can pause to evaluate and speculate about certain practical implications of the conjoint family therapy approach. We can ask first whether or not in individual therapy Mrs. S. would have been able to sustain motivation for sufficient length of time for the change to occur. From the initial clinical impression of seven experienced individual therapists, this seemed to be an unrealistic expectation, especially since her overt reason for therapy was to help her sick daughter exclusively. Furthermore, we may wonder what would have happened to the marital relationship if Mrs. S.'s change had occurred in the course of individual therapy. She has obviously de-invested some of her old neurotic relationship patterns and has struggled with the concomitant painful frustration. What enabled Mr. S. to adjust to the fundamental changes occurring in the marital relationship? The therapists have found themselves being used by both Mr. and Mrs. S. as transference parental objects and as rewards for attempted change. More recently, Mr. S. too has been able to talk about his transference needs, at least in the form of a denial: "I will remember these sessions but you, Doctor X, won't remain my father and you, Doctor Y, won't be my brother." To all appearances, one partner's movement toward a better defini-tion of herself as an autonomous person seems to have prodded the other partner to utilize, however ambivalently, the available therapeutic opportunities.

Although the family members are far from having reached the

limit of their potential for growth and individuation, they have unquestionably changed. In conventional, individual-based terms the following changes have taken place: Mrs. S. has stopped most of her intrigue to play husband against daughter and has developed an ability for introspection. Mr. S. has become more independent and secure in his decisions. Apparently, he has also intensified his social activities. In therapy he is now able to listen to and reflect on interpretations. Mary has stopped acting out in a desperate fashion, finished high school, and has not shown any true signs of psychotic disorder for over two years. Frankie seems to have achieved an increased feeling of security and is more able and willing to speak up for himself.

INTERPRETATION

The entire process of family therapy has to be understood in its complex interrelationship, including the interactions occurring between family and therapists and between the two therapists. In the preceding account and excerpts of the treatment of the S. family, the emphasis was on the family's multipersonal system of pathology. Such a system concept of family dynamics is certainly the most distinctive of the contributions of the conjoint family therapy approach. Yet one cannot underestimate the therapists' extensive utilization of their experience with individual psychotherapy and related phenomena of developing patient-therapist transference. Finally, the deeper dynamic implications of the intrateam relationship are perhaps the most difficult to understand because of the delicate balance that the two therapists must maintain between their professional and personal relationships on the one hand and their own family experiences on the other.

The family's "pathology" can best be described in terms of individual and familial system concepts. A system is a dynamically regulated set of processes, distinguishable through its structural and homeostatic properties. It is a truism that the ultimate locus of psychic experience is the feeling and perceiving individual, the person, and also that for certain purposes the motivations and actions of a person can be regarded as a self-contained and self-centered universe. But it cannot be questioned that much of what we do is regulated by the feedback between our actions and our own reactions to the effects of our actions. An important motivational feedback system exists between the self and its introjects. Another segment of our motivations and actions, however, is patterned in accordance with the feedback effects of all motivations and experiential reactions of significant others. Such multipersonal system patterns naturally encompass those aspects of our living which are non-individuated.

As we have seen, certain motivations are vicariously shared among the members as parts of one whole pathological system as, for instance, in the case of postponement of mourning over lost objects of the past. These non-individuated amorphous facets of a person's psychic make-up represent an increasingly recognized source of what in the individual framework has traditionally been termed psychopathology or illness.

It is important to realize that it is the *state of undifferentiatedness* itself, and not any particular shared fantasy or "folie à deux," that constitutes the essence of family system pathology. Undifferentiatedness regarding the members' sense of identity and role attitudes is a dynamic structural system property, maintained by the economy of the participants' fixated needs (see the pertinent dialectical conceptualization in Chapter 2). The ambiguity of the parent-child or dependency differential is an important example of these structural aspects of motivational-experiential system pathology. In the case of the S. family, the initial rendition of the family myth by Mrs. S. presents a good illustration of the multiple layering of conflicting dependency differentials in a family system. On one level Mrs. S. identifies herself (perhaps for vicarious gratification of her own needs) with Mary's dependent needs for a father. On another level, however, Mrs. S. seems to be blaming Mary when she states that she and her husband have found it necessary to point out to Mary that their arguments were "on account of her," implying that Mary has the power and responsibility with which to regulate the parents' happiness and contentment. On this motivationally more fundamental and relevant level the parent-child differential is implicitly reversed: the parents become the children. The simultaneously contradictory structuring of relational templates amounts to cancellation of the parent-child boundary.

In order to understand the pathological family system, we have to recall the dialectical concepts concerning the role of relationships as contexts for the individual's sense identity (see ch. 2). From a dynamic point of view, family systems are based primarily on deep existential and experiential structures, and only secondarily on communicational and other observable transactions. The family system validates a member's identity only if he can experience the other member(s) as a fittingly antithetical background to his own relational need template. In a functioning reciprocal (mature) relationship the spectrum of the constantly alternating role complementations is broad and adjustable to the requirements of relational growth. In a marriage, for instance, one can be parent to the mate in one moment and child in the next moment. On the other hand, in a "pathological" relationship the members must continually repel each other because of their fixated, mutually non-complementary need configurations.

The early loss of one or both parents have created in Mr. and Mrs. S. fixated, life-long dependency attitudes. One can hypothetically assume that if the parent is prematurely lost as a component of the child's identity delineating ground, a fixated "bottomless" craving for trust becomes his permanent character trait. The natural tendency of all parents to at times parentify their child will be increased in a parent with such a life-long dependency attitude; the child will be caught between the two controversial role definitions or demands: that of being a child and that of being a parent (see also Schmideberg, 1948).

Nevertheless, in accordance with the belief of many family therapists, I am convinced that individually non-mutual and non-complementary relationships add up to homeostatically maintained systems. The fact that such systems cannot progress by changes occurring in one participant only is one of the basic rationales of conjoint family therapy. The individual therapist may be at a disadvantage of being unable to distinguish between definitive intrapsychic change and relational change of the patient's switch into another fixated relational role. Ryckoff, Day, and Wynne (1959) have described, for instance, the rigid stereotype of the schizophrenogenic family's fixated role system. They have described how corresponding alternating role changes are made by other members when one member switches to another role previously occupied by another member. As long as each of the component roles is filled, the system remains unchanged even if every member changes as an individual. In summary, from our point of view no true change of role or definitive working-through can occur in any single family member without a corresponding change in the system itself.

In contrast to being exposed to a simultaneous ambiguous involvement in two contradictory roles, a person's boundaries can be confused through not being clearly and meaningfully invested by others. In the four-phase acting out sequence of the S. family, for instance, Mary is first exposed to simultaneous demands to be a grown up "non-pretending" individual on the one hand, and a child in need of protection against her father on the other. Subsequently, however, interest in the child is dropped and the parents enter their own battle, each trying to make a parent out of the other. From here on Mary's role in the family becomes completely undefined. She is not used even as a target for transferred dependency needs, let alone permitted to gratify her own dependency needs. It is conceivable that this pattern of overstimulation and subsequent withdrawal of relationship may have contributed to the causes of Mary's self-destructive patterns of behavior.

In the course of family therapy, it is chiefly the relational rather than characterological implications of a member's relationship with his own introjects which is explored. When, for example, Mrs. S. reported certain emerging memories or dreams about her parents, efforts were made to connect their implied intrapsychic attitudes with observable tendencies toward distortion in her current relationships with family members and therapists. In individual or group psychotherapy the therapist must rely on the patient's reports about his relationships with significant others; the family therapist, however, can actually observe how insights gained from intrapsychic exploration or cathartic outbursts actually affect important current relationships.

The conflict among members based on their unconscious and dimly conscious relational needs resulted in a protracted cold war-like situation. Unmitigated hot war could have erupted and manifested itself in physical violence, but this did not occur. At times, however, an open battle of needs has come to the surface and become the subject of verbal argument over one or the other parent's rights to be taken care of, as in the case of Mr. and Mrs. S. in a family therapy session during the ninth month of treatment. The following moving, cathartic exchange must have altered Mrs. S.'s relational orientations rather deeply and probably irreversibly.

MRS. S.: You said something very, very important . . . *which* has been in my mind ever since I married you. You have always felt that I had a wonderful childhood. I had parents, which I didn't from thirteen years on. He didn't. He had a hard life. So now that we are married together, I am supposed to give everything to him because he never had nothing. I am supposed to shower everything on him, which I do; I am trying to make him happy. I try to give him a lot of affection and show him that I care for him. But where is *my* thirst coming in? (cries) *I am thirsty too.*

MR. S.: You're not thirsty.

MRS. S.: Yes, I am.

MR. S.: You are not. You're not thirsty.

MRS. S.: (desperately) No . . . no . . . I am not thirsty! I am not supposed to have any love and affection from you . . .

MR. S.: You don't. You can't get it.

MRS. S.: You don't consider me a bit.

The open battle brings the individual members close to expressing their deepest needs. Mrs. S. is a crying, hungry infant, and Mr. S., the other hungry infant, says: There is no milk. He even denies her the right to her feelings ("You are not thirsty"). Perhaps he is expressing the hard inflexibility of the fate of the deserted child: there is no hope, you just starve. After all, he had lost his parents before he was ten and nobody listened to his hungry crying. Thus, finally, the intense, deep-lying marital conflict could emerge clearly from behind the mask of complex parent-child-parent conflicts.

In their frantic efforts to cope with the pain of early, structurally uncompensated object-loss, the family members tend to rely on certain defensive measures to a "pathological" degree. Some of these defensive efforts can be classified in terms of the six *relational modes* described in Chapter 2, Figure 1.

1) *Intrasubject Boundary.* One can create within himself the illusion that his self is internally divided by an *intrasubject* boundary into two entities, without a consecutive self-other dichotomy. This intrapsychic maneuver may manifest itself as a narcissistic pseudo-dialogue, exemplified by Mr. S.'s customary prefatory saying, "As I said before." It is as though he wanted to validate his own veracity, using others merely as an audience to his soliloquy. Hypochondriac delusions and ideas express a quasi-relationship between the mind and the body. We presume also that under stress the organism "responds" with psychosomatic compliance to symbolic conflicts within its "mind."

2) *Internal Relatedness.* Reliance on purely internal relatedness between self and introjects is manifested in hallucinations or in persistent dreams, e.g., when Mrs. S.'s dream about her mother became so real that she had to remind herself of the fact that her mother was dead. Depressions, or intensive feelings of guilt in general, represent an internal relatedness between the self and the superego. In addition, internal relatedness constitutes the structure of masturbation fantasies.

Internal relatedness can intrude into seemingly unconnected external situations and produce deceptive effects. Real and transferred relational attitudes can overlay in a complex pattern. What appears to be a true feedback between two partners may actually be programmed by their internal relational events. Many marriages are essentially lived between each partner and their respective introjects. Two members' acting-out behavior can be effectively supported or maintained by a third member's relational needs regarding his introjects. A mother, for instance, has been seen to unconsciously encourage an incestuous relationship between her husband and daughter, without having their incest "on her mind." It is possible that the mother's wish to possess two real parents is symbolically fulfilled through "marrying" her husband and daughter who represent her transference parents.

3) *Merger.* Another method for dealing with deep object hunger consists in an imaginary merger with the wished-for gratifying (parent) object. This technique is reflected in slips of the tongue, for instance the one in which Mrs. S. equates herself with her

dead mother. The S. parents made many slips in which they unconsciously equated each other with Mary, whom they frequently placed in the role of a wished-for parent for themselves. Deep-lying, unconscious, wishful expectations for fusion may constitute the dynamic basis of one member's vicarious participation in another member's acting out of an unconsciously shared impulse. Fusion-like undifferentiatedness characterizes the early, pre-object-relationship phase of ego development. Partial manifestations of such fusion survive in the adult's tendencies for projection or introjection, especially in psychotic conditions. Fusion is usually described in a dyadic relational framework. However, we have to understand the fusion aspects of an entire family system, especially in an amorphously symbiotic family. Often one member cannot interact with another without imaginarily fusing himself with one or several others. Mrs. S., like many other mothers, has shown a tendency to fuse herself and her children into a "we" while arguing with her husband. In the battles of a married couple one can often sense the presence of two warring families.

4) *Being the Object.* What was described in Chapter 2 under "being the object" is vividly represented in the "pathology" of the S. family. The concept is different from being a mere re-statement of the passivity of transference neurosis. Although the nature of the expected gratification is dependent and passive, the act of assigning someone a transference role is based on an active though partly unconscious choice. In this sense the one who assigns a transferred parental role to another family member assumes an active position, and the one who is willing to *act* the assigned role accepts being the object. For instance, the S. family's four-phase acting-out sequence would not be possible without Mr. S.'s willing compliance to play the assigned role of a reprimanding parent opposite his wife. His compliance with the assigned object role also shows in the form of slips of the tongue, e.g., ". . . my wife would say to me, *Dad* . . . Frank . . ." Also essential for being the object in the "parentification" of children is the child's acceptance of the assigned role of being a replica of his parents' parents. A wish for such transference may be detected in Mr. S.'s slip: ". . . when the child *corrects* . . . embarrasses the parent . . ." Unconsciously, the father expects to be corrected by the (parent-like) child.

Being-the-object is a relational position that can be assumed toward a multipersonal family system, instead of single individuals. The inner abhorrence of loneliness, object-loss, or lack of dialectical Self-delineation (Chapter 2) makes one comply with the role demands of a "pathological" family system even when there is little chance for a reciprocal dialogue of give and take. The existence and perpetuation of a shared family myth is proof of the members' compulsion for accepting certain object role assignments in the interest of maintaining and at the same time masking the deeper underlying dynamic systems of the family. An example of this type of compliance is provided by Mary's participation in the four-phase acting-out patterns in which she behaves according to Mrs. S.'s expectations. Mary first produces a behavior which provokes reprimand from her father; then, upon receiving the appropriate message, she switches to the role of the unjustly hurt, defenseless child, anxious to receive the mother's protection, and then, as soon as the two parents resume their usual bickering, she is ready to leave the scene. In many families, being the "patient" is accepted by the designated member as an object role. The act of designation may take the form of double-binding, scapegoating, etc. (see in this connection Spiegel, 1957).

5) *Being a Subject.* If we consider the passive aspect of being a captive object opposite to an accusatory and paralyzing parental introject, it is easy to realize the advantage of being a subject who assigns a transference parental role to another person. However, despite their active component, transferred role assignments do not usually initiate a reciprocal role dialogue because of their strong internal (narcissistic) component. The ensuing interaction can usually go in one direction only: the Other is expected to impersonate, for instance, a reprimanding parent.

As described earlier, assignment of the parental role can be implemented through a "negative" or "passive-aggressive" role behavior which provokes reprimand. An example of successful object role assignment is also implicit in what is called neurotic secondary gain. Secondary gain connotes the satisfying dependency aspects of a relational situation, resulting from the fact of one's being sick. An implicitly parent-like, considerate, and supportive role is assigned to others as a result of the social impact of another's illness. A somewhat more complicated mechanism is manifested in the triadic structure in which one member acts out vicariously another's dependent needs for a reprimanding parent-like third person. In this regard, it is interesting to speculate whether Mary would have acted out in a more self-destructive fashion if Mr. S. had not been so willing to accept the assigned reprimanding parental role.

Transition from the role of being an object to being a subject is one component of Mrs. S.'s therapeutic change, as illustrated by her reaction to her dream about her mother. She has turned from a captive, guilt-bound object into an actively and critically repudiating subject. Now even her husband's willingness to offer himself as a reprimanding but caring father has not diverted

Mrs. S. from her newly found active attitude. It is as though emancipation from her oppressing introjected mother enabled Mrs. S. to give up her need for projection. One member's progress toward individuation may catalyze and has to dovetail with the progress of the family as a dynamic system. A new pattern of interaction must now be found.

6) *Dialogue.* Despite unquestionable changes in the S. family members, however, their relational situation has not yet reached the level of genuine dialogue. Both Mr. and Mrs. S. have become more capable of facing or perhaps even actively promoting painful changes, but they have not achieved a true give-and-take relationship. Perhaps they have come closest to a meaningful dialogue in the excerpt in which they try to distinguish between their own parental attitudes and Mrs. S.'s parents' attitudes. However, any gain toward individuation appears to be undone when Mr. S. becomes drawn into stating his position in a way which is almost identical with the neglectful, pseudo-liberal attitude that Mrs. S. has begun to accuse her parents of.

Although it is instructive to define pathology and its change within the dual frameworks of intrapsychic and dyadic interpersonal dynamics, the members' behavior eventually will have to be interpreted from a triadic and, hopefully, a four- and six-member system point of view. For example, the fact that it is Mary who has become psychotic can be interpreted from a more complex system-based viewpoint as an indication that she has been used in a covert but working alliance of the parents. Despite their bickering, the parents have been in collusion regarding their wish to retain Mary as a captive, substitute parental object. In this respect, her psychosis, of course, also represented an escape from the threatening bind, especially when the bind began to involve her awakening adolescent sexual impulses. Yet Mary's rebellion was only partial, since she could not have given up all the gratifications that the system provided. Individual therapy has probably taught Mary to value it as a model of a close relationship, if only to strain the overly tight symbiosis of the family system. This strain has brought out another collusive pattern between the parents. Their eagerness to ally with the therapists amounted to a move to push Mary aside insofar as possession of the therapists was concerned. Once the therapists had broken into the family's closed relational system, they became natural heirs to the object roles that previously were assigned to Mary.

A recurrent family resistance phenomenon can be used as illustration of the multiple layering of system dynamics in what may appear as a two-person interaction. We have observed repeatedly that one member's efforts at recovering past memories is encouraged by the other members only as long as they remain unsuccessful. At the point when one member is able or innerly compelled to explore his internal relationships, one or several others usually intervene with distraction or filibuster or even overt discouragement. The mechanism of these resistances to letting the other proceed with self-exploration is extremely complex.

In the case of Mr. S.'s resistance to letting Mrs. S. develop new insights into her past relationships, we assume that he was deeply enough committed to the projective family system in order to resist its change. He must have welcomed the removal of punishing projections. But what was the change he tried to resist? Did he resist his wife's renouncement of disputes or did he resist her deep-going personality change? Some of his references indicated concern about the alteration of the children's relationship to both parents as disciplinarians. Furthermore, the therapists' rewarding attention, given to any member who was struggling with significant insights, could have been the most important motivation for Mr. S.'s obstructionism. Like any rivalrous sibling lacking the ability to out-perform the other, he wanted to interfere with the successful attention-getting device of the other sibling. Thus, in addition to the member's transference to the therapists, the therapists' actions and comments themselves became parts of the complex system of growth and resistance to growth.

One of the most difficult tasks is to describe what the therapists actually did to actively help bring about a change in the family system. In addition to inevitably, though intangibly, injecting their own life attitudes as points of reference, they have evolved a pattern of balance between receptiveness and directiveness. The initial offer of individual therapy certainly made a significant inpression in the family system. Although individual therapy for the designated patient by itself may only have helped to endlessly perpetuate the pathologic family system, in combination with family therapy it has helped to build up a rivalrous force within the family's fixated libidinal system, forcing the father to seek his own transference parental figure in the person of the other family therapist, while Mrs. S. related to Mary's therapist through what she alleged were her daughter's needs. With the therapists' decision to stop individual therapy the whole existing family system was shaken up. This decision meant a threat of renewed separation trauma. In the process of working through, however, a reorientation of the family system has become possible. Mrs. S. has learned to relate to the former individual therapist without the subterfuge of Mary's presumed needs. Mr. S. has become more accessible to secondary process communications. Mary has acquired a capacity to face the depression caused by her maturation and necessary object-relinquishments instead of masking the depression with acting out and shallow intellectualization. Frankie has acquired a capacity to say no. In all likelihood, these people could not have developed deep enough relationships on an individual therapeutic basis necessary for change. Instead they would have drifted away from the therapist under the forces of the family's symbiosis.

To take on the family members' wishful (transference) object assignments required no effort on the therapists' part. In fact, each had to struggle to avoid being swallowed up in the role of substitute parental object, a role that the parents assigned through childish behavior and through an enticing gratefulness and respect. On the other hand, the therapists realized that, in order to exert a therapeutic influence, they had to represent parental objects who could remain discrete individuals, thereby impelling the family members to extricate themselves from their wishful symbiotic fantasies.

It is interesting to note the ways in which the family tested the therapists' strength. One criterion of therapist strength was the ability to stay united and not let the family play one therapist against the other. Also, the therapists would be weakened if they could be made angry enough as parents in retaliation against their "runaway children." If they could be made anxious enough to intervene in the family's real life decisions (as it happened once in the question of Mary's school attendance during the first year of family therapy), they would become like weak, insecure, and overprotective parents. The therapists realized that they should guide but not take over real life decisions. They should help make sense out of the chaos; they should interpret where there is projecting, filibustering, denial of manipulations, and a variety of other resistance games. Finally, the therapists should reward the pursuit of mourning and serious exploration of the introjects by taking notice of these efforts as they occur. They must act as good parents through their incorruptible strength and their constructive empathy.

Prior to the major therapeutic change, the members of the family had been engaged in a seemingly never-ending, over-invested struggle to possess each other as substitute parental objects. Their wishful fantasies pictured the other member as a caring, correcting, reprimanding, and strong parent. This vicious circle was broken when the therapists became the strong substitute transference parents. Gradually, the "empty cup" was perhaps filling up, providing Mrs. S. with borrowed strength which enabled her to use her latent potential for self-reflection. Of course, it took almost two years before the old patterns of neurotic irresponsibility and dependency could be given up by the parents to effect a reversal of the distorted parent-child differential. The parents began to learn other means of control than refusal of autonomy. In fact, they began allowing Mary to be the child without immediately retaliating against her demandingness. Finally, Mrs. S.'s dream showed that her trust in the therapists had enabled her to re-evaluate her desperately clinging internal allegiance to her mother. As it turned out from examining her dream, Mrs. S. harbored a repressed resentment based on her perception of her mother as a non-caring, guilt-making, selfish person.

To some readers it may appear that the repeated stress on parentification needs is a reductionistic oversimplification of the family members' motivations. The purpose in stressing the importance of this deep motivational source is not to exclude other determinants from consideration, but to emphasize the usefulness of an internal object relations-based, most comprehensive framework for interpersonal "inappropriateness." The fixed intensity of the family members' internal relationships corresponds to these individuals' defective capacity for neutralization, sublimation, and redistribution of libidinal investments. A somewhat similar conceptualization to our parent-seeking motivations is E. Berne's (1964) transactional use of the concept of a "child ego state," potentially present in any person.

Goals and Rationale

Family therapy has complex implications for the goals of psychotherapy in general. Its criteria for cure are even less "operational" than the criteria for psychoanalytic cure. Eissler (1963) has observed that technically uncured psychoanalytic patients may improve their social adaptational function as a form of acting out of unresolved conflicts. Thus, a sweeping change in one's whole adaptational life style may result from *resistance* to rather than acceptance of structural change. What in the individual patient are referred to as criteria of structural change will have to be translated into the conceptual framework of family "pathology" and health. In addition to the criteria of individual structural change, the family therapists will have to become acquainted with the criteria of changes in overt and covert multipersonal patterns and processes. It is possible that the phasic relational process (described in Chapter 2) is the most reliable measure of therapeutic as well as developmental change in a family. As the family's style of interactions moves from symbiosis toward individuation, the capacity of the offspring for genuine encounter increases. The practical goal of family therapy is a more meaningful marriage relationship for the parents and separation and meaningful marriages and parenthood for the offspring.

Confronted with the complex dimensions of (a) individual needs, (b) kinds of family structure, and (c) stages of family process, the family therapist finds difficulty in answering the simple question, "What is the goal of family treatment?" Nevertheless, in the interest of scientific clarity, we must make every effort to define technical guidelines for the implementation of help through family therapy. In this chapter it has been my intention to outline such general guidelines rather than give a catalogue of specific therapeutic techniques.

The most fundamental premise of the answer to the above question lies in the fact that relational events can only be evaluated in terms of other relational events. Generally, it is assumed that the therapist has lived through sufficient familial experiences to have a relational vantage point for his work. Since he is not going to work primarily with symptoms, or with persons motivated for self-explorative individual therapy, he will have to muster relational strength for his work. He has to exemplify and *live* in trust and confidence in the frustrated and often hateful family atmosphere. It is hard to predict the relational strength of the family therapist even if he has been analyzed. He has to remain open to deep, primary process clues in the context of an actual family drama. In piercing the defensive façades of one family, he may suddenly be reminded of the pathology of his own family life. Unless he is helped by a colleague in the co-therapy relationship, he is apt to selectively ignore defensive façades that resemble those of his own family. In other words, the therapist's guide toward goals derives from his constant honest effort toward self-awareness and his willingness to inject his relational styles into his professional work as a model for family members. Since he has to rely on his personal relationships as a gyroscope, it is inevitable that his personal family relationships will also become affected in the course of his work. As in many other fields, professional and personal growth will have to balance each other.

The most general guidelines for the technical goals of family therapy issue from the theory of the phasic relational process (Chapter 2). According to this theory, all relationships go through phases of unrelatedness (autistic phase), affiliative overinvolvement (symbiotic phase), growth of autonomy in members (individuation phase), and dissolution (separation phase) leading to re-involvement in new groups. The family therapist has to be aware of two important relational processes, each following the phasic rule: (1) family process and (2) therapy process. Characterization of the phases of the family process was given in Chapter 2, and only a few therapeutic applications will be added here. The family therapy process is somewhat related to the process of individual psychotherapy, but it is complicated by the family aspects and, if applicable, by the relational aspects of a therapy team.

The "operational" validation of relational phases in the family as well as in the course of psychotherapy is difficult because phasic changes may take place in the members' fantasy, i.e., in their inner relational configurations, as well as in their observable behavior. Further, the intrapsychic (object) representations of outward behavior may undergo a phasic elaboration without any concurrent outside manifestations. Transference-distorted behavior is one of the well known outside manifestations of these hidden phenomena. The experience of a mother, for instance, whose symbiotically bound 22-year-old daughter had abruptly moved to a separate apartment, was painful at least on three levels: (1) real-life fact of diminished contact with the daughter; (2) the daughter's hostile behavior, which served as the latter's defense against her own symbiotic longings; and (3) the mother's reactivated feelings of loss and ambivalent longing transferred to the daughter from the objects of her own past (internalized) relationships. In other words, the mother's experience of an actual, interpersonal separation conflicted with inner, ambivalently longed for, partially given up, past love objects. A trial separation in one relational process activated a feeling of loss in at least one additional process.

I do not intend to revive the old debate of whether or not individual psychotherapy depends mainly on relational or intrapsychic, insight-like factors. Our perspective regards intrapsychic as well as interpersonal relational factors as co-determinants of psychotherapeutic change. It is commonly assumed that the less autonomous the patient's personality (ego) structure, the more the approach has to rely on supportive techniques, and the more important the actual, interpersonal relational component becomes. However, any psychotherapeutic help can be conceived as offering a new relationship to one or several persons who are arrested in their relationships and would like to involve themselves in other relationships. Formal psychotherapy or analysis is often called jokingly a paid friendship. Freud was very sensitive to the danger of the analyst's (or therapist's) own needs for involvement when he advised neutrality and caution regarding counter-transference attitudes. Temporarily, the patient is expected to develop a capacity for a reinvolvement in a new object, the therapist (transference), at the expense of the current transference involvements of his everyday life. Finally, the patient is expected to give up his internally fixated involvements, as well as his real relationship with the therapist, and to become individuated, capable of reinvolvement with others on a more autonomous and satisfactory level. The individual therapists cited below seem to concur, at least implicitly, in a phasic relational process point of view of psychotherapy.

Otto Rank (1950) emphasizes three steps of therapy: (1) the initial engagement phase, (2) the middle phase requiring a total surrender of the patient's self to the therapeutic experience, and (3) the third phase in which the patient learns to "will" the giving up of the therapist for other reality relationships. Whitaker and Malone (1953) in their penetrating book give new emphasis to the crucial significance of the patient's and therapist's mutual accessibility to each other's unconscious dynamics. In what these authors call the main or "core" stage of the therapeutic process, this accessibility transitorily reaches a level of "psychotic involvement" or "therapeutic psychosis" (p. 96). Searles (1961) describes what he calls the "overall pattern of the psychotherapeutic course" of treatment of schizophrenia. He traces the process from an "out-of-contact" phase through phases of symbiosis to a phase of individuation. Therapy, if successful, will eventually provide the patient, through new attachments, with an increased ability, for lessening the concomitant feelings of loss and privation after relinquishing old attachments.

Freud (1919) explicitly emphasized the threapeutic importance of controlled frustration in the psychoanalytic relationship, a subject which requires fuller understanding. The inevitable privation, built into the nature of the transference relationships of psychoanalysis, is the relational condition of achieving a durable change in the ego. Family therapy, too, exposes the members to privation experiences, and the defense against them is often carried out by the multi-person family system. According to our dialectic concept of ego identity, every ego structure is based on a subject-object (relational) configuration. In order to obtain a new ego-orientation, an old subject-object delineation will have to be replaced. To give up an old ego-configuration, one would have to struggle also with the concomitant loss of the intrinsic relatedness of the ego to its delineating object or ground. In other words, without the possibility of forming a new internal or external relationship, one cannot be expected to be able to change his ego attitudes.

Incomplete relinquishment of past relationships constitutes the basis of neurotic behavior patterns in a broad spectrum of individual and multipersonal manifestations. The lingering presence of important attachments to partly introjected, partly reprojected past relationships constitutes the constellation of what in its familial context amounts to a multipersonally acted out deferment of mourning. In the developing transference to the family therapist the therapy relationship becomes perfused with the same lingering internal dispositions which have contaminated the family members' relationships.

In the final analysis the chief advantage of conjoint family therapy may lie in its offering of a chance for completed or accelerated object relinquishment in an atmosphere of collectively catalyzed support. Although family members may have the basic motivation to undertake this painful step toward growth, they may recoil from it out of fear of frustrations, retaliation, or threat of loss, unless professional help is provided.

Our emphasis on the advantages of exploring the complex relational systems of multipersonal pathology should not create the impression that the realm of intrapsychic dynamics is of any lesser significance in family therapy. To be sure, individual therapy and psychoanalysis are the preeminent methods for understanding of and focusing on the distortions of a person's internal relational world. What should be stressed here, however, is the probability that even in individual therapy it is the relational context rather than a detached genetic curiosity in the patient's internal world that produces the most significant changes. In its deepest implications, coming to grips with issues is a relational rather than conceptual struggle even in individual therapy or psychoanalysis, because it involves the decision to either interrupt or to deepen the therapeutic relationship at each new point of resistance. Conjoint family therapy cannot and should not avoid dealing with the intrapsychic sources of (transference) distortions; besides, it has the advantage of doing so in the relevant context of close real relationships. Certain fixated intrapsychic constellations can only be revealed in the field of personally demanding interactions. To hear a mother describe her relationship to her child is very different from observing the mother in interaction with her child. Generally, individual psychotherapy and psychoanalysis are the best suited methods for the exploration of stress phenomena while the patient develops personal demands toward a relatively non-demanding professional. Family therapy provides observation of "patients" while they are exposed to intensive personal demands from each other.

Intensive family therapy, as described here, is only one variant of a whole new armamentarium of psychiatric treatment methods. No doubt the individual interview will be maintained for those patients who can best obtain benefits from it. Especially, those people should utilize psychoanalysis and individual psychotherapy who have made forceful moves in the direction of individuation and responsibility, yet feel neurotically inhibited in their growth. But the recognized value of the individual method should not hamper the development of freer therapeutic approaches which explore the multiplicity of relationships. Some people do not tend to develop a strong transference relationship with the therapist because of the nature in which their relationships with members of their family are transference-distorted and symbiotic. Furthermore, they cannot relate to a therapist who attempts to be neutral. In fact, even in most cases of family therapy therapeutic progress can only be maintained if the therapist knows how to pose appropriate demands to the family for change, e.g., to alter detrimental sleeping arrangements or the distribution of male-female roles, etc.

The theory of the phasic relational process enables the family therapist to design somewhat more specific therapeutic goals, depending on the stage in which the particular family is fixated. The autistically unrelated family may need a suffusion of trust. Its members may have little or no capacity for picturing the world as a place for enjoyment. Paradoxically, the therapist's anger with the mistrusting members or expressions of therapeutic despair (Farber, 1958) might convey his inner belief in the existence of some goodness in life. On the other hand, the symbiotic family, submerged in a meshwork of overinvolvements, will first require a careful study of the unconsciously collusive and vicarious ways in which individuation is blocked and undermined. Often absent members need to be brought into the family sessions as a requirement for progress. The multiperson mechanisms will have to be understood in terms of the participants' distortive needs and interpreted in these connections. Individual needs are best supported by catalyzing the development of one-to-one dialogues in which clear individual positions take the place of a previous meaninglessness. Once individuation and separation become a tentative possibility, support is needed for members who begin to experience the pain of object-loss because of change in the other member. This is usually where the process of mourning reaches a point at which important relationships to the member's introjects can be extensively revised, often with the "assistance" of multipersonal resistances as clues.

One more concrete goal of family treatment is, naturally, the *removal of symptoms* and consequences of a mutually destructive mode of living. This is usually the overt motivating goal of most family members for participating in conjoint therapy. The therapist should be careful, however, to detect any member's underlying wish for changing *other* members in order to "get" more out of family life, without relinquishing his own commitment to the pathological system of acting out.

A more dynamically central goal of family therapy is related to enabling children to obtain "workable" *models for identification.* In terms of the dialectical theory, such a model must be based on a reciprocity of empathic abilities. Quite frequently, the conflict-ridden family members are unable to utilize even their existing potential for empathizing with an adolescent member who is desperately hungry for understanding. Often the basis of emphatic inability lies in the members' transference-distorted view of each other.

A more specific goal for conjoint family therapy is the *removal of specific obstacles* which stand in the way of the family's relational growth. Often, without any deeper understanding of the family's rational dynamics, the therapist notices certain familial pecularities of communication, stale repetitiousness of conversations, fixated habits of living, secrets, unspoken emotional separations. The therapist can directly ask or even instruct the members of the family to alter these habits as conditions for the therapy. Besides testing the depth of the family's motivation for change, such demands may produce communications on a more meaningful level.

A related goal is the achievement of a *freedom for raising and resolving controversial issues* within the family. Often the fixation of the family's life process is manifested in a rigid avoidance of all sharply formulated points of view or, in extreme cases, of all meaning (Schaffer *et al.*, 1962). Yet, according to the theory of dialectical synthesis, growth can only be achieved by manifest presentation of both thesis and antithesis. An unspoken or too generally stated resentment, for instance, cannot be resolved. Often the obstacle to a clear statement of issues is a habit of loud, repetitious, and personally destructive arguing among members.

Another goal implicit in family therapy is the improvement of the family's dynamic *exchanges with the larger community*. More realistic and active community attitudes will probably follow a basic relational improvement within the family. The therapist will have to be careful, however, not to expect only good community "adjustment" from the family members, even if the referral was made by some corrective agency of society. Yet, in expecting changes in a family, the therapist has to use good judgment and not set his goals too high. There are areas in which it is humanly impossible to aim higher than a *compromise*.

Problems of Therapy and Therapists

Confronted with interlocking systems of pathology, the family therapist has to design a suitable strategy. He must not be trapped into wanting to save one member from another. Yet it is obvious that each member's autonomy is not only threatened by his own regressive needs but also by the needs of the family system. No family member is able to develop a strong, self-sustaining, autonomous ego organization if his "partner" in a complementary pathology is reluctant to change. One marital partner cannot alone switch from a sado-masochistic sexual pattern to genitality without a corresponding change in the other partner, unless one partner leaves the relationship. The family therapist must be alert, however, to notice the variety of complex ways in which the partners are "grounded" in each other's personality.

A new strategic approach evolves logically from the conceptualization of the therapy situation as based on a dynamic of two opposing alliances: the therapist's alliance with the autonomous aspects of each family member's ego on the one side and the family system of allied pathologies on the other. One is reminded here of Guntrip's (1960) formulation, according to which the individual therapy relationship has to compete with the power of the patient's pathological internal object relationships. In addition, in family therapy the therapy relationship has to compete with all complementary pathological relations within the family system. However, on the positive side is the fact that the family therapist is in a better position to empathically reinforce the available life- and growth-oriented (autonomous) interactional resources among family members than is the individual therapist who has to rely on purely intuitive reconstruction of family interactions.

Multipersonal systems of family relationships can be considered a complementary identity delineating context as well as a powerful field of external influences. Rapaport (1958) has emphasized the need for extending the concept of ego autonomy to include an executive freedom opposite to stimuli from the outside world. For the family therapist the external stimulus, limiting the autonomy of the patient, can be equated with the motivational impact of the needs of complementing, perhaps symptomless, family members. In this regard, the mechanisms so perceptively described under the name "superego lacunae" by A. Johnson and Szurek (1952) were noted with great interest at the early stages of our family therapy work. Although initially only certain family members seemed to be involved in these confining and pathologically vicarious complementarities, further experience has taught us that most of the seemingly asymptomatic and non-involved family members are also components of what we now call the "family system" of pathology.

In every family therapy situation it might seem temporarily as though the primary patient or some other member were in favor of changing the system. However, at the point when genuine change begins to disrupt the system, the primary patient, who had seemed to be helpful in enforcing regular participation by all members, might himself start missing sessions, stifle relevant discussions, etc.

This discovery is one of the most shocking disappointments that can occur in view of the inexperienced family therapist's rescue motivation toward and wishful identification with the primary patient. A single, schizophrenic female patient encouraged her therapist to endorse her viewpoint within the family, namely that living with her father in his bachelor apartment would amount to a "suicide" on her part. When the therapist endorsed this point of view, however, the patient turned around and joined her family in a vigorous rejection of such odd concern on the psychiatrist's part.

The beginning therapist may not be aware of the inherent conflict between his traditionally learned individual psychotherapeutic approach and the requirements of the family-based method. There is a tendency to be preoccupied with the "productive" members' contributions. The member who produces conflictual behavior, slips of the tongue, or dreams during the conjoint family session may, usually unknowingly, form a perfect complementarity with the therapist who is himself most secure on the grounds of individual therapy. In his efforts to reach the dynamically most relevant family system of pathology, the therapist, especially the beginner in the field of conjoint family therapy, can often be distracted by seemingly meaningful "individual" dimensions of pathology. In one family, an allegedly honest effort at recalling of and associating to dreams was practiced by previously psychoanalyzed family members. It was revealed later that this was a device for resisting exploration of the parents' painful marital problems.

Even if the therapist is convinced of the necessity for ultimately dealing with the system-based forms of family pathology, he might be lured into paying undue attention to a demanding family member. He may, of course, sense correctly that the most unreasonable member can lead him to the core of the family's dynamic system. The family therapist must indeed find at least one member capable of a level of communication whereby he can reach and eventually manipulate the core of the family system. However, it requires experience to recognize the system-relevant aspects of individual symptoms, and it is advisable to search beyond verbal expression. If one presumes that that which is never verbalized is a more crucial part of family pathology than the manifest behavior, one has to assume also that the silent members often hold the key to the more resistant facets of the family pathology. A seemingly passive victim may turn out to be the shrewdest manipulator of another member's feelings.

The assumption that any one family member might be the key to the family system should not be confused with rigid single-cause-oriented thinking, according to which certain members' contribution is secondary (victim-like) to other members' primary contributions. Genetically, of course, it has to be assumed that the parental marriage and its pathology precedes the children's contribution. However, once the children's personalities have become adapted to their roles in the family system, their investment in maintaining the system may become as active as that of the parents. The therapist may need help from his supervisor or therapeutic team partner to realize the distortion of his own transference-based biases in selecting the "main" patient.

PROBLEMS OF THE THERAPIST

Space does not permit a truly systematic elaboration of the complexities of the role of the therapist in conjoint family therapy (see also Chapter 8). The therapist's personal contribution to the conjoint family therapy situation may turn out to be even more crucial than the individual therapist's unconscious contribution to his therapy. In our experience the chief difference between the two therapies lies in the team approach of family therapy with all its hidden intra-team relational implications.

We have found the personality fit of the two therapists a far more significant therapeutic factor than the interprofessional gap regarding training, role, and status in our group. Often, two professionals of the same category (e.g., psychologists) have had more difficulty in aligning their approach than have teams of a more heterogenous combination. Yet an automatic alignment and sharing of points of view is not necessarily the ideally desirable team attitude. The recognition of differences in work attitudes is bound to be followed by the recognition of deeper, often conflictual or ambivalent attitudes. We have found that the teams are more successful in resolving their conflicts if they periodically bring problems before the membership of the entire project of eight therapists.

The most fundamental aspect of the "technique" of family therapy relies on the healthy emotional survival of the therapists in the midst of incredible tensions, generated by what can be called the family members' unconscious manipulation of the therapists into resolving the family's covert incestuous and murderous conflicts. For example, considerable temporal foreshortening can occur as a result of the activation of long dormant grief processes through the quick alternation of object cathexes within the space of ninety minutes of conjoint family therapy. The need for possessing good and for rejecting bad love objects in succession motivates the family members to reject the therapists at a point when they feel most securely accepted by the family. It is the depth and trusting quality of the team relationship which can help the therapists to survive these sudden changes without resorting to neurotic defensiveness.

The frequent treacherousness of the family's acceptance of the therapists in conjoint therapy is illustrated by an example of therapy with a 19-year-old schizophrenic girl's family.

The parents' pathological possessiveness of their daughter was initially evident from their negotiations with the physician responsible for the girl's individual therapy in the hospital. It soon became clear that the parents wanted the therapist to commit himself to hospitalizing their daughter for at least one year. One the other hand, as the parents began to accept family therapy, in the course of several months they showed signs of a strongly ambivalent and regressive transference toward the family therapists. Concurrently, the daughter's symptoms diminished and she began to express interest in continuing her studies, out-of-town. The parents' combined possession of daughter and therapists became threatened; a choice had to be made. After considerable inner conflict, both family and individual therapy were rejected by the parents under the pretext that they wanted to respect the daughter's occasionally expressed vague wish for another individual therapist. Paradoxically, in the heated atmosphere of the last session the mother, who herself rejected the therapists, blamed them for cruelty and lack of willingness to help. Soon the daughter was back in another hospital following several comparatively serious suicidal gestures.

It follows from the above and similar examples that the "primary process" desires of family members may aim at retaining the therapists in therapeutically ineffective yet prolonged "feeding" roles. The therapists' effectiveness regarding genuine personality change is an undesirable by-product, as far as the resistant members' internal need constellation is concerned. This state of affairs places the therapists in a dilemma over whether they should themselves carry the principal motivation for change. Most therapists are, of course, emotionally committed to be successful in their work. Motivations of rescue may, unfortunately, become reinforced by the therapist's unconscious needs for acceptance and approval by those to be helped. Yet the family therapist may be rejected for that which he wishes to be accepted for, i.e., for wanting to help the family change. On the other hand, he can be increasingly accepted and therefore rewarded on a deeper, primary process level for forsaking his professional aims. If he chooses to concur with the family's stagnation game, he is seduced into giving up his professional integrity; if he opposes the game, he loses acceptance and support on the part of those for whom he is struggling. Without a good and openly communicative co-therapy relationship, the therapist may lose unnecessary amounts of sleep at this stage. The fate of the therapy clearly does not depend on what is being communicated verbally but on whether the family's relational system can be made to yield or not. The therapists' relational strength has to survive the pathological familial strength that it challenges.

Concluding Remarks and Outlook

Before conclusion, I believe I owe the reader a few statements regarding results or effects of our family therapy venture. A systematic, controlled evaluation of the results of the approach is naturally even less possible at this time than is an objective evaluation of intensive individual therapy. Lack of sufficient time and number of cases is but one reason for the difficulty. The lack of a consistently accepted framework of pathology and of its descriptive application constitutes a more serious reason for the dearth of publications on results of family therapy.

From the point of view of ultimate scientific progress it is small consolation, although it is encouraging, that the practitioners of parallelly conducted individual and family therapies have gradually become encouraged rather than discouraged to consider the latter as the more promising approach, *in depth* as well as in numerical coverage per therapist hour. We are aware of the need for a fuller communication of the observed familial changes to the professional community, but the completely non-verbal, multipersonal, and often imponderable quality of the results makes the task exceedingly difficult and probably premature on the present level of conceptual clarity.

The fact that at least in families with schizophrenic and delinquent designated patients, our therapists have become increasingly convinced of the usefulness of the family approach, suggests that work on this level might contribute significantly to an emerging relationship-based (psychiatric) evaluation of individual maturity per se. Schizophrenia is just one instance of the whole range of phenomena suggesting that man's emotional security is based on the quality of his close relationships. Further progress will be required for the development of specific indicational criteria for the dyadic versus conjoint psychotherapeutic approaches as treatments of choice. Evaluation of the outcome of treatment is equally difficult in both approaches. The only conceivable controlled comparison would be one based on large numbers. A further question remains regarding the choice of the type of family therapy. Certain goals can be reached through a mere support for the realignment and clarification of communication channels. The more serious the members' personality stagnation, the more obvious is the indication for the exploration of interpersonal distortions and their intrapsychic roots. The *system aspect* of interlocking and mutually reinforcing distortions, however, can best be explored in conjoint family sessions. Ultimately, the depth and intensity of any therapy approach is regulated by the extent of the patient's motivation.

Although one could anticipate rapidly growing professional acceptance of the family method of intensive psychotherapy, resistance against the serious undertaking of change through this treatment approach can be expected to parallel the initial reluctance to accept psychoanalysis as a valid treatment of "serious" nervous conditions. The sacrosanctity of the individual and of the family will be used as arguments by some critics of the approach. The intrusion of family therapy into the unconscious facets of *collective* neurotic mechanisms will often be resisted in the guise of righteous indignation over the therapist's presumed "unfair" implications of willful irresponsibility or destructiveness on the part of the "well" family members as *individuals*. Temporary increase of symptomatology will be deplored just as much as it is in psychoanalysis. Behind a presumed lack of understanding of the system-oriented aspect of the family approach lurks what really amounts to a dynamic resistance against changing the system itself.

The battle for or against acceptance of family therapy will only highlight the confusion regarding the role of the family in modern life. The significance of family life is probably undergoing a profound change, a change which is dynamically connected with social transition. As industrial-mechanical organization de-individualizes interpersonal interactions, the rise of the scientific-rational outlook tends to replace the previous dependency on a religio-ethical world order. The life of the individual increasingly resembles a rational proposition of calculable material gains and limitations. It is natural to assume that modern man's major outlet for emotional dependency and opportunity for personal growth continues to exist in family life.

It is probably erroneous to assume that the family's dynamic equilibrium can be understood without its relationship to grosser societal phenomena. Few would question the value system and rites of the adolescent society as complementary and often diametrically opposed to the traditional values of the family. Furthermore, it is obvious that seemingly ubiquitous outlets for hostility, such as prejudices, dictatorial political systems of aggressive domination, and hostile competition between the sexes, tend to hold a dynamic equilibrium with gratification through relatedness opportunities within the family. The child can threaten the parent with separation and can shift to reliance on the values and attractions of the adolescent society for emotional support, and the parents can in turn react with unconsciously defensive, conserving maneuvers directed at the children, the latter being viewed as deserting parent-like transference objects.

The broadest question of family pathology pertains to the role of the family in modern society. To what extent does contemporary societal development overtax the resources of family living? The "system" characteristics of the emerging family of the future seem to undergo certain modal changes. Buehler (1962) concludes that the overt mutual dependence of parental and filial generations has decreased in the course of the last decades. It is possible, furthermore, that the parental techniques of our age have diminished the extent of physical contact between mother and infant with a consecutive decrease in development of basic trust. One can postulate that a decrease in basic trust in combination with the de-individualizing effect of modern mass communication media contribute to new patterns of communication in families with the result of a decrease in intimacy and closeness of interpersonal relations. Will children of subsequent future generations be exposed to an increasing extent of confusing double-bind messages along with an increase of superficial sophistication of social habit patterns? Are society's existing alternate choices for the non-familial gratifications of emotional needs of adolescents both sufficiently attractive and sufficiently growth-supporting? It can be predicted that the "therapy" of the family can succeed only if society does not place an insurmountable demand upon family life and parental roles.

³ The author gratefully acknowledges Dr. Oscar R. Weiner's significant contributions as co-therapist and conceptualizer of the dynamics of the treatment process of the family reported in this chapter. Dr. James L. Framo did a painstaking job in reading and reviewing the manuscript in great detail; he as well as Mrs. Geraldine Spark and Mrs. Geraldine Lincoln have made many helpful suggestions to improve this chapter.

References

BERNE, E. (1964). Games people play; the psychology of human relationships. New York: Grove Press.

BOSZORMENYI-NAGY, I., AND FRAMO, J. L. (1961). Hospital organization and family oriented psychotherapy of schizophrenia. Proceedings of the 3rd World Congress of Psychiatry, Montreal.

BOSZORMENYI-NAGY, I., AND FRAMO, J. L. (1962). Family concept of hospital treatment of schizophrenia. In J. H. Masserman (Ed.) Current psychiatric therapies, vol. II. New York: Grune & Stratton.

BRODY, M. W., AND MAHONEY, V. P. (1964). Introjection, identification, and incorporation. Int. J. Psycho-Anal. 45, 57–63.

BUEHLER, C. (1962). Values in psychotherapy. Glencoe, Ill.: Free Press.

DEUTSCH, H. (1942). Some forms of emotional disturbances and their relationship to schizophrenia. *Psychoanal. Quart. XI*, 301–321.

EISSLER, K. R. (1963). Notes on the psychoanalytic concept of cure. *Psychoanal. Study of the Child. 18*, 424–463.

ENGLISH, H. B., AND ENGLISH, A. C. (1958). *A comprehensive dictionary of psychological and psychoanalytical terms. A guide to usage.* New York: Longmans, Green & Co.

FARBER, L. H. (1958). The therapeutic despair. *Psychiatry 21*, 7–20.

FREUD, S. (1919). Turnings in the ways of psychoanalytic therapy. In *Collected papers.* New York: Basic Books (1924), pp. 394–402.

GUNTRIP, H. (1960). Ego-weakness and the hard core of the problem of psychotherapy. *Brit. J. med. Psychol. 33*, 163–184.

JOHNSON, A. M., AND SZUREK, S. A. (1952). The genesis of antisocial acting out in children and adults. *Psychoanal. Quart. 21*, 323–343.

KANZER, M. (1957a). Acting out, sublimation, and reality testing. *J. Amer. Psychoanal. Assn. 5*, 663–684.

KANZER, M. (1957b) Acting out and its relation to impulse disorders. Panel Report. *J. Amer. Psychoanal. Assn. 5*, 136–145.

RANK, O. (1950). *Will therapy and truth and reality.* New York: Knopf.

RAPAPORT, D. (1958). The theory of ego autonomy. *Bull. Menninger Clin. 22*, 13–35.

RUBINSTEIN, D., AND WEINER, O. R. (1964). Co-therapy teamwork relationships in family psychotherapy. (With collaboration of Boszormenyi-Nagy, I., Dealy, M., Framo, J. L., Lincoln, G., Robinson, L., and Zuk, G.) Paper read at Conference on Family Process and Psychopathology: Perspectives of the Clinician and Social Scientist. Eastern Pennsylvania Psychiatric Institute, Philadelphia, October.

RYCKOFF, I., DAY, J., AND WYNNE, L. C. (1959). Maintenance of stereotyped roles in the families of schizophrenics. *Arch. Gen. Psychiat. 1*, 93–98.

SCHAFFER, L., WYNNE, L. C., DAY, J., RYCKOFF, I. M., AND HALPERIN, A. (1962). On the nature and sources of the psychiatrists' experience with the family of the schizophrenic. *Psychiatry 25*, 32–45.

SCHMIDEBERG, M. (1948). Parents as children. *Psychiat. Quart. Suppl. 22*, 207–218.

SEARLES, H. (1961). Phases of patient-therapist interaction in the psychotherapy of chronic schizophrenia. *Brit. J. med. Psychol. 34*, 169–193.

SPIEGEL, J. P. (1957). The resolution of role conflict in the family. *Psychiatry 20*, 1–16.

WHITAKER, C. A., AND MALONE, T. P. (1953). *The roots of psychotherapy.* New York: Blakiston.

4

JAMES L. FRAMO

Rationale and Techniques of Intensive Family Therapy

Expository writings on psychotherapeutic techniques have traditionally possessed the virtue of daring and the hazardousness of exposure.
Some very experienced therapists have questioned not only the ad-
visability of publishing books and articles on technique but honestly
believe that it is futile to attempt to put into organized language
what a therapist does or should do. It is their legitimate belief

The writer is indebted to Dr. Ivan Boszormenyi-Nagy, not only for being an
innovator in leading the Family Therapy Project toward the insights of family
therapy, but for providing the organizational machinery and overall inspiration
which helped to promulgate many of the ideas in this chapter. Cross fertilization
of concepts and opinions which have occurred in ongoing conferences are also
reflected in this chapter. Special thanks are owed Dr. Oscar R. Weiner for
participating with me in many discussions which resulted in ideas borrowed consciously and unconsciously. Drs. Boszormenyi-Nagy and Weiner have both read
the chapter and offered useful suggestions. The author acknowledges those
mentors and friends who influenced his personal and professional development:
Drs. James R. Frakes of Lehigh University, Joseph J. Rubin of Pennsylvania
State University, Wayne H. Holtzman of the University of Texas, Leslie Phillips
of the Worchester State Hospital, Sylvan S. Tomkins of Princeton University,
and Morris D. Galinsky of Philadelphia.

that the attempts to convey and analyze the therapeutic process always suffer in interpretation, and that the vital communications in all forms of psychotherapy are intuitive, felt, unspoken, and unconscious. Much of what transpires between patients and therapists is expressed by tone, gestures, expression, sensory impressions, feelings, and a host of other almost incommunicable states. Only a small part of therapeutic commerce takes place via words. Therapy supervisors have long known, moreover, that a wide discrepancy frequently exists between what a therapist says he does and what he actually does do. For example, one therapist may believe he is dealing with very deep material, but its impact on the patient may be quite shallow; another therapist may believe he is only doing supportive psychotherapy by dealing exclusively with reality problems, yet discover to his astonishment that the patient has become thoroughly involved. A further argument against defining techniques is that all therapists vary widely in personality, style, amount of activity, quality of focusing, goals, etc., even within the same psychotherapeutic school. Moreover, no amount of reading on technique will make an effective psychotherapist. It has long been known, but rarely stated, that meaningful psychotherapy demands from the therapist the necessary personality equipment (admittedly difficult to specify) capable of development under personal treatment and competent, detailed supervision. This supervision, in order to be effective, should take place in a free "therapeutic" atmosphere which permits exploration of the feelings of the student.

There is another line of reasoning that argues against technique-oriented writings, that is, the nature of psychotherapy itself. From the writer's viewpoint we still know very little, in a definitive sense, about what happens in psychotherapy, why it happens, how people are helped, and what really constitutes help. From the subjective standpoint of the patient, the critical, therapeutic ingredient in psychotherapy, whatever theory it is based upon and no matter what the therapist does or does not do, may simply be that the patient comes to feel that *someone cares*, however he interprets caring or "love." When the patient feels that someone cares he can begin to care for himself. Sometimes the patient can feel "loved" on the basis of a transference dream. From the viewpoint of the conceptualizer who is obliged to explain the therapeutic factor in psychotherapy as a dynamic, explanatory mechanism, love, it is said, is not enough. Other elements are presumed to be involved: the uniqueness of the therapeutic relationship, the uncovering, the well-timed interpretation, the careful working through. But it takes a very mature patient to realize that what the therapist *can* give—technical skill, reliability, relative objectivity, sense of trust, relatively unambivalent interest in the patient's growth—truly amount to love. What patient, in a moment of unguarded honesty, has not asked the therapist, either verbally or non-verbally, "Tell me, would you be interested in me if this were not your job or you were not being paid?" What patient has not watched, with super-acute alertness, for signs that the therapist is doing something "extra" for him outside the structure of his usual giving, or for indications that the therapist is being a real person to him? Sensing these patient needs, throughout the entire range of psychopathology, every therapist, whatever his orientation, at each check-point (i.e., how to present an interpretation, whether to reveal his feelings to the patient, which part of the patient's productions to respond to, etc.) has to make a choice along the dimension: should I gratify or should I frustrate? will the patient benefit more from my giving or from my withholding? Is the therapist so sure that the effect of his activity or non-activity can be as non-specific as, for example, feeding or not feeding? If we take away the patient's distorted fantasy that he was "loved" as a child, do we replace it with something else, or do we encourage the acceptance of his loss? These questions go beyond considerations of technique.

Though criticisms of technique exposition are cogent and valid, it is nonetheless encumbent upon practitioners to open the door to the treatment room and attempt to convey to colleagues information on how they conduct treatment sessions. Otherwise, practice, theory, and research would proceed along separate paths, uncoordinated and unintegrated, without a systematic discipline of therapeutic structure ever evolving.

It is especially important to reveal procedures whenever a new area of therapeutic endeavor is introduced. For example, in family therapy a host of new variables peculiar to the family approach must be considered in addition to the already incredibly complex variables of individual and group psychotherapy. However, this chapter on techniques of family therapy is not intended as a how-to-do-it treatise. A list of instructional rules would not only be premature but presumptuous. Rather, a statement of principles derived from our own practice in family therapy and a description of the development of techniques found to be useful, promising, limited, or anti-therapeutic will be communicated. The views expressed in this chapter are an extension of those previously describing our work (Framo, 1962). The present statements reflect our learning experiences, shifts in conceptions, and, it is hoped, a greater sophistication in the approach to families since the previous publication.

It must be emphasized at the outset that the rationale and techniques to be described were developed under certain conditions within a particular setting. This setting and the history of development of the unit are described in more detail in Chapter 3. Our unit is one of the few in the country where *long-term* family therapy is conducted. We believe that there are certain deep parameters of the family system which can be revealed only by extended work with the family.

Although many of our observations were originally based on work with families with a female schizophrenic member, several years ago we began treating families which included designated patients of both sexes and varying ages and whose symptoms covered the scope of psychopathology from character and personality disorders to neurotic, somatic, and psychotic reactions. More accurately, however, we are no longer diagnostically concerned with psychiatric categories or symptoms. Symptoms in the designated patient often change from week to week, and symptoms, as non-specific responses to accommodations in the family system which is undergoing therapeutic review, can shift from one family member to another.

Our criteria for admission to therapy is applied to the family instead of the individual patient. For a detailed discussion of criteria for selection of families for family therapy, see Chapter 7, Wynne. There are certain concrete guidelines we have followed: families referred to the project are seen for several evaluation sessions, not only to obtain a preliminary estimate of family dynamics but also to determine the kind of motivation which is operating within the family. It is extremely rare for a family to unanimously express motivation (i.e., "We need help as a family"), and when this does occur we usually discover that other stratagems are at work. For instance, several families were referred by an expensive private institution which allowed patients to stay only a limited time, and the parents, upon learning that we could provide hospitalization if the families agreed to participate in the treatment, could then easily "see" the problem as a family problem. The initial motivation in such cases was to save money and find a hospital in which to place the designated patient.

In our early work we tended to accept families on the basis of whatever motivation existed (most typically oriented solely around getting help for the designated patient). Because of lack of knowledge, we tied our hands and went along with the variety of excuses which were given for the absence of an important family member: one of the children could not get out of school, or grandmother would be too upset by the meetings, or father's job prevented him from attending all the sessions, etc. Gradually, we learned from our mistakes and, more significantly, gained more confidence in what we were offering; we have come to demand more from families by asserting conditions for acceptance into the program early in the evaluation process, conditions which give us maximum maneuverability. At the first evaluation session, and sometimes even before that, all family members are requested to sign an application for evaluation, which introduces the family concept that the entire family participate regularly in the treatment; a fee was established for the family sessions (previously none had been required); during the evaluation sessions we determined, on the basis of the family dynamics, what was to constitute the "family" we would be working with (i.e., all those immediate and extended family members as well as extrafamilial persons who exert a demonstrable influence on the total family system); the designated family members had to agree to arrange their schedules so they could all be present for weekly sessions; and, finally, in response to exploratory questioning, the family had to give some indication during the evaluation sessions that they could give more than lip service to family problems *other* than those having to do with the designated patient. Even though it may not be posible to get the parents or "well" siblings to admit that they have problems, the question should be raised and discussed in order to put the family therapy on a more realistic therapeutic basis. The therapists should ask each family member, "What changes would you like to see in the family that would benefit you?" or "What changes would you like to see in yourself that would make your life better?" Questions posed in this fashion avoid blame or accusation of sickness with all its moral and value judgments.

Whether or not to hospitalize the designated patient came to depend on the family dynamics as well as on the psychiatric condition of the patient. (After a patient is hospitalized, the presence or absence of symptoms do not determine whether or not he stays in the hospital. We sometimes send patients home with active, psychotic symptoms if this procedure is more likely to provide leverage in dealing with the family system.) From this position of strength we not only had a basis for dealing with the "absent-member maneuver" (Sonne, Speck, and Jungreis, 1962) by retaining the option of having any family member on call, but later we were able to be more flexible by allowing certain members to stay away with legitimate excuses and also by preserving the freedom to work with family sub-systems. We had learned earlier that the greater the family's resistance in bringing in a particular member of the family, the more that member's presence was necessary to understand the total system. Of course, our early drop-out rate increased; families telephoned to say, "We decided we really don't need help," or "Everything is a lot better now," or "My husband can't take time off from work," or "You doctors didn't tell us how to handle our sick daughter," or "We decided to send our daughter to a psychiatrist, or to another hospital." Nonetheless, we have learned that the families who persevere in the evaluation process are not as likely to terminate once they perceive the full impact of what is really involved in family therapy. Inasmuch as family therapy requires more than ordinary commitment in personnel and time, a weeding-out process is necessary. These, then, are the methods we have developed for dealing with motivation problems in those asymptomatic family members who would ordinarily never have sought psychotherapy for themselves inasmuch as their intrapsychic conflicts are acted out intrafamilially. With the advent of family therapy, for the first time we are beginning to reach the people who bring other people in for treatment. It is a mixed blessing that family therapy brings in as patients these kinds of people who, while they have a great impact on others, are often beyond the reach of treatment.

Despite our built-in filtering system, however, it needs to be stressed that we are still in the early stages of estimating motivation for family therapy. We have treated families who, motivationally speaking, initially looked like very poor prospects and later profited a great deal from therapy; there are also those who looked very promising during the evaluation process and made little or no progress.

Initial evaluation sessions are observed by the entire staff of eight therapists. Using their global human reactions as a guide, two therapists who have chosen to work with each other will volunteer to treat a particular family. The distinctive basis for a family's capacity to evoke an encountering response in certain therapists, and the reasons we use two therapists who select each other are interesting topics which will be elaborated upon later in this chapter. We are unable to determine, of course, how a different setting and a different set of conditions would have led to other techniques and conclusions.

As a further caution to the literal interpretation of our techniques, it must be recognized that techniques develop out of an ongoing process and are always incomplete. Only a small part of what we actually do in day-to-day treatment is described in this chapter, which may partly explain the paucity of writing on technique of family therapy (Ackerman, 1960; Bell, 1961; Bowen, 1961; Jackson, 1961; Midelfort, 1957), despite the growing literature on family therapy itself (see Ch. 1, bibliography).

This chapter is arbitrarily divided into the following sections: rationale; early phases of family therapy; middle phases of family therapy; resistance in family therapy; marriage problems in family therapy; the "well" sibling in family therapy; transference and countertransference; co-therapy team relationship; terminal phases of family therapy; and, finally, a subjective evaluation of family therapy. While organizing the chapter it was found that these subdivisions fell naturally into place as important dimensions of the family therapy process.

Rationale

It must be recognized that techniques are designs or contrivances which implement a rationale of therapy. We are in the earliest stages of developing a conceptual understanding of family disorders, and, of course, the techniques for dealing with these family disturbances lag behind the comprehension of them.[1] The rationale of our therapeutic approach to families is based upon subsequent observations, which represent a distillation of our learning. Since our early experience has been with families with a schizophrenic member one could question the generality of these findings to family dynamics in general. However, our more recent experience suggests that pathogenic system processes should be used to diagnose families, and that such processes cut across diagnostic categories. All families have system properties, whatever form the manifest symptoms of one of its members may assume. Some of the following statements may appear contradictory, but they apply to different levels of inference and are regarded as valid at those different levels.

1) Unless one has had the experience of seeing family members together over a period of time, it is difficult to grasp the full implications of the notion that the *substance* of psychiatric disorder can be a family manifestation, and that the designated "patient" is only the most obvious symptom through which the family system manifests its pathology. When one first sees the family of a schizophrenic, for example, it is difficult to conceive of schizophrenia as a family disorder, since the patient appears so different from the other family members. The interconnected quality of the family problems can often be dramatically confirmed by observing a family session after a period of treatment and trying to pick out the sick member.

Some of these ideas can perhaps be illustrated by contrasting the individual and family approaches to the same problem.

---

[1] Although there is a long history of interest in family conflicts and methods for handling them, particularly on the part of the social work profession, the specific dynamic, *clinical* emphasis on the family, dealing with the interactions and transactions themselves, and treatment of members of the family conjointly are largely phenomena of the last decade.

A patient was referred to our unit with the following symptoms: she was suspicious and felt persecuted at the office where she worked. She was a dispatch messenger and believed that she was relaying messages of ominous intent. Ordinarily, in a good psychiatric set-up she would be interviewed, perhaps hospitalized, undergo psychological testing, and be presented at a staff conference. There would be involved discussions of diagnosis as to whether or not she was schizophrenic, and if so, how malignant the process was; there would also be some speculation about her dynamics in intrapsychic terms. A social worker might report on interviews with the parents who were able to give detailed accounts of the patient's developmental history and background. Following a factual account of the parents' backgrounds, the social worker might make some incidental observations about the parents, perhaps commenting on their individual oddities or on how concerned and responsible they seemed. After such a staff conference, a program of individual psychotherapy might be instituted for the patient, with perhaps one or both parents being seen by the social worker.

Now, contrast this typical approach with what we learned after a few sessions with this girl and her family meeting together.

After resisting efforts of the parents *and* the patient to talk about the patient's symptoms and difficulties at work, we learned that the designated patient was caught in the middle of a family-wide paranoia, that her symptoms were but one component part of a network. Out of all the intricacies and levels involved, one set of facts clearly emerged. Several years ago the father became extremely jealous, suspecting that his wife was having affairs with every man she met, and he would constantly follow and check up on her every movement. The patient was sometimes employed as the father's emissary on these missions. His jealousy then abated and, more recently, the mother, basing her suspicions on the flimsiest of evidence, erupted into the same kind of irrational and violent jealousy which had occurred with her husband earlier. The patient was again called upon to act as mediator between her parents, a role which she ambivalently accepted, displacing her rage, suspiciousness, and excitement onto her work situation.

We learned from the transactions of this family, as with every other one we have seen, that a part of the problem resides in each family member, like separate aspects of a multi-layered riddle.

2) The system of the family has regulating mechanisms of its own which control the collective mechanisms of its individual members. More is involved than the unconscious dynamics of each person; the complicated processes of the ongoing system govern the individual motivations. Despite numerous plots and sub-plots, the family remains a unity. Each family member uses every other member to balance his own pathology. Still, it is not one person acting upon another person; it can be any one person who affects the

whole transactional structure. Although an event such as psychosis or delinquency, *if it disturbs the family system*, can introduce great strain and upset the existing equilibrium, it can sometimes be quickly absorbed into the system and become a part of the family's way of life. Sudden psychosis in one member can occasionally create enormous family anxiety of the kind generated when a dangerous fantasy or game threatens to become real.

3) Each member of the family has to fit in with the rules of the family game (Haley, 1959). Deviation from this fitting-together on the part of any one member leads to a graduated series of injunctions, the most extreme of which is threatened abandonment (a punishment which is almost never meted out in any permanent form because each part is necessary to the whole). The members of undifferentiated families have never learned that it is better to have the voluntary love of a free, separate human being than the "love" resulting from emotional enslavement. At times a family member tries to fight his way out of his role: the father usually goes through his sequence of futile protestations and then gives up; his needs are too great for him to stay away if he separates. Frequently what seems like a separation gesture by an adolescent is actually an effort to get the parents involved (e.g., the daughter's indirectly letting her parents know she is having an unhealthy love affair). On rare occasions someone, usually one of the so-called "well" siblings, does manage to break free to some extent, but the "break" is typically of a violent sort, and the old conflicts are carried over into the new relationships. Many people delude themselves into believing that if they physically move far from home and never see their family again for the rest of their lives, they are no longer involved with them.

In the large majority of the families seen (especially the tightest family systems, those with an only child), all the significant emotional exchanges are contained within the closed, complete social system of the family, and there is little or no contact with the outside world. A minority of the families we have seen constantly explode distress signals and over-involve others in the community. Neighbors, police, social workers, psychiatrists, etc. are frequently called to give outside control or supplementary "feedings" to these deficient "family egos."[2] Every community is familiar with these

---

[2] The author recognizes that a number of technical terms ordinarily used in other theoretical frameworks (particularly psychoanalytic) are carried over into the area of family therapy (family ego, family resistance, etc.). In going into a new area one naturally depends on familiar terms, even though they retain a specific, restricted meaning within a theoretical system. The creation of new technical words, however, would have less communication value at this time.

families, who are registered with nearly every social agency in town; some of the members of these families are known to many of the psychiatrists in the city, the family having consulted each of them at one time or other.

4) In the more poorly differentiated family, it is more likely that the parents cannot see or act toward their children or each other as they really are but, instead, as screens to project on or as imagoes through whom they can work through past, unsatisfied longings and hurts which stem from their original experiences with their own families. Each family, then, has its own fossil remains which are preserved from past generations and largely determine what goes on in the present. Though a one-to-one representation is rare, there is some merit in trying to discover which key figure or fusion of figures in each of the parents' background the patient represents. Since they need to be seen as good parents, however, the mothers and fathers will frequently show obsessive concern about some aspect of the patient—her physical health, I.Q., pimples, weight, speech, clothing, etc.

5) The designated patient half willingly accepts her role as the scapegoat and sacrifices her autonomy in order to fill in gaps and voids in the lives of her parents or in her parents' marriage relationship, to conform to some preconceived notion of the parents as to what she should be, or to preserve the stability of the parents. She cannot evade any of the assigned roles of wife, husband, friend, mother, father, grandparent, sexual substitute, sibling to parent, pal to parent, object of ambition, or object of revenge. The designated patient, moreover, has been subjected to what we call the "yo-yo" syndrome; she is pulled toward the parents when they need her and pushed away or ignored when her own needs come to the fore. Outright rejection is never expressed, and if it were it could be better handled than continually teasing the patient with promised love which is never quite delivered or sustained. (During the course of family therapy we have learned that the parents, too, had similar yo-yo experiences with their own parents.) The designated patient tries to ward off her allotted role at the same time that she is enticed by its exciting qualities; she is constantly asking through her behavior, "What do I have to do or be to be accepted?"

The family concept of therapy clarifies the process of reality impairment. Ordinarily children develop the capacity for abstract thinking along the natural lines of genetic intellectual endowment. However, when unrealities prevail in the minds of the parents themselves, the child has little choice but to conform to these unrealities. Powerful guilt pressures and implications of treason or disloyalty can be brought to bear upon the child if he persists in pursuing reality. These pressures can not only force the child to renounce reality but they can block off the higher levels of reasoning which are associated with abstract thinking. After a while the unreality of the parents becomes the unreality of the child. Gradually, through the years, the designated patient is "trained" to be the living embodiment of the projected image. To be on the receiving end of a projection of someone else's internal image can be, however, a particularly frustrating and perplexing experience if that someone else is a vitally needed person; you must be seen as malevolent, spoiled, prematurely grown-up, deceitful, or what have you, and nothing can be said or done to change this view. One of the most baffling and painful emotional states results from having one's decent or autonomous motive twisted into something evil or unhealthy.

One patient in individual and family therapy was beginning to become autonomous; she confided less in her mother and would no longer allow her mother to set her hair. The mother, perceiving the withdrawal and threatened by the loosening of the symbiotic tie, responded with, "You must be getting sick again; I'd better take you back to the hospital." The patient, already painfully vulnerable about being labelled "sick," then became bewildered and anxious, especially since she found it so tempting to confide in the mother or allow the mother to fix her hair.

On the basis of such data we can perhaps understand more fully the genesis of some of the classical symptoms of schizophrenia (perplexity, disharmony of affect, etc.). Whereas the symptoms of the designated patient can sometimes be translated psychodynamically as an expression of some family phenomenon (e.g., the patient's expression in exaggerated or symbolic form of the sub-clinical symptoms of a parent or some oblique commentary on the nature of the marriage relationship), at other times the symptoms have little or no meaning in either family or intrapsychic terms, and eventually prove to be epi-phenomena or non-specific "noise." Often the designated patient gives the SOS signal by such misleading symptoms and actions as stomach pains, stealing a car, locking herself in a room, truancy, or hallucinations. It is unfortunate that so many years have been spent on developing accurate nosological categories for individuals with specific treatments for specific conditions. Even family therapists have gotten into the habit of characterizing families by the overt symptoms of the designated patient (e.g., schizophrenic families, acting out families, etc.). One of our tasks for the future, on which some preliminary efforts are now being made, is to try to develop more meaningful transactional diagnoses for families.

6) Ordinarily, those who have achieved a relatively clear distinction between self and non-self realize that awareness of a need

does not guarantee satisfaction of the need, and also that willing an external behavior on the part of someone else cannot magically bring about the behavior in the same way as one wills one's hands to move. Yet, in families where the individual members' ego boundaries are diffuse and where they have great difficulty distinguishing among each other, there are indeed occasions when one family member has only to wish or will the satisfaction of a need and it is met. The mother who feeds her child when she herself is hungry may addict the child into responding to her unspoken needs, and this phenomenon may spread into a family-wide magic and omnipotence which can be exceedingly difficult to dislodge. Why should these deep gratifications be traded for reality? The perpetuation and "stickiness" of these pleasurable-painful, pre-verbal needs constitute the main resistance to change in the family. When attempts are made to modify or eliminate them, the alternative ways of relating are perceived by the family members in terms of the ultimate horror—the agonizing state of unrelatedness. They dread reaching the point where nothing they do or are or become matters to anyone. In some ways families who argue openly or relate to each other in hurtful or humiliating ways are better off than they would be in a state of futile nothingness.

7) Whenever there are disturbed children there is a disturbed marriage, although all disturbed marriages do not create disturbed children. In some poorly differentiated families the marriage exists largely on the basis of what the children provide. The parents have long since given up on each other and live side by side with little or no sense of real relationship, except to serve each other as objects of projected hostility or as representatives of introjects. To avoid the intimacy-aloofness conflict, various arrangements may be worked out to maintain the emotional divorce: absorption in television viewing when they are together; the husband taking jobs which keep him away from home; the wife or husband getting overinvolved in causes, organizations, or clubs; the parents intensifying their relationship with members of their families of origin, etc. Some of these marriages would be quite workable if there were no children. There are occasions when the parents' relationship to one child, usually the designated patient, can be stronger and more meaningful than any other relationship. The patient, her own Oedipal feelings realized under these conditions, finds that anything offered by anyone outside the family can in no way compete with or match the stimulation promised by the primary love objects. By offering themselves, the parents can inculcate a life-long, built-in persuader against the patient's ever finding a life outside the family. Since the parents' real sexual satisfaction with each other is limited or non-existent,

they may turn to the children for sexual love. The more children are involved in the marriage and used by the parents the greater the threat of incest and the greater the chance of development of psychosis in the child. The expression of sexual feeling toward the child may range from overt seductive behavior to a preconscious or unconscious sexual temptation against which the family members must defend themselves by threats or sudden withdrawal. Families in which actual incestuous sexual expression occurs are uncommon. Severe sexual inhibition in a permanent atmosphere of great temptation is more characteristic. The family members cannot allow even normal affectionate displays or playful sexuality; some never even dare to touch each other.

The patient is almost always enmeshed in the marriage, although in a few situations we have seen she has been excluded from the marriage twosome; under these circumstances she is regarded by her parents as a misfit, a poorly designed piece of machinery which does not work properly. Though the patient may have been a "victim" in her early years because of an immature ego, by the time she reaches adolescence she ceases to be a victim because she is certainly part of the family system by that time. For example, she does not feel she can make a life for herself unless her parents have a life of their own with some degree of satisfaction with each other; on the other hand, she is likely to become more anxious if her parents do achieve greater closeness.

8) Traditional psychoanalytic views have stressed the following intrapsychic phenomena as fundamental hypotheses in the etiology of schizophrenia: a disturbance in the relationship of the libido to objects; a defect in the ego as a problem-solving agent; a defect in the ego as an experience in relation to the object world—past, present, and future; the existence of a greater than usual destructive drive; an abnormally great degree of anxiety; and a failure of integration and synthesis of all of the foregoing factors. From the standpoint of a transpersonal family concept, schizophrenia, or any other kind of mental illness, despite its protean manifestations, can be looked upon as the only logical, adaptive response to a deranged, illogical family system. Despite the tempting gratifications provided by the parents and despite a symbiotic orientation, the designated patient has the most life to lose; she therefore sometimes "develops" the psychosis as a way of signalling for help and change, while at the same time offers herself in the sacrificial role and denies responsibility for wanting change in the family. In this connection it is interesting to speculate how often an act of juvenile delinquency can be looked upon as the only "safe" way of calling attention to an intolerable family situation. The patient feels too guilty to

be disloyal to the parents, as every therapist learns when he tries to interpret the obvious discontent. Still, when the patient does try to identify reality in the family distortions, this effort is often labeled by the family as "sick," and when she is hospitalized the doctors (and society, in effect) reinforce and confirm the family's diagnosis. Such considerations have led us to avoid hospitalization unless absolutely necessary.

The symptoms of the designated patient, while restitutional and regressive, do create numerous other problems. It has long been known that certain kinds of symptoms provoke attitudes in other people which can affect the course of the disorder itself (e.g., passive withdrawal often promotes mothering; obsessive dawdling forces others to urge and push; paranoid twisting or aggressive behavior can make others punish or reject; delusions can fascinate or repel; depression arouses mixtures of pity, helplessness, and anger; sexual acting out provokes envy and disgust; etc.). Then, too, the intact portion of the psychotic patient's ego is painfully aware of the stigma of mental illness; some of the patient's motivations and behavior can be understood as various means of handling the intolerable burden of shame and feeling like an outcast.

Mental illness can also serve as the means of obtaining secondary gains for the designated patient, primarily as a strategem of gaining some intrafamilial advantage. All anti-family symptoms are regarded by the parents with horror; those which are not are looked upon as minor annoyances, tolerated, or even indirectly fostered. Generally speaking, if the patient is giving the parents what they need, she is not regarded as sick (one father said, "Doctor, this lovely girl *can't* be sick; she kisses me with such feeling!"). Characteristically, once the anti-family symptoms disappear in the designated patient the parents are demotivated to continue family therapy.

Because therapeutic efforts are usually directed toward the young life which is hurting so much and seems especially vulnerable, and because the designated patient seems to possess a greater capacity for change (although this is not always due to the flexibility associated with youth), it has become common practice to conduct individual treatment in conjunction with family therapy. There are family therapists who have a deep conviction, based on their prior individually-oriented experience, that resolution of conflicts with introjects can only take place through transference work on a one-to-one basis. They reason, too, that in individual treatment, hopefully, the therapist can meet some of the patient's needs, although long-term individual treatment alone with the psychotic frequently threatens to develop into a lifelong-dependency attachment with the therapist (Hill, 1955). The prospect of this outcome may be the reason why so many therapists shy away from commitments to treat psychotic patients. Some therapists have come to believe that it is necessary to almost adopt the schizophrenic in order to teach him how to live (Szasz, 1957). Others, particularly the therapists at Chestnut Lodge, feel that the symbiotic attachment between patient and therapist is a necessary phase in long-term treatment and that any resulting complications are capable of resolution (Searles, 1958, 1959a, 1959b).

Many aspects of psychotic behavior have the quality of a two-year-old's provocative testing of its mother. This behavior may be oriented toward testing a mother's or father's concern and a commitment to see them through and care for them, no matter what. This testing-out behavior may also occur in the hospital with nursing staff and ward personnel in the roles of parental substitutes of the patient (Boszormenyi-Nagy and Framo, 1961, 1962). If a therapist stands by the patient through a stormy psychosis and follows through afterwards, then the patient can begin to trust others and build up ego-constitutive goodness. From time to time, however, the therapist's true concern will have to be proven. If the therapist withstands the patient's tests, he gains a place in the patient's relational world and can assume at times more importance than the parents. Not many therapists can endure this testing, which can get very nasty at times, taking the form of direct physical assaults, escapes from the hospital, furious rages, gifts, seductive pleas, hunger strikes, etc.

Experience over the years has led us to de-emphasize individual therapy for the designated patient in favor of working with the interdependent family system. The member of the therapy team which was seeing the designated patient in individual therapy, because of his special relationship with the patient, frequently found it more difficult to see and maintain the family system point of view. We learned, further, that the individual therapy had a diluting effect on the family therapy and came to be used as a resistance to exploration of family dynamics. The parents were usually eager to have the doctors deal with their sick daughter, rationalizing that it is the doctor's responsibility to take care of the sick person. We have found it more realistic that the parents rather than the therapists assume the responsibility of raising the child. The termination of individual therapy is usually followed by an increase in the intensity of family therapy. There are, of course, still occasions when individual therapy is indicated for the designated patient as well as other family members.

9) Do people really do things to other people or do they do things to themselves? The extent to which psychopathology is purely

an internal, intrapsychic affair and the extent to which it can come about, be attenuated or modified as a function of how people in close relationship affect each other has been and will continue to be one of the central theoretical and practical issues of our time. (The two polar positions on this issue are taken by traditional psychoanalysts on the one hand and by family therapists on the other.) An ultimate theory of personality, it seems to us, will have to consider an intricate but appropriate combination of both the individual and transpersonal points of view.

People who do not successfully resolve problems that arise with each step of growth carry over to each successive developmental stage a series of conditions and handicaps which limit their capacity to relate to others except in the light of their own needs (see Ch. 8, Erikson, 1950). Narcissistic relating, however, is never total; people in a relationship of long duration (e.g., husband and wife) also respond to each other on the basis of their accumulated experience of mutual accommodation, even though their relationship is intermingled with and framed within past transference relationships. That is, there are occasions, even in the most symbiotic relationships, when the persons concerned see and respond to each other as separate individuals. Nevertheless, in our experience we have seen that the family cannot undergo deep or meaningful change if the therapists deal only with current, immediate interaction among the members. The most powerful obstacle to successful treatment is the individual members' libidinal attachments to their parental introjects, no matter what the parents were like in real life (Guntrip, 1953); it is necessary for each individual to work through the struggle with the incorporated internal objects (Fairbairn, 1952) which are being acted out with the other family members. The unconscious clinging to the disturbing internal object world is associated with the endless attempts to change real others into unconditionally loving parents. (The need to help parents become better integrated people is probably based on the belief that if the parents were better integrated they could give more.) One of the most pathetic situations arises from an individual's lifetime efforts to obtain something from a mother or father that can never be obtained.

There are also important parameters in the family concept which are only beginning to be realized—that introjects are not only based on a one-to-one relationship to the mother and father as individuals, but on the nature of the marriage relationship between the parents; on the *psychological* mother and father of the family; on the family itself, including the sibling system. In other words, a whole family system—its emotions, its codes, its style—is sometimes introjected. In introjection of family emotions, for example, at one extreme there are families where affect is open and explosive and at the other extreme where intense emotions are muted or never expressed; such methods of handling affect can have drastic consequences for the personalities of the children of such families. Further, people are strongly motivated to experience specific emotional states or combinations of emotions in specific sequences under specific conditions; the relevant motivational formulae always bear a lawful relationship to the emotional network within which the original family drama was enacted.

10) Professionals in the area of family treatment have discovered that because of the vital stakes involved for each family member, dealing with the family system in any meaningful way is always much more threatening to the family than dealing with a single individual's defenses and conflicts. Therapists have long sensed that a patient in individual psychotherapy or analysis has not changed and has developed great resistance because the transactional elements of his family life (what analysts put under the category of "reality problems") have not been under direct observation or dealt with directly. The "resistance" of the patient often resides in part in someone else. The uncommunicativeness of adolescents in individual therapy is often mute testimony to their inner recognition that the wrong person is being treated. Therapeutic work with a child is often undermined at home, and work with an adult patient is often sabotaged by a spouse or parent or sibling with both the patient and the other member often conniving to maintain their bilateral and pathologic fantasy "game." How often have individual therapists heard their patients say explicitly or implicitly, "I will change if so-and-so also changes," or "What good would it do for me to change if so-and-so doesn't change too?" When the therapist counters with, "But we don't have so-and-so in this room; you are the one we have to work with," the patient may overtly agree but silently feel, "You can say what you like, but I have too much to lose from somebody important to me if I really do change." The purely intrapsychic approach has often failed for these reasons, and the therapist is often at a loss to explain why. When the silent but powerful outside influences are brought within one therapeutic setting more factors can be observed and controlled, but, of course, the therapeutic task is made none the easier. Techniques for dealing with these system defenses are next discussed.

Early Phases of Family Therapy

As stated earlier, in our recent work we have selected for family therapy only those families who met the minimal conditions of agreeing to meet weekly with all those immediate and extended family members specified by the therapists, and those families who could see problems in the family other than those having to do with the designated patient. Consequently, the accepted families are already a selected group, and presumably there would be some degree of uniformity among them in their approach to undertaking family therapy, but such is not the case. Anyone who anticipates that families will come to the treatment sessions and relate their difficulties in living as, for example, a well-motivated individual out-patient might do, will be considerably disappointed. All people, of course, have to present their problems in the only way they know how. Problems are usually set forth inferentially by the family—by their behavior, by non-verbal "acting out," by their family style. The dilemmas can be exhibited by a myriad of forms which are rarely meaningfully constructed with genuine affect, such as helpless silence, bickering, half-concealed smirks, a flood of words, the patient's "standing on her head," intellectualized abstractions, constant over-agreeing with the therapist to avoid listening to him, etc. Most families cannot put into words their need for help.

Some families present their pathology in a striking way from the first contact. They over-reveal their dynamics. In other families it is much more difficult to see the pathology at first; everyone except the designated patient may seem reasonable, conventional, and psychiatrically well-balanced. The parents seem to have remarkable insight into their daughter's illness and to be able to accept easily their own share of responsibility and contribution. The marriage seems fairly healthy, and even when the therapists listen carefully they can detect nothing grossly unusual in the family's description of its past or current modes of relating. Everyone seems to say the right thing, and it all sounds like they've read the textbooks. It may take a long time to perceive the extremely subtle strains of pathology which are interwoven through the system; the "sweet" sacrifice of mother, suppression of autonomy in the child, competition of father, or a concealed alliance between two family members may all hide behind multiple covers or be only delicately apparent. It takes the proverbial "sixth sense" to detect the specific sources of pathology; one knows one is close to these sources when the family tries to avoid the topic or gets anxious as it is approached. Both the open and closed, or expressive and repressive, family systems present their own kinds of resistance to exploration.

The quality of near public exposure is one of the most striking attributes of family treatment, in contrast to the privacy of individual treatment. Communication is naturally freer between a patient and his own doctor in the privacy of the office. The sanctity of the doctor-patient relationship in psychotherapy is unquestioned. To most therapists, treating a family together seems not only an unwieldy and chaotic prospect, but also one which would thwart any attempts to work with defenses and explore underlying motivations. It would seem to be impossible to keep track of all the factors involved. Therapists ask: "How can you deal with five people talking all at once?" "Do you really think people will open up in a situation like that? Everytime something is said, everybody hears it; how can you possibly expect to elicit anything but superficialities to work with?" Further complications arise from experience in family therapy; much of the family's defensiveness revolves around not only self-protection but also the "protection" of other family members. When people in close relationship are under therapeutic surveillance this interesting protection phenomenon always appears and seems to be related to the guarding and preservation of vested interests and vital needs which are fulfilled in the relationship. The protection may appear in a variety of ways, most often in the form of one member blocking therapeutic exploration of the other (interruptions, completing the other's sentences, diversionary tactics, etc.). Resistance against change in oneself as well as disturbance over the possibility of change in the other—even a change which is desperately desired consciously—always elicits protection ploys as each member attempts to restore the previous balance in the relationship because the old gratifications, no matter how much pain goes along with them, are at least familiar. Not only will whole families conspire to keep family secrets and prevent revelation of the family plot, but because of the public nature of family therapy it is often difficult for one member to acknowledge even a consciously defended painful feeling. For example, when it is interpreted to a mother that she is jealous of her husband's preference of their daughter to her, how can she react, even when the implication is made explicit? In individual insight therapy she may come to admit it after defenses are softened, perhaps proceed to wonder why it bothers her so, and then trace its roots to the past. But does she want her husband and daughter to know she feels jealous? Her final response to the interpretation (denial, evasion, etc.) is determined not only by her resistances, but by the added factor in family therapy of having to make a public admission, sometimes in front of the very people she'd least want to know.

In the face of these almost insuperable difficulties, then, what can be done, what techniques promise to make the process one of actual therapy, rather than the recurrent actualization of repudiated and projected motives? As in all therapy, one has to be selective, depending, among other bases, on the current constellation of individual and system defenses and the possibility that the family is listening to and making use of therapeutic intervention. Naturally, many things are missed, but if they are important they will re-occur in some form.

We regard the entire family unit as a patient, usually structuring the treatment situation as an opportunity for the family members to explore problems with each other. When parents are told that we work with the entire family, they initially accept the idea with equanimity, saying, "Yes, doctor, we understand. We want you to know that we will do everything in our power to cooperate to get our daughter well. No sacrifice is too great." In our early years of operation we used to allow discussion about the designated patient to go on for a number of sessions; our rationale was that the sessions should begin with what most concerned the family, which obviously would be the illness of a member of the family. A typical exchange at that time was as follows: The parents would turn to the patient with the words, "Tell us what is wrong, dear. Why don't you talk to the doctor? Don't be afraid to say anything; we can take it. Would you like to tell us off or hit us? Will that make you feel better?" The majority of the time the patient, sensing the concealed injunction that she'd better say the right thing or at least avoid self-incrimination, would respond, "Nothing's bothering me," or she would behave in some irrational way to confirm the view of her as a demented or inept person. If the patient, particularly if she has undergone individual psychotherapy and feels the support of her therapist, actually reveals what's on her mind, for example in the form of "disloyally" commenting on the parents' unhappy marriage or angrily passing a judgment on mother (thus violating family dictum number one [Jackson, 1959, p. 138]) a series of events follows very quickly. Father quickly changes the subject, a sibling begins to laugh, and mother, after a dumbfounded look, hits her hand on her thigh, turns to the doctor, and says, "See, doctor, this is what I mean. She's getting sick again." We have repeatedly noticed in most families that the mother can never consider her daughter well until the patient no longer manifests anger or deep resentment toward her.[3]

---

[3] An interesting counterpart to the parents' shock when the patient begins to open up after being pressured to talk is seen in the individual psychotherapy of schizophrenics. As Searles (1961) put it, "Not infrequently one hears from fellow therapists and ward personnel of how 'stunned' or even 'shocked' they were at seeing dramatic improvement in the long-ill patient, and I have felt this way many times myself . . . Noteworthy, also, even among the most technically capable of therapists, is the initial reacting with dismay and discouragement to a patient's new-found ability to express verbally the depths of his despair, loneliness, confusion, infantile needs, and so on."

As we gained more experience we felt more comfortable about probing into other family problems early in the therapy and deflecting discussion away from the problems of the designated patient. Families are usually unable to deal with the general question, "What are the problems in the family?" Such a question usually gives rise to embarrassed silence or clichés or the statement, "We don't have any family problems except for our sick daughter here." Instead, we sometimes approach indirectly by asking each of the family members in turn to talk about their experiences in this present family, their views about each of the other members, their ideas about the family life, in order to get the history of the family from the vantage point of each member. In the course of the recounting there may be frequent interruptions as other members may dispute a characterization of themselves or some event, or react with astonishment to some statement with: "John, I had no idea you've felt this way all these years." We also ask the parents to talk about their families of origin, significant losses and trauma, their own parents and their parents' relationship with each other, as well as a history of the present marriage. In the beginning only expurgated, well-defended, and distorted accounts of people and events are divulged, but that is not important at this early stage. The children are usually avidly interested in hearing about their parents' backgrounds and marriage, sometimes hearing some secrets for the first time. Our strategy in opening up all these areas consists not only in obtaining outlines of the parental introjects in order to understand problems in the present family, but also to uncover the underground psychological elements in the family. As these various views and opinions are discussed, new issues arise, the family members interact, and the patterns, divergencies, coalitions, forms of influence, cross-complicities, persuasive techniques, motivational struggles, status hierarchies all begin to emerge. A dawning realization of the real meaning of the family therapy procedure emerges out of this intensive mutual exploration, usually precipitating marked anxiety. The anxiety may be manifested in a variety of ways: there may be renewed, frantic efforts to bring the focus back to the patient ("Now, just a minute, doc, it's our daughter who's the sick one"); there may be an attempt to withdraw from family treatment, using a diversity of rationalizations; or the patient may become the spokesman for the family fear and say, "I don't think family therapy will help. My problems have nothing to do with my family," hoping all the while that she will not be taken seriously.

An unexpected occurrence at these times is when one of the parents edges his chair close to one of the therapists and begins to recite a detailed history of unfilled need and disappointment, thereby displaying himself as the hungriest and angriest one of the family. The patient is usually surprised by an occurrence of this type, which may confirm a dimly perceived, long-held suspicion that in some ways her parents are worse off than she. Sometimes, when the patient is acutely psychotic, she may be so intent on making the sacrificial gesture by rescuing her parents or calling attention to herself that she will attempt to block exploration of the family by such diversionary tactics as psychotic rambling, screaming, responding loudly to hallucinations, wandering around the room, etc.; it is necessary at times simply to shut the patient up, occasionally requesting that the parents control her. We have seen a few occasions where the psychotic patient, from the privileged sanctuary of her psychosis, would try to humiliate her parents, making them perform like trained seals, or try to force them to deny reality and go along with her delusions. The parents, embarrassed in front of the therapists and intent on showing them that they love their daughter, will, despite their helpless rage, often try to go along with the unreality because after all, "you can't get angry at someone who is sick." Their behavior is often explained as "humoring" the patient. On a deeper level, however, the patient is caricaturing the important role she has in her parents' life; parents and child have made a deal: "Let me possess you and I'll be your slave." The master-slave role alternates between the two. When the designated patient is loud and noisy, the therapists must skillfully follow both the primary process level of the patient and the mostly secondary process level of the rest of the family, especially since at these times the psychotic productions are frequently burlesques of some deep aspect of the family dynamics.

There are also problems in the handling of sessions when the designated patient is quietly psychotic. The less dramatic near-mute passivity which follows a period of overt disturbance in the psychotic patient always bothers the therapists more than the family; the parents are likely to be more diffident about the quietness than the "well" siblings, explaining their apparent unconcern with, "But she was always like this before she got sick." It is very difficult to prevent parents from settling for the premorbid non-person status of the patient, and since it is at this point that families frequently want to terminate therapy, the necessity of the patient's role as an incompetent in maintaining the economy of the family system is confirmed. We have found it important at these times to try to bring the quiet one into the discussion and to create dissatisfaction in the parents about their child's condition. Such efforts, however, do not always succeed because they threaten one of the essential cogs of the family system. Many of these parents feel adequate only if their child is inadequate; therefore one of the tasks of the therapists is to help raise the parents' self-esteem so that the inadequate child becomes dystonic to the system. It is sometimes very difficult, however, to want more for people than they want for themselves.

When the therapists sense that the balanced family arrangement is too tenuous to be dealt with, it is sometimes useful to spend the early phases of the family therapy doing individual therapy with the member who is hurting the most or who is most accessible. It is surprising how often someone other than the designated patient, usually the mother or father, presents himself for this purpose. Although this "individual" therapy takes place in the presence of other family members, the latter frequently benefit from it even though they may seem not to participate in it. Sometimes it is necessary to eliminate the pressing problems of one person or an alliance from the treatment scene before one can deal with the whole transactional system. For example, a family could not begin to examine a mother's non-existent relationship with her husband or her overinvolvement with her delinquent son until the mother was better able to understand that her real struggle was with her own mother.

Rather early in the treatment, the therapist may combine exploration with confrontation or low level interpretation, setting the stage for future family therapy and commenting on the essence of the family dynamics, saying, in effect, "These are the things we have to work on." As the therapists give their impression of the dynamics, some of the following hidden coalitions and family myths are exposed: lack of commitment to the marriage relationship, the deep attachment of the parents to the families of origin, how the symptoms or acting out of the designated patient are related to what is going on in the family, etc. When reality is brought into these forbidden areas the shock of disbelief, half-recognition, or fear appears on the faces of the various family members. Family secrets are often exposed, and it is interesting to note how often these secrets concern sex (illegitimate births, affairs, previous marriages, etc.). There may even be some work done with introjects during the early phases, but at this time the discussion is largely intellectual and only later are some of the emotional connections established. Much of the material uncovered in the early phases is repeated in the middle phases but with more detail and more emotional substance.

During the early phases especially, acting-out behavior outside the sessions and emergency problems are likely to appear, necessitating greater activity on the part of the therapists. The therapists frequently find it necessary to keep one foot in the reality problems and one in the fantasy system. There are times when flagrant misrepresentations, scapegoating, or exploitation of a victim need a controlling hand. For example, when one set of parents would argue vehemently and then turn to the two young children for the final decision as to who was right, the therapists stepped in to interpret their use of the children as parents and pointed out the consequences of their behavior. However, when one of the parents said to these same children. "We were all right until you kids came along," the therapists were angered at the gross unfairness of this statement. The handling of acting-out outside the sessions (e.g., sexual or delinquent behavior on the part of the adolescent who is intent on "saving" the family) is a broad topic which requires extended separate discussion.

It is difficult to generalize about the early phases of family therapy because of the wide differences among families, differences in the way problems are approached or presented, and variability in the styles of the therapists. But the preliminary stages of family therapy are largely characterized by the accommodations and adjustments which must be made between the family and the therapists, the harmonization of the co-therapy team, the jockeying for position as well as at least partial apprehension of the interlocking quality of the family pathology. There are many paths to these goals, and some families remain in these early phases for a long time without ever advancing into the real core of family therapy. Most succinctly, in the early phases the therapists are trying to break into the family system and the family is trying to keep them out. If the middle phases are reached, the therapists are *in* the family.

Middle Phases of Family Therapy

There are centers in the country who see a family for only several months, offering a family therapy program which does not go beyond what we would consider the preliminary phases of treatment. The real test and serious work of family therapy, in our judgment, resides in the laborious working through and building of trust in the therapists, a process which takes time. There are, to be sure, numerous difficulties which have to be overcome, some related to the nature of the family, some to the nature of the therapy team, and some to the unique quality of family therapy itself. What follows in this section is an attempt to deal with some of the problems which come up in these middle phases of family therapy, which comprise the heart of the process, as well as some of the techniques which have been developed for handling them.

The one overriding goal of these intensive middle phases, once the therapists are part of the family, consists in understanding and working through, often through transference to each other and to the therapists, the introjects of the parents so that the parents can see and experience how those difficulties manifested in the present family system have emerged from their unconscious attempts to perpetuate or master old conflicts arising from their families of origin. In general, the parents impose the same acts of unfairness and overburdening on their children that were once imposed on themselves. The parents in these families have each had their own grievous betrayals and shortchangings, and in order to make any real progress in family therapy they have to be led gently to remember and face them. It is a great deal to ask of any person to reopen old wounds and re-experience old guilts which have been shunted aside, discounted, ignored, or lived through with someone else. In an atmosphere of trust and reliance toward the therapists, established over a long period of time, this sometimes anguished self-exploration can take place. The essence of the true work of family therapy is in the tracing of the vicissitudes of early object-relationships, the varieties of human experience, and the exceedingly intricate transformations which occur as a function of the intrapsychic and transactional blending of the old and the new family systems of the parents, as well as the contribution of the children. The process is long and arduous with many levels; intense feelings are aroused, and progress is by no means in a straight line. When one person moves ahead the whole family equilibrium is disturbed and many painful adjustments have to be made; there may be frantic efforts to resume the status quo and re-establish old patterns. For example, after the wife has faced some of her anger toward a parent, she may no longer need to use her husband as a bad object of transference rage, but the husband may continue to "ask for it," even after complaining about it for years. Not many families can achieve this level in therapy, but when it is reached it is very impressive, and, unless it happens, we believe there can be no real hope of resolution of conflicts or meaningful change in the individuals or the family.

Once the early stages of blaming are past and questions directed toward the therapists are deflected back to the family, the members do try to interact with each other, and, as a general rule, the therapists attempt to expose the hidden feelings underlying the manifest interactions. There are families, however, who find it almost paralyzingly difficult to talk to each other in the presence of the therapists. These sessions begin with the therapists asking, "How are things going with the family?" (focusing on the family as a unit).

Father or mother reply, "Everything is all right." A long silence follows and one can sense the fear. Then one of the parents will turn to the designated patient with, "What have *you* got to say?" The patient, aware that any meaningful statement may incriminate her, will usually say, "Nothing." The therapists usually become more active at this point. Sometimes it isn't discovered until the end of the session that there has been a violent scene at home, or that between sessions a bitter, silent war was being waged at home. It usually takes a great deal of probing and pressure to find out what actually transpires at home between sessions. We have tried the technique of maintaining, along with the family, silences which last as long as half an hour, and everybody, including the therapists, finds these silences unbearable. We have occasionally fallen into the trap, through clever interpretations, of doing the thinking (and the "feeding") for the family by telling them what their problems are. In these middle phases of therapy the family members, because of the transference feelings which by then have been established, are usually less interested in exploring their difficulties than they are in sitting back and getting something from the therapists. This presents the therapists with the dilemma of whether to supply nourishment or to provide a free atmosphere of introspective inquiry. It is perhaps under these conditions of mixed therapeutic motivations that the therapists become more active and interpretive. It is now our conviction that those techniques which promote family interaction are the most productive in the long run.

A useful technique in therapy is to focus on the immediate situation, rather than get lost in abstract formulations, and specifically point out to the family those characteristic behaviors and mannerisms of which they are unaware (e.g., "Have you noticed, Mrs. Jones, that you complain about your husband's not talking enough but every time he tries to speak here you stop him from talking or you finish his sentences?" or, "You both keep nodding your heads in agreement with what we say, but I don't really think you're listening to the words," or, "Don't you think Suzie handles her skirts poorly, exposing her legs?" or, "Have you all noticed how often you all exchange with each other those secret smiles?"). These behaviors, when brought to the attention of the family, almost always precipitate embarrassment, denial, evasion, and rationalization. But sometimes they make an impression and the family begins to wonder about them. It is especially useful to concentrate on here-and-now feelings; this method usually penetrates much deeper than dealing with feelings described in retrospect. The technique is particularly useful with intellectualizing families who isolate affect. (e.g., "Mr. Jones, your daughter just told you to get out of the room, yet you smiled and ignored her statement and then got angry about something else").

Every family has its own unique practices, customs, and myths, which, because they have served the needs of the family system for a long time, seem logical, right, and comfortable to the family members, but to outside observers (in this case, the therapists) they may not only seem weird and incomprehensible but often bewildering and even outraging. Sometimes the family myth is some glaring injustice which has been isolated from everyone's awareness. For example, in one family the mother, instead of wearing her husband's wedding ring, wore the ring of a fiancé who had been dead for 30 years. One of the co-therapists, a female, astonished by this state of affairs, said, "This is crazy! Why do you stand for this, your wife wearing on her finger the ring of another man?" In another family it was revealed that the wife was the sole breadwinner, handled all the money, gave her husband an allowance, and had her husband sign the house over to her as sole owner because of his "incompetence." One of the male therapists turned to the husband and said, "For God's sake, why did you allow this to come about?" Sometimes the therapists are prompted to comment about some feeling which has been massively excluded from the family arena: "This whole family seems to be dead. Don't any of you ever have any fun?" The interjection of the therapists' feelings frequently helps as a powerful stimulant in opening up issues and areas which had long been closed and walled off by the family. There are other occasions when the therapists seem to step out of their roles as professionals and use themselves as real people. This maneuver occurs most often in response to the drastic violation of semantic meaning which some families present (Schaffer *et al.*, 1962), although it must be remembered that every therapist will find strange and disturbing things in every family, depending on how different they are from his own family experience. At such times we have tried the technique of admitting ignorance or perplexity as to what is going on; one therapist adopted a "playing dumb" attitude and kept pleading to the family that he didn't understand, saying "I'm lost; find me." The co-therapists may even interrupt the interaction, turn to each other as islands of reality in the room, discuss their confusion, and speculate about the meanings. Sarcasm and impatience may be used to make the family defenses more pliable; also reassurance, physical touching, sympathy, empathizing with the family all have their place. The therapists may also openly admit to having personal taboo feelings, which the family cannot express; they may admit, for example, to having had sexual or hostile feelings toward their own parents, siblings, or children.

Rarely does one observe overt seductiveness or direct sadism, or full expression of socially undesirable feelings in the sessions, not only because no family ever fully relinquishes its loyalty to the family code, but also because the approval of the therapists is greatly desired. The same person who says of a family member during the session, "I admire her courage and perseverence and wonderful personality" or "He's kind and tender and sweet and like a rock for me," has been quoted as saying in the privacy of the home, "I'll knock your teeth down your throat, you stupid bastard!" or "You're just a piece of shit." Goffman (1956) has beautifully illustrated how people present themselves to outsiders, in contrast with their behavior at home. After several years, as the family begins to feel that the therapists are really with them, there is a deepening of confidence and an increase in spontaneous behavior, but, of course, the degree of openness can only be conjectured.

As we gained experience in working with families we became less hesitant about taking more forceful, active positions in order to help the family become unshackled from their rigid patterns. Sometimes these procedures are used in the early phases. At times, we would insist that loud, disorganized families who jumped from one topic to another focus on one issue and discuss it in minute detail. On other occasions, especially with the more regressed families, we have found it useful to make certain demands calculated to cause a shift in the intrafamilial dynamics. For example, in one family the father had lived away from home for a number of years and the therapists insisted that he move back into the house; with several families, we have suggested that the parents, who had not done so for years, sleep together in the same bed; in another family situation we referred a father, long unemployed, for vocational training so that he could gain self-respect by working. In one family the parents never made a joint decision; decisions had always been made by a steamroller of a mother who felt she had to handle everything. The designated patient, an only child, had exploited this situation by driving a wedge between her parents and manipulating them against each other. The father made his futile protests, often complaining that he had no authority, and was envious of his daughter's capacity to exact favors from his wife by constant demands. At a certain point in the family therapy, the patient had been discharged and was sitting around the house being waited on by the mother; we insisted that the parents, then and there, jointly discuss and decide what daily chores the daughter should carry out. It was interesting to watch the anxiety build as all three family members repeatedly misinterpreted these simple instructions; the parents avoided discussion between themselves and kept addressing their statements to either the daughter or the therapists. Without proper timing, these active moves by the therapists may result in meaningless, ritualistic conformance.

Some of the therapeutic procedures utilized have been frankly experimental and occasionally accidental. On several occasions when one of the co-therapists could not attend a session another member of the staff would sit in in his place. We were surprised to note that when this happened the family would often adapt to the change with extreme docility and passivity, continuing their discussion from the week before as if nothing was different, not raising any objections, and frequently not even asking about the missing therapist. This type of reaction has made us wonder about the extent to which therapy is perceived by some families as a non-specific absorbing and feeding process wherein the therapists, whoever they may be, are faceless dispensers of nurturance. There have been instances when the therapist replacement, because he has not been so involved in the countertransference, has been able to "see" and deal with the family and co-therapist on new terms and with a new perspective, thereby helping to break up a long-standing logjam. The use of a visiting therapist has been a standard procedure at the Atlanta Psychiatric Clinic (Whitaker *et al.*, 1956) where a member of the staff is routinely invited to sit in on problem therapy situations as a consultant.

One procedure which has proven its worth is temporary work with family sub-systems. There are certain family systems with built-in sets of conditions which make it extremely difficult to work with the system as a whole. One such family situation is where divided loyalties are operating, for instance in a family where a man is torn between his wife and his mother and paralyzed in the presence of both. We have found it useful in situations of this type to approach the system at its weakest point by dealing with one segment of the total system. In the aforementioned family, after meeting for some time with the entire psychological system of father, mother, two children, and paternal grandmother, we learned that the father called his mother every day and confided in her, while at the same time his wife resented his lack of closeness to her but felt unable to verbalize her feelings because she, too, needed her husband's mother as a substitute for her own dead mother. When we met with just the father and his mother together we were able to make some inroads into the problem of their symbiotic relationship; for the first time in his life the father was able to get angry at his mother, especially when she uttered her familiar guilt-provoking statement, "Don't worry about me, I'm going off to an old ladies' home. Go back to that wife of yours." The work with sub-systems, of lesser or greater duration depending on the nature of the dynamics, must sooner or later be tied in with the larger picture. There is the possible handicap of creating anxiety and suspicion in the family members who are transitorily excluded, but this newly created anxiety itself may also be an avenue for the opening up of new areas.

There are a number of typical family problems which appear repeatedly. One of the most common results from the parents being so overwhelmed with their introjects that there is essentially no marriage and the children, for their own survival, are engaged in attempts to save their parents' marriage. Another common problem is when the mother identifies with the child and obtains fathering through the child and the father identifies with the child and obtains mothering through the child; then their complaints about their mates as *the* mother or father relate to themselves. One usual pattern is for the mother to be overinvolved with her own mother and, from this hostile-dependent alliance, the two women use the men as scapegoats, so that when a child gets psychiatrically ill it's because father "was not a father to the children." In such a situation the father has derived vicarious satisfaction from his wife's involvement with her family and frequently seeks the projected, scapegoated role. Some of the complexity of scapegoating as a transpersonal, rather than intrapsychic, phenomenon is better understood when it is observed in its family context. In one family the mother had strong feelings of unrecognized hostility toward her daughter who to her represented a hated sister. The mother constantly reminded her husband of the daughter's misbehavior, and the husband would punish the daughter by whipping her. Then, after the beating, the mother would comfort the daughter and, in the daughter's presence, would accuse the father of being brutal and lacking in understanding. Family therapy sessions dealt with the theme of father's "brutality," and the father, confused by the double bind, could only sputter helplessly and defensively about how his daughter's bad behavior deserved punishment. Father and daughter argued and mother, skillfully scapegoating her husband, remained in the background, concealing her role in the transaction by quiet and righteous comments. These situations are further complicated by the fact that every family member scapegoats every other family member behind camouflaging maneuvers. Sometimes the scapegoating involves a network of collusion with a dyad against a larger number (e.g., both parents unconsciously allied against the children's autonomy, by, perhaps, trying to turn the children against each other).

The dominating-aggressive mother and inadequate-passive father stereotypes have become part of the folklore of family psychiatry, and like all stereotypes there is a bit of substance to the over-simplifications. Our initial experiences with the mothers of this type led to considerable difficulty because we tried to meet them head-on. This type of woman projects all of her undesirable qualities onto the other members of the family or the therapists. She does not "hear" anything that does not agree with her own notions and she can be bafflingly infuriating. Interspersed between the servile flattery of the sycophant are belittling statements such as, "What psychiatric textbook did you get *that* out of?" and cutting, retaliatory enjoinders which raise the small hairs on the back of one's neck. These women have a vital need to engage in emotional in-fighting and a compelling talent for getting the therapists involved to the extend that much therapeutic time has been spent by the co-therapists in rescuing each other from the engulfment. In our early experience the co-therapists struggled to maintain tight control by working together, but in extended work with these women we learned to avoid noticing what they did and pay attention to what they missed in life. This procedure helped to slacken their defensiveness so that sooner or later there would emerge from behind the awesome pseudo-strength the deprived, frightened little girl who had always felt worthless and unloveable. When this step was reached the rest of the family reverberated to the change, initially with fear of loss of the powerful parent and later by having to make necessary accommodations.

Despite the frustration in dealing with the aggressive mother, however, we soon learned that the passive father presented a more formidable challenge. First of all, some degree of humiliation and admission of failure on the part of the father is contingent in coming for family therapy. And although the therapists make every conscious effort to build him up during the sessions, some double-binding is inherently operative when either the "sick" child is taken over by a therapist in concurrent individual therapy or when the father observes the therapists dealing with his wife in a way which he has never been able to. Inasmuch as some of the built-in procedures may reinforce the father's inadequacy, we have wondered whether the therapists unconsciously subsidize the powerful forces from wife, children, and the father himself which synchronize to maintain the system. An additional obstacle the therapists have faced is that sometimes it just doesn't seem cricket to question such a nice, reasonable guy. A number of techniques have been tried in dealing with these predicaments: forcing more interaction between the husband and wife; assigning tasks (e.g., insist that for a given period of time the father make the decisions at home, right or wrong, and that his wife give unquestioned support); having a female therapist give encouragement in a flattering way; occasional individual sessions with the father. Metaphorically speaking, we have not been as successful in giving the father a "penis" or getting him to use it as we have been in removing it from the mother. There are many dynamic bases for the adoption of passivity as a defense; in our experience one common one is that it serves the purpose of warding off murderous feelings. More accurately, however, we find greater success in dealing with the system aspects by focusing on the struggle for ego strength between the parents, how the mother and father represent dissociated aspects of each other, and how the children often help reinforce the internecine conflict.

In the exploration of the entire family system, the problems of the designated patient, the spark which precipitated the referral for family therapy, should not be ignored. It is necessary for the designated patient to accept her own share of responsibility for her behavior. One of the most instructive experiences for the family, however, occurs when they can recognize the connection between one of the designated patient's symptoms and a glossed-over family situation or long-avoided characteristic of one of the parents. One of the patients kept saying, "There's no sense in living when you can't talk to people." Her parents tried to reassure her that her ideas were foolish, that she *could* talk to people, etc. Afterwards we learned that in this family nobody talked to each other at home; the parents, in particular, never meaningfully discussed anything with each other. One father had been complaining for months about his son's stealing, accusing him of being a "loner," and holding himself up as a paragon of virtue; he finally sheepishly admitted that he used to steal and had never had any close friends. In their ramblings, psychotic patients frequently use the words "phony" and "counterfeit," referring not only to themselves but also to their parents. We have had to spend much time dealing with duplicitous behavior. One can tell that the family is making progress when the members become more honest about their feelings about themselves. The motives of the parents can usually be hidden behind conventional views which no one could dispute. The father who complained about his daughter's aimless wandering through the streets at night stated his realistic fear that something sexually dangerous could occur; yet he revealed another motive besides fatherly concern when he said, "As long as she does this sort of thing, there can be no real intercourse between us . . ." When their daughters date obviously undesirable men, parents feel justified in objecting and can safely conceal from themselves their wish to keep the daughter bound to the family and free from enduring heterosexual attachments. The patient, by going out with objectionable men, cooperates with the motives of her parents. Only when she begins to date eligible men in a realistic way can the reluctance of the parents to liberate her be unmasked.

Actually, when family therapy has really begun its effect, the problems of the designated patient, which used to be the exclusive preoccupation of the family, have long since receded into the background. Each of the parents has had the sobering experience of struggling with his own inner world, of having taken back some of his projections inside himself (a process usually followed by depression), of having had to re-examine his whole manner of existence and outlook on other people, and, especially, of having had to re-evaluate his feelings about his own parents or siblings. There are always mixed feelings about the process of decathecting from introjects. One father who badly needed to sustain the illusion that he was loved as a child brought in a picture of himself as a baby, sayings, "See me smiling there? I *must* have been happy then!" One mother burst forth with, "All right, my mother never gave me anything that counted and never appreciated anything I tried to do for her. What can I do about it now? What do you doctors want me to do, go to her grave and scream and curse at her?" The children are usually quite moved and sympathetic to their parents during these revelations; it is not uncommon to see them cluster around a mother or father and hug and kiss them as their parents cry over past hurts or disappointments. The designated patient or one of the "well" children may even develop symptoms or act out outside the sessions in order to save a parent from suffering. These later sessions are usually quiet, punctuated by sudden realizations, connections between the past and the present, and, occasionally, of turning to a mate or a child and really seeing him for the first time. Such revelations of the parents brings to them that curious combination often seen in those who have gained some true emotional insight: a new-found sense of relief, sometimes accompanied by omnipotent feelings as to their limitless possibilities as people, plus a sense of depression and regret over partial loss of the introjects and, in addition, some guilt over the way family members and other people have been "used." Sometimes the changes of the parents are evident in their increased interest in their appearance and in extrafamilial matters; we have even noticed marked changes in voice quality and other physical characteristics. The most important change which occurs, however, is the strengthening of the marital tie, a topic discussed in greater detail in the section on "Marriage Problems."

In family therapy as in all forms of therapy, there seems to be a great deal of wasted time, lost motion, and empty chit-chat before the few dramatic moments occur, when a meaningful connection is made, or an honest exchange of feeling is expressed. However, it is hard to tell when something internal is happening even though on the surface everything seems the same. The seemingly empty fill-ins may be necessary in order for the significant changes to take place. Personality change is very subtle. Sometimes even the therapists do not recognize the change in one of the family members or the family patterns; occasionally it takes the observation of some outsider, like another member of the therapy staff, to direct the therapists' attention to the change. There are many levels on which change can take place. Frequent regression to old patterns occurs, sometimes precipitated by real change in one member, sometimes by separation anxiety when the therapists go on vacation or talk about future termination.

As the families begin to consider the idea that they *can* change their feelings about each other they will become more unguarded, and their behavior in the treatment setting will more closely approximate that which may occur at the dinner table when, for example, they have an argument. In fact, some families will unwittingly exaggerate their feelings in order to provoke more interest from the therapists. It must be remembered, though, that the motivation for change in most families is dissociated. At the deepest level they continue to attend sessions in order to get the therapists' assistance in restoring things back to how they used to be. During the course of the therapy they become more dependent on and involved with the therapists, and when positive change takes place it occurs almost despite themselves.

We have been describing thus far the kinds of families who make the most effective use of family therapy by achieving the ability to open up, to relate, to reflect, and to change. There are other families, of course, who are unable to use the structure of family therapy as a means of growth. These families frequently require constant transfusions in the form of more explicit parental-like roles taken on by the therapists and even by bringing into the sessions extended family members or significant peripheral persons who could contribute added strength to the main family. These are the families who provoked some of the more active and experimental techniques described earlier; they seem to need concrete action rather than words. We have realized with some of these families that they cannot be forced to change; you sort of have to go along with them.

What has been called in this section the middle phases of family therapy may be a misnomer since there is insufficient knowledge of the therapy process to be able to delineate regular phases or whether a particular aspect belongs in one phase or another. Although the problems of resistance, marriage, the "well" sibling, transference/countertransference, and co-therapy team relationship are here included as sub-sections of the middle phases, they will make their effect known at any stage in the therapy process.

RESISTANCE IN FAMILY THERAPY

Resistance, the opposition against attempts to expose unconscious motives, can assume many different guises in all forms of psychotherapy. Sometimes even professional therapists slip into thinking of resistance as contrariness or stubbornness because the blindness of people toward recognizing what they are doing may seem like obstinacy. Conscious resistance (e.g., fear of rejection, shame, distrust of the therapist) creates particular therapeutic problems, but unconscious resistance, which is dealt with most carefully in classical psychoanalysis and is at the root of all conscious resistances, is far more complicated, not only because the unconscious of the therapist can dovetail with that of the patient, but also because anything can be used in the service of unconscious resistance (e.g., silence or too much talking, lack of affect or too much affect, acting out or inability to act, etc.). These, then, are the intrapsychic resistances of individuals which operate within the relatively non-threatening setting of one-to-one psychotherapy.

Different kinds of resistances come into play in traditional group therapy, largely as a function of the defenses of the individual in the group situation (Varon, 1958) as well as the nature of the group resistance itself (Redl, 1948). The individual in the group situation not only has to protect himself from knowing certain aspects of himself, but he has to conceal his deeper motives from others while at the same time he is attempting to adjust and accommodate to other members of the group. Here we have one of the key differences between group and family therapy (Handlon and Parloff, 1962). The family comes to therapy with a long history of fit, private understandings, highly predictable responses, and deep feeling for each other; group dissolution at the end of treatment is highly unlikely. In group therapy the culture is created *de novo*, and the members do not expect real satisfaction of needs from each other. Family therapy and group therapy both provide the opportunity for the members to master in a socially real situation the types of near-refractory experiences which produced the particular kinds of pathologic defenses in the first place—group therapy by providing sibling and parental surrogates and family therapy by the presence of the original figures. However, because of the unique quality of the family group and the special bonds of relationship and familiarity, both conscious and unconscious resistances have a distinctive quality and life all their own in family therapy and operate *in addition* to the familiar ones seen in individual and group therapy. It is selected aspects of these latter endemic transactional and system defenses which this section describes.

Once we felt in our early years of operation that we had made important discoveries about the validity of the transactional and shared psychopathology viewpoint in diagnosing what was going on in the family which eventuated in overt disturbance in one member, we optimistically believed that all we had to do was bring the members of the family together regularly, utilize our knowledge of psychotherapy, and we would then be in a position to alter the total structure in a therapeutic way. This kind of naïveté about the enormous complexity involved in bringing about change in people probably accompanies the development of every new psychotherapy approach. At any rate, our therapy teams not only ran into types of resistances which were unlike any previously encountered in prior experience with individual and group therapy, but occasionally the therapy teams were surprised and disappointed when they began to realize the formidability of the therapy task before them. For example, they learned that a massive resistance phase is encountered with every family once the preliminaries are out of the way; although this phase should have been expected, in our early experience it still came as a shock. One therapy team said at that time, "I can't understand it; the family was working so well, we were really getting somewhere, and now suddenly they don't want to come in anymore." We learned two lessons from this experience: (1) to be wary when things seem to be going too well in therapy, and (2) that families will manipulate when they sense that the therapists want them too much, just as they will respond by withdrawal when they feel that the therapists do not like them. Families can evoke feelings of jealousy and possessiveness in therapists much more powerfully than can individual patients.

There are some people who start family therapy with great enthusiasm because they have a strategy in mind, and when the therapists do not fit in with their strategy they are quickly de-motivated. One mother, who had abandoned her children for many years after the break-up of her first marriage, remarried and then tried to make a home for her children. This second husband was seen by her and the children as a monster who was strict and arbitrary. The mother persuaded her reluctant husband to attend the initial evaulation session and was hoping to get her children and the therapists to see what a bad man he was. As the therapists saw the situation, however, this man was a better parent to her children than she was; his so-called strictness showed genuine care for the welfare of the children. Her strategy became more clear: to use her husband as scapegoat and convince everyone that she had not abandoned and rejected her children. By the end of the initial evaluation session, the mother did not want to continue family therapy and her initially reluctant husband was pushing for it.

The massive resistance phase usually follows when the immediate crisis presented by the designated patient is past and the family system is not hurting so much. There then ensues a "don't rock the boat" attitude. The resistance makes its appearance innocently enough when the family spokesman (usually the father, urged to speak by the mother) requests that they come in every other week instead of every week. Or there may be complaints from the children about missing school. In their early experience with families the family therapists used to meet the resistances head-on, engaged in controversy, and even attempted to persuade families to continue, citing reality reasons (e.g., "Now which is really more important—that the family continue with this sick kind of living or that Johnny misses his class in English?"). There was something about the quality of family therapy and the anxiety aroused which subtly provoked therapists to by-pass their usual precautions in working through resistances and making confrontations palatable. These early kinds of activities caused such narcissistic pains that the families often terminated the therapy. At any rate, by using the security of the co-therapy team relationship we learned to deal with the fears of loss and all the other unconscious reasons which lay behind the resistance. As in all matters of technique, more depends on *how* something is said rather than on *what* is said.

Resistances in family therapy can assume many different shapes and forms, and in the final analysis it may become a question of whether the therapists can tolerate them over a long period of time. One type of resistance that is particularly frustrating is a kind of passive mastery practiced by the family whereby they come in week after week, produce little or no material, and do not relate their feelings. After making valiant efforts to stimulate and get the family to move, the therapists frequently end up feeling useless and wiped out as people.

Another test of the therapists' tolerance occurs after many months of treatment when the families seem to go round and round, fixated in an immovable rut with each other, recognizing that much distress is created but being unable to do anything except repeat the same pattern over and over, even though they say they want something different. When it is interpreted that they must want it this way, that everything they do perpetuates the situation, and that essential needs are being filled through this manner of torturous relating, they always deny it. We have speculated that perhaps, given the inner and outer circumstances, this is the best that the family can do, that perhaps they are settling for what they have rather than what they really want because they view the alternative as an even greater danger (e.g., abandonment). Many problems are encountered in the process of resolving such massive resistances. Occasionally interruptions or hiatuses in treatment, whether planned or accidental, have often helped a family to surmount these seemingly endless repetition compulsions.

Whether or not treatment sessions should be held without all specified family members being present is one issue on which there seems to be some division among family therapists. Sonne, Speck and Jungreis (1962) first pointed out the absent member maneuver as a major resistance in family therapy. They suggested that one member of the family would absent himself from the therapy sessions in order to preserve fixed paired relationship patterns in the family, and that this maneuver, entailing the cooperation of the whole family, occurs in order to avoid the anxiety of a triangular heterosexual growth experience. The maneuver is generally handled by insisting on the presence of the absent member. Another point of view, set forth primarily by Bowen (see ch. 5) is that the family approach can still be utilized by seeing the family members in any combination. Bowen maintains that there are occasions when the therapist can, at certain stages in the treatment process, see one family member in family therapy and that this procedure is not individual psychotherapy because the raising of the level of differentiation of one member is oriented toward serving a therapeutic need for the entire family. The contradictions between these two viewpoints may be only superficial since they both stem from increasing recognition of the way family system resistances operate. When it is the therapists, rather than the family, who control the situation and decide who should be included, many resistances can be anticipated and managed. Further understanding will be needed before family therapists can decide with a particular family when to approach the family system through one member or a pair, or when to insist that all members be present at all times.

Several other controversial issues have confronted family therapists: whether or not children should be present when parents discuss their sexual relationship; or how old children should be before they are to be included in the treatment sessions. These decisions should be decided on the basis of a particular family's level of integration and dynamics. In general, in families where the children have al-

RATIONALE AND TECHNIQUES

ready been overexposed to sexual talk or behavior between parents, we have tended to have children present, largely in order to help clear up distortions in their minds. Some therapists are more reluctant to follow this procedure and are more convinced that children should be protected from this aspect of the adult world. Also some family therapists can work comfortably with pre-school children present during the sessions, whereas most would prefer including only children of at least six or seven.

Resistance in essence revolves around the question of change inasmuch as the unavoidable, powerful forces which protest and try to maintain the pathologic arrangements are most operative when the therapy begins to deal with conflictual areas which, if fully faced and resolved, could result in growth and change. Searles, in a very penetrating report (1961), has written about some of the reasons why individual schizophrenic patients are so afraid and unable to change (many of his concepts could be applied also to neurotic patients and character disorders in psychotherapy and analysis). Families, too, conceive of change in terms of deprivation rather than enhancement, and, at the deepest level, they fear change in the family system which will result in loss of some vitally needed form of relationship, even if the relationship has its hurting aspects. Family members are threatened to the core of their beings by the prospect of having to abandon infantile needs provided by or hoped for from other family members, and they will jointly resist efforts to reveal these motivations, much less give them up. It is the theory of psychoanalytic treatment that when infantile needs are frustrated (unconditional love, sympathy, indulgence, total acceptance, comfort, fondling, nursing, etc.), the analytic patient reaches the turning point of renouncing them in their literal, infantile form and can seek gratification of these needs in more mature and realistic ways (Menninger, 1958). The much deprived members of the families we have seen, however, seem to need to pursue gratification of their infantile needs in a very real sense and have great difficulty renouncing any of them, despite the fact that they are chronically frustrated. Each family member participates in the resistance, moreover, for each member has an investment in a role which serves a system function and maintains family homeostatic balance. Efforts made by dissatisfied members to change the system have had the paradoxical effect of perpetuating the system.

There are, of course, many other reasons for resistance to change other than the inability to abandon infantile needs, which we consider the most fundamental. Although on one level each member of the family recognizes the necessity for changes in someone else in the family, rather than in himself, on another level each member unconsciously suggests that he would feel a burden of guilt if he himself changed. For example, the designated patient signals trouble in the family by developing symptoms or acting out; then, once family therapy is undertaken and the parents get upset, the designated patient begins to feel guilty over disturbing the parents and then makes efforts to terminate the therapy. (One wonders, in this connection, how many individual psychotherapies and analyses have failed because the patient would rather keep his particular symptoms than to feel guilty over maturing and making someone else suffer in the process.) When we see parents blocking each other's therapeutic explorations we know that they fear that if their mate matures they themselves will be seen as they feel they really are (unlovable, childish, hateful, etc.) and, therefore, they will lose them. It is very difficult for people to realize that ultimately they can only change for themselves.

Sources of resistance are complex and varied: parents' use of the sessions to report on the designated patient's crazy behavior; avoidance of discussion of the marriage relationship; exaggeration of the therapists' comments to the point of absurdity; motivation for family therapy expressed in order to screen and deflect from intrapsychic exploration; particularly strong injunctions against family disloyalty; family members' "protection" of each other; intense feelings of family honor and position; reciprocal scapegoating. Other sources of resistance are based on countertransference factors such as fathers who are important members of the community; "well" siblings who have managed to free themselves to some extent from the family embroilments; social standards about the sanctity of the family; sweet, grey-haired mothers; the fragility of some families (e.g., those in which there has been a great deal of trauma); wide cultural differences between the family and the therapists. These are all examples of resistance factors which can operate, sometimes very subtly, to thwart exploration and change. There are occasions when the therapists learn relatively late in the therapy process about some very significant peripheral person (friend, neighbor, extended relative, lawyer, doctor, religious advisor) who exerts a great influence on the family but whose existence is concealed. This special relationship can act as a strong resistance and it is advisable to invite such a person to the sessions. Resistances are always a function of an intricate interplay between variables in the family and variables in the therapists (e.g., conflicts in a single therapist or between the co-therapists). As Carl Whitaker once remarked, is there really resistance or is there something in the therapist which prevents exploration?

MARRIAGE PROBLEMS IN FAMILY THERAPY

As we acquired experience working with families, one functional goal of family therapy gradually evolved: to separate the generational differences which had been breached extravagantly and emphasize that parents are parents and children are children. We soon discovered that this goal cannot be approached until the parents begin to meet each other's needs. Our implicit set of values may, as anthropologists have pointed out, be an anomaly of Western society; apparently, there are parts of the world where parents are not expected to raise children alone or to fill all their important needs in each other. We would agree with Bell (1962), moreover, that the family should not be viewed as a "self-contained unit existing in a social and cultural vacuum" and that one should not neglect the extended family and surrounding society network as the framework within which the family develops. From a practical clinical viewpoint, however, our approach of strengthening the marriage has paid off the greatest dividend in terms of freeing the children to have lives of their own. The impact of extended family relations and the wider community, in terms of what they mean to a particular family and how they are used, is an inherent part of our daily therapeutic work.

Attempting to create a marital bond where there has never been a husband-wife arrangement, however, is no small task. Before recounting our experiences in handling marriage problems in family therapy, some theoretical considerations about marriage will be discussed. It has been said, with some justification, that the greatest happiness which can be achieved in life emerges as a by-product of a "good" marriage and, conversely, that an incredibly varied range of human misery can result from a "bad" marriage, ranging from legal divorce, emotional divorce, perpetual bickering, destructive acting out, psychosomatic and psychological disorders, and their pernicious effects on children, society, and the human spirit. Another truism is that the greatest gift which parents can bestow on children is to give them the security of two parents who love each other.

It is very difficult to determine, nonetheless, what constitutes a happy or even a workable marriage. The writer, while preparing this chapter, looked over a number of books on marriage and was surprised to discover the number of contradictory statements made by equally experienced professionals in this area. It has been said by some that no one ever cured himself of a neurosis by marrying and that the neurotic problems of the two marriage partners are cumulative; on the other hand, others say that a marriage by virtue of its being unhappy can mask or prevent the emergence of a neurosis, or that the marriage relationship may embody compensatory mechanisms for seriously disturbed partners. One group of investigators maintain that the personality is fairly well fixed by the time a person marries and that marriage partners are doomed to disappointment in their eternal efforts to change the personalities of their mates; other practitioners say that marriage partners can help each other to grow and mature.

These contradictions are probably not as incongruous as one may suppose when some of the intricate complexities involved in marriage relationship are examined more deeply. One could start with Kubie's chapter in what is probably one of the best publications in the marriage field, *Neurotic Interaction in Marriage* (1956, ch. 2). After stating his initial point that there are neurotic ingredients in every human personality, and, consequently, in every marriage, Kubie goes on to present his major thesis that the main source of unhappiness between husband and wife is found in the discrepancies between their conscious and unconscious demands on each other and on the marriage, as expressed first in the choice of a mate and then in the subsequent evolution of their relationship. Congruent with this thesis, Kubie describes how unconscious forces derived from the family of origin and based on the need to "wipe out old pains or pay off an old score," can create profound marital discord and estrangement, particularly when the partners can be so misled by the illusory romantic tradition. One finds, then, that individuals unconsciously seek parents instead of spouses, that they marry those with whom they can prove or correct something about themselves, those with whom they can duplicate or master an old conflictual relationship, etc. Since the unconscious demands cannot be met without conflicting with reality and conscious considerations, lack of marital integration is the rule rather than the exception. The foregoing helps explain why martial prediction studies, which rely on conscious report, are so limited, why the pre-marriage courtship relationship is no predictor of marital happiness, why agents which may help one marriage relationship may serve to destroy another, why hasty marriages can be as successful as those made with serious foresight, why reading marriage manuals or books on sex instruction can make matters worse, and that, as Kubie says, a happy marriage may be a happy accident.

The preceding considerations represent insights into the dynamic aspects of marriage difficulties which orthodox psychoanalytic thinking has given us. Although this thinking does stress the importance of unconscious motivation and there is some recognition of complementary patterns, it remains essentially an individually-oriented emphasis. What is not taken into account is the interlocking collusion which occurs on an unconscious level, a bilateral reciprocity which has only been discerned through exploration of the transactional operations between people. When the interacting relationship of a couple has been studied as the partners were treated together as a dyadic unit (Whitaker, 1958; Haley, 1963), the fit of the contours of their internal object relationships was observed for the first time, no matter how other factors served to obscure the unconscious mutuality. In order to clarify the implications of this finding, it is necessary to discuss some of the dynamics of mate selection.

Whenever professionals in the marriage field have wanted to point to one factor as being responsible for marital difficulties, romantic love has been cited as the culprit. Kubie, for example, defines "being in love" as "an obsessional state driven in part by anger." Still, romantic love as a psychic reality must be reckoned with since, in our culture at least, it is a powerful tradition reinforced by advertising, popular songs, movies, plays, and novels. (One can cite such fine British films as *Brief Encounter* and *Room at the Top* and such contemporary American plays as Chayevsky's *Middle of the Night* and *Marty* which portray how profound the effects of sentimental love can be for even the unlikeliest matches. As one character put it, "Why should I give this up? When I feel like this there aren't enough hours in the day!") The process whereby a woman and man become attracted to each other and fall in love is an intricate almost magical one. In order to achieve that subjective, inspirational, pleasurable-painful state of "being in love," an extremely complex and subtle blending of conscious and unconscious conditions must be met: the loved one must have a certain combination of physical characteristics associated with sexual appeal, and certain mannerisms, style of relating, quality of affect, etc., which will stimulate the re-creation of the childhood, idealized family romance with all its promise of unconditional love; at the same time the prospective mate must be enough like the bad inner object to allow for eventual penetration of old hatreds. The ego may say: "I want to marry a man who will be strong but gentle, who can make me feel like a woman, who will be dependable, who will be successful, who will be faithful, who will control but not dominate me, who will make a good father for my children, who will be easy going." The unconscious may seek "a man who can *almost* love, who lies or cheats or drinks, who is undependable, who will make a good father for *me*, who will keep me guessing, who will be unsuccessful, who will be weak and helpless, whom *I* can control, who will be difficult to get along with, who will be detached." The forthcoming marriage promises to make everything right that has always been wrong, and part of the function of the romantic ritual of courtship is to deny recognition of the bad object in the partner which will provide confirmation for the inner role model. The unconscious confirmation and dovetailing, moreover, is a two-way process; each partner has had his signal from his emotional radar system which recognizes the other as closely fitting the internal object needs. During the courtship and honeymoon period each partner, for the first time in his life, accepts the other and feels accepted for what he is, with all his different selves, all the residual part objects; the two merge into a satisfying oneness; the couple are "in love." It is no wonder that at times of stress during a long-lasting marriage the partners will try to recapture the feelings of the courtship and honeymoon period, the time when they felt united and fulfilled, each by the other.

Gradually, however, a spouse begins to feel that rather than having his real personality confirmed he is being trained to conform to and behave like the mate's projected internal image; at the same time he is unwittingly doing this to his partner. Each spouse begins to maneuver the other, unconsciously, into fitting the mold of the despised, exciting inner imago. The more the partners behave like the anticipated bad internal object, which is compounded of real, sometimes partially disowned traits of one's own plus the unreal projections of the mate, the greater the likelihood that a new kind of confirmation will take place, one that has been unconsciously sought and consciously dreaded. Each partner will begin to sense vaguely that some old ghost has risen to haunt him. This is the reason why spouses' complaints of each other, while containing some irrational elements, may be quite justified; the mate can give numerous instances of their validity ("She is not affectionate," "He nags," "I can't count on her," "He runs around with other women," "She doesn't really know me," "He is no longer passionate," "She is too jealous," "He is untidy," "She puts everyone before me," "He never listens to me," "She can't love," "He doesn't really care for me," "She's too bossy"). What is not recognized by the complainers is that this is what they "asked for." When disillusionment sets in, as it does in all marriages in some form ("You're not what I thought you were") the individual "remembers" the faults disregarded during courtship, feels betrayed, and then transfers to the spouse the reactivated hatred originally felt toward the split-off bad object of childhood. The disappointment occurs most frequently in the early part of marriage as the partners test each other out with their infantile ambivalencies, which is why so many divorces occur in the early years of marriage. (The problems of legal divorce, multiple marriages, and inability to separate are probably different aspects of the same dynamic.) The crises of disconfirmation may occur later, however, during crucial check-points and stages of the marriage: the arrival of children, economic insecurity, involvements with in-laws, acting out by one or both partners, the separation of the children from the parents, retirement, etc. The greatest test of emotional maturity is the ability to make the exceedingly complex adjustment to another person in marriage, to tolerate in each other the working through of hated, ambivalent internal objects, and to permit each other's regression, all of which infantile strivings are embedded in the context of bonds of affection, the process of give and get, the acceptance of adult responsibility, and the overflow of love to the children. Feelings of outrage and frustration will be greatest in those couples whose own parents could not resolve the universal marriage struggle and who were themselves subject to deprivation, resulting in low self-esteem, a weak sense of identity, and a polarization of their love-hate conflict. These partners have even higher expectations of marriage, and they feel even more keenly a sense of treachery and having been cheated.

In the more chronic, prolonged kind of marital disharmony situation that we see in family therapy, the "can't-live-with, can't-live-without" syndrome is the most common. Dicks (1964), some of whose thought is represented in the prior statements and whose concept of the "shared internal object" as a bond between marriage partners is very intriguing, has made the following incisive statement on the question as to why unhappy couples stay together: " . . . social values and duty to the children apart, there is a need in each partner to wring out of the other the response that signifies to the unconscious the typical interaction model with the internal object or objects which have come to be vested in the marital relationship" (p. 269). When these kinds of marriages persist through many years the mates are caught up in a relentless open or silent warfare, obtaining their gratification by using each other or the children almost purely as bad internal object representations. The real personalities of the family members have long ceased to exist, and we witness a marriage characterized by absence of sexual relations and the partners' almost exclusive use of each other as child or parent, far beyond the occasional alternation of roles seen in all marriages. One system aspect of the marriage problem is that the roles of each of the children can reflect the partners' ambivalence about their marriage, one child often representing the good and one the evil. Or, the children may be ignored, punished, or become the battleground of an unhappy marriage.

Clinical counterparts of the previous theoretical notions are seen in our work with couples during the course of family therapy. With the goal of "remarrying" the parents, we attempt to explore the relevant motivational formulae in each partner, help them come to terms with their introjects, and explicate the interlocking nature of the meaning of their marital bond. There is considerable diversity in the capacity of couples to work along these lines, as well as variability as to the stage of family therapy in which the marriage relationship can be approached. Many couples are very fearful of having their marriage relationship explored and use the problems of the children as dilatory tactics to ward off exploration of themselves. Sometimes we have found it useful in these situations to make a direct confrontation of the unspoken horror: "How long have you both felt that this marriage hasn't really existed?" After exploration we usually find that these couples have long ago abandoned honesty in their relationship. Early in the marriage attempts had been made to relate real feelings to each other, but these talk sessions ended in great frustration because neither could get the other to see his point of view. Communication had become impossible because each was using the language of his own background where words of love, closeness, jealousy, intimacy, and aggression had different meanings. The partners then arrived at a *modus vivendi* whereby they wrote each other off and played a role by not letting the other know their real feelings. By mutual unspoken consent their problems with each other no longer existed, although they could be quite concerned about problems in the children. As these marriages are probed by the therapists, their implicit contract of "I won't tell on you if you won't tell on me" (Carroll, 1960) can be violently ruptured. The mate who breaches the contract and begins to "tell" can expect a vitriolic counterattack, such as, "Okay, brother, if that's how you're going to play, now watch me!"

Other couples' marriage difficulties are in the open from the first session, as each partner pours forth upon the other a welter of grievances and bitter recriminations. They turn to each other with accusations and counter-accusations as they recount obsolete injuries, blame each other's families and ancestors, using the therapy sessions to gain allies for their cause. Curiously, though, a dispute of this sort may suddenly cease and the parents will point toward the designated patient as the real problem in the family; their controversies with each other appear to them to be extrinsic and isolated from the problems presented by the designated patient. At times they give the impression that they're relieved to have their child's illness to contend with so that they won't have to face fully their despairing, terrifying, and potentially murderous feelings toward each other.

Although in both types of marital discord problems—the silent and the open—there are threats of divorce, the real possibility of separation or divorce is almost non-existent; in the unconscious separation means psychic death. When the therapists wonder, in view of so much obvious discontent, whether they have thought of leaving each other, a partner may say, "He does this and that cruel thing to me, but deep down I know he loves me." The variety of meanings given to the word "love" is legion. Note the universality of the statement: "I love you so much I wish I liked you." Or take the following interchange: *He:* "I wish you could be as kind to me as you are to strangers." *She:* "But I'm not in love with *them!*" For some people, sad to say, it is true that, in the words of the popular song, "You always hurt the one you love." Of course, the children *must* feel their parents love each other because if they don't there is no love in this world and what hope would exist for them? While it can be said that love which is never demonstrated becomes an abstraction with no content, on another level deep attachment can be revealed during extreme emergencies or loss, for example through death, as witness the depression in a sado-masochistic partner when his mate dies. A man and woman who have touched each other, had sexual intercourse and children together, argued, smelled each other, and shared experiences and reminiscences together do become a part of each other. When there has been intense emotional investment in each other, people can only separate savagely. Note, for example, the vituperation and acrimony which surrounds divorce proceedings; the bitter quality of the exchanges shocks even experienced lawyers (Nizer, 1961, ch. 2).

In many marriage situations one of the partners acts out in some gross fashion (e.g., alcoholism, unfaithfulness), and we often learn how the objecting partner's needs are being served by the acting out. Very frequently, the partner who brings the erring mate to treatment ends up being the more seriously disturbed member. There is an old saying, "Be careful about what you say you want very much; you may get it," or, in converse form, "Be careful about what you say you don't want; you may lose it." We have seen spouses begin to change in the direction demanded by their mates, only to find the fulfillment of their wishes followed by severe disturbance. And we have seen "objectionable" behavior cease in one mate, followed by acute anxiety in the other over its absence.

As we work with the parents' past life, their deprivations and confusions, how they misused and were misused by their own parents, how they have misused their marriage partners, and how their pathology interlocks, they frequently develop a more empathic understanding of each other and thereby increase their capacities of giving to each other. There is a level of communication between husband and wife which is unobservable even by trained therapists; the medium of exchange is subliminal and may not be detected during the sessions because it occurs when they are alone with each other. In other words, improvement in the marriage may be seen only by its side-effects; for example, the parents may still argue, but the children are less involved in the arguments.

Does family therapy, however, end up being couple psychotherapy conducted in the presence of the children? Why have the children present at all? Is it possible that the therapists are subsidizing the family pathology by implicitly or explicitly calling on the assistance of the children in "marrying" their parents, thereby again parentifying the children? We have found the presence of the children helpful because when the therapists assume the responsibility for bringing the parents together, the children can be children again. If the therapists do not bring this union about, the children feel that they have to; the children have been trying unsuccessfully for years and the therapists help free them from the healing task. As my colleague Oscar Weiner says, what the therapists are doing, essentially, is kicking the children out of the parents' bed. Sometimes the designated patient or one of the other children will develop symptoms during this process because they are losing the familiar, cherished but ego-disruptive role. Children also get upset when they see their parents suffer over past hurts, but in the long run it is comforting; they have always sensed unhappiness in their parents, but they didn't know why. As the uncertainty becomes more understandable, the parents seem more real; the ultimate in the relationship with parents, as Oscar Wilde put it, is when you come to forgive them.

THE "WELL" SIBLING IN FAMILY THERAPY

The chief questions, raised by both professionals *and* the family, against the concept of interrelated pathology in the family and against the view of parental contribution to the illness of the designated patient are: "If the parents are to blame and it's the family atmosphere that is responsible, why aren't the other children in the family sick? How can children from the same family be so different?"

Several investigators have attempted to answer these questions by interviewing patients, siblings, and parents, but unfortunately these studies were restricted to the one syndrome of schizophrenia and were, with one exception, based on separate interviews rather than observation of family interaction. Yi-chuang Lu (1961) found that schizophrenic patients had concentrated all emotional investments in their parents, especially in mothers, whereas the normal siblings had wider emotional investments and avoided either a strong attachment or repulsion toward the mother. Prout and White (1956), utilizing separate interviews with schizophrenic patients, their siblings, and their mothers, concluded that the schizophrenic patient had been different from his siblings since infancy; they maintained, *on the basis of reported recollections*, that the patients had been more sensitive, unhappy, and less social than their healthier siblings. They further suggested that since the pre-schizophrenic child was so dependent and needed such an unusual degree of support and attention, the mother's overprotection was invited; the mother was merely meeting the needs of a weak child. The shortcomings of these studies are fairly obvious; they accept the statements of family members at face value, exclude fathers, and are oblivious to family interaction and system factors. A far more sophisticated approach was undertaken by Lidz *et al.* (1963) who utilized repeated intensive interviewing, home visits, projective testing, the reports of friends and teachers, and observation of family interaction of sixteen families. The problem of the differential effects of the family on siblings was examined by these comprehensive methods with the following considerations: the effects of changing family circumstances, the mother's capacity to provide nurturing care during the patient's infancy, the child's role in the family dynamics, the sibling's gender, idiosyncratic problems in the parents' relationship to the schizophrenic offspring, and the interaction between siblings. They found, first of all, that the so-called "well" siblings were not so well when studied carefully. As many siblings were psychotic as were reasonably well integrated, and all except five or six of the twenty-four siblings had serious personality disorders. Those siblings who had made a good adjustment did so by the defensive maneuvers of constriction and flight from the family. They found that in half of the families the patient was raised under conditions quite different from those under which the siblings were brought up; the family circumstances were so deviant in several cases that the patient seemed to have been born into a different family than the one into which the siblings were born. Moreover, a child of one sex may be more vulnerable within a given family than a child of the opposite sex. They found, further, that the child who becomes schizophrenic often lessens the impact of the parental pathology upon the siblings by serving as a target of the parents' intrusiveness, as a scapegoat, or as an example for the siblings to avoid. By identifying some of the dynamic elements which are involved in the differentiative forces which operate on children in the same family, Lidz *et al.* have advanced knowledge considerably in this area. However, although it involved some observation of family interaction, their work could not explicate the deeper levels of learning which can be revealed in extended family therapy.

Before relating our experiences with "well" siblings in family therapy, a few thoughts about the relatively neglected area of the sibling world are appropriate. Important learning and emotional experiences take place among children in the same family. Siblings learn to test strong love and hate feelings toward each other which are too dangerous to express toward parents because of the stakes involved and because a brother and sister cannot do much to you in any lasting way; the siblings know who stands where with what parent and they learn how to win, lose, or draw. When children play together they learn how to have fun; they see each other receive punishment or favorite treatment and have to deal with the resultant guilt or envy; when siblings quarrel they learn how to deal with their conflicts, and when parents quarrel the children can vent their frustrations on someone only slightly weaker or stronger. The siblings protect each other against parents or any extrafamilial threat; they can find an ally of like size in times of crisis; they master the skill of getting along with someone they don't always like; they struggle with the conflict between sharing and wanting everything. The sibling world, in brief, is a powerful family sub-system with a culture all its own. Excluding this sector of the family from treatment would result in an incomplete picture.

Inherited random variation of the genes has always been assumed to be the basis of personality differences among siblings, and it was not until the advent of the family concept that other factors began to be more fully appreciated. For example, role inculcation can contribute diversified personalities in the children which serve family system needs. Wynne *et al.* (1957) have reported on a set of monyzygotic quadruplets whose roles within the family social organization accounted for differences in personality development and variability in the forms which their schizophrenic illnesses took. The various children in the family come to represent valued or feared expectations of the parents, based on the parental introjects; sometimes roles of the children are chosen for them even before they are born (e.g., the child who is conceived to "save the marriage"). Sometimes one child can represent the super-ego of the family and one the id. In every family of multiple siblings there is "the spoiled one," "the studious one," "the conscience of the family," and "the wild one;" the assigned roles are infinite. The "well" siblings frequently fill in gaps in the family and act as more successful interpreters between the parents than does the designated patient and are often highly valued for this purpose. Certain kinds of impulses (e.g., sexual or hostile) are considered to be pe-

culiar to particular children in the family; these children are sometimes seen in these fixed ways even when their basic nature presents
evidence to the contrary. Every therapist is familiar with the mother
or father who continually anticipates that the girl is going to "get
in trouble with boys," so much so that daughter finally "cooperates"
by getting in trouble with boys. Roles can be so fixed in a family
that when role exchange takes place between two siblings the family
may perceive the change as tantamount to psychosis in one or both
children; Ryckoff et al. (1959) have illustrated how "good" and
"bad" daughters acted out conscious and unconscious pressures
from their parents by exchanging roles, an exchange which precipitated violent upheavals in the family. It is not uncommon to see
in the family of the schizophrenic one rebellious child who acts
out a destructive role complementary to the patient's over-conform-
ity; the same core conflict can exist in both patient and sibling
but may be handled oppositely.

The aforementioned considerations partially account for several
striking phenomena which we have observed during the course of
family therapy. Those "well" siblings who managed to adjust by
not dealing with the crazy contradictions of their family and who
utilized the defenses of isolation, constriction, repression, and
amnesia in order to survive, did become more disturbed as past
trauma and the family ways unfolded in therapy. These siblings
frequently began to display some of the same symptoms exhibited
by the designated patient. Even the super-adequate, successful sibling
shows deep pathology when the surface is scratched. For years one
mother had been blackmailing her family into giving to her by
constantly threatening to leave the house and go back to her mother.
The only way this dire event could be thwarted was for one of
the children to get sick. When the designated patient began to improve, the mother stated her threats again and one of the children,
who had previously been considered the most outgoing and healthy
one in the family, began having some of the same symptoms which
the designated patient had shown earlier. This kind of experience
is the basis for the statement of family therapists that the symptoms
which shift from one family member to another represent relatively
non-specific accommodations to stresses in the total family complex
and have a system value.

As a general rule, although some "well" siblings reflect the family
system during therapy sessions, conceal it, or go along with it, most
of them almost act as assistant therapists or observing egos because
of their willingness to expose the system, reveal family secrets,
comment on the pathologic communications, and expose the du-
plicities (e.g., one child said, "Now, mother, you know darn well

you hate these meetings and you don't like what the doctors say to you, yet when the doctors ask you you say you like them"). Because they are usually willing to expose the family system, the "well" siblings are particularly directed toward the "absent member" role. It is more rare for the designated patient to risk being considered the family traitor. Some of the siblings, while they bear the imprint of some of the family pathology, are sufficiently sturdy to offer rescue to their ill brother or sister. We have seen siblings manage the psychotic one in a far more reasonable way than do the parents, thereby providing a bridge away from the family entanglements.

There is one possible drawback in utilizing the openness of the "well" siblings in family therapy sessions. Sometimes it may seem that the therapists are allied with the children against the parents. Great conflict of loyalty can develop in the children when they perceive that the therapists can have more realistic concern for them than do their own parents. And the parents may indirectly encourage the children to oppose the therapists or may even take retaliatory measures against the children. It is very necessary for the therapists to convey the message that they are interested in helping all the members of the family, even though they may temporarily seem to favor the view of a particular one. Sooner or later the parents have to be helped to take over the role which the therapists have transitorily adopted.

Initially we were hesitant to include in family sessions the "well" sibling who managed to escape the pathologic family, but since we began to insist that the siblings do attend we found that progress increased. Besides, we learned that in the long run the siblings benefited themselves and felt deprived and excluded when they were left out. The whole question of the "well" sibling is an intricate one which needs to be elaborated as further experience in family therapy is accumulated.

TRANSFERENCE AND COUNTERTRANSFERENCE

Any attempt to cover the multitudinous aspects of transference and countertransference in family therapy in several pages is destined to be incomplete. Since the transference distortions in these complicated family therapy situations become extremely involved, only a few components which seem important to us can be identified. The topic of countertransference is presented in greater depth in Chapter 8 by Whitaker, Warkentin, and Felder.

Freud discovered the phenomenon of transference as an ubiquitous human quality whereby people displace feelings, thoughts, and fantasies which are applicable to significant others from the past onto others in the present; the psychoanalytic treatment situation creates the conditions for this process to occur with greater intensity and specificity. The very nature of any therapeutic situation has regression built into it. It is almost impossible for any person not to feel child-like and not to have certain unique and deep transference expectations *vis à vis* the therapist, no matter what the therapist is like and what he does or does not do. The affects which are transferred are most commonly complex mixtures of fear, hope, hatred, admiration, contempt, wonder, humiliation, love, shame, etc. These transference anticipations are so compelling that the actual personality of the therapist often does not begin to make a difference until fairly late in the therapy process; the feelings are so powerful that they can override personality differences between co-therapists. In general, transference interpretations tend to be made relatively late in family therapy, not only because transferences have become more fixed and the therapists are differentially responded to, but also because it is more difficult for the family members to utilize the interpretations when they are only peripherally engaged in the therapy in the early phases.

Transference certainly does not occur in the same form in individual or family psychotherapy as it does in orthodox psychoanalytic therapy. The family therapy situation is complicated by the simultaneous presence of two or three generations plus the therapists. When emotional attitudes are repeated from the past and roles are assigned to each other and to the therapists, one has to distinguish between the real family member being responded to and the introject of that person. In other words, the transference distortions of the family members not only are manifested toward therapists but toward each other. While the therapists are reacted to as grandparents, mother, father, siblings, etc., by each of the family members, additional complexity arises from the fact that the transference paradigms are perceived and apprehended by each other, resulting in feedback effects. Moreover, the transference distortions all occur within the context of the conventional social role expectations of patients and doctors as well as other reality considerations. The therapists, of course, introduce their own transference and countertransference misconstructions. It is, therefore, an understatement to call the subject of transference in family therapy complex. Its intricacy may account for the absence of literature on transference in family therapy, but does not lessen its importance. Indeed, as in all forms of therapy, transference phenomena are crucial, and techniques for dealing with them are indispensable if one is going to do the kind of intensive, protracted family therapy espoused here.

Family therapy has also revealed a new kind of transference, that of the family system as a whole, which is more than a collection of the individual distortions. The "sicker" the family the more obvious the family transference; more integrated families can play their "normal" role much better. As mentioned in the beginning of this chapter, two therapists who select each other choose a particular family to work with; the initial evaluators of the family may or may not end up as the therapists. The basis on which the therapists choose a family undoubtedly has its roots in the early family life experiences of the therapists as individuals as well as in the nature of the co-therapy team relationship. While this instinctive response to a patient occurs in individual psychotherapy, when it happens with a family it has an entirely different quality. The following are some aspects of the family which may attract or repel therapists: the family's physical appearance, their manner of dress and bearing; how they come to grips with their feelings, their style of relating to each other, how disorganized or tight they are, how the parents handle the children and each other; whether they seem insatiable or whether they are capable of being filled; whether they make the therapists feel that they can give them nothing or whether they are hungry for too much; the depressed or the paranoid family; whether the hostility is too naked or whether the therapists sense murder in the family; how they respond when someone cries; how drastically they violate meaning. Further, we have all had the experience of initially disliking a family and then growing to like them, and vice versa. When certain aspects of the family appeal to particular trends in the therapists, which are derived from the therapists' own internal imagoes, the therapists are able to make an encounter and thereby select the family for therapy. These transference elements of the therapists are often unrecognized, but they are certainly part of the process which determines how the therapy will proceed. The subjective, often unconscious attitudes of the therapy team probably have more to do with the outcome of the therapy than the nature of the family problems. The one source of transference or countertransference that is the most loaded emotionally, and about which little is written, with the notable exception of the group at the Atlanta Psychiatric Clinic (Whitaker and Malone, 1953), has to do with the needs of the therapists and how their own personal family relationships, both current and past, affect the therapy process.

The fact that countertransference is an unconscious phenomenon is often overlooked; when therapists react with their own irrational biases and preconceptions, *at the time* they do not know it. They may recognize the exaggerated feeling or response later when it is pointed out to them by a co-therapist or by the observing group of therapists. Family therapy is particularly disposed toward eliciting inappropriate responses because of the charged quality of the inter- actions. One cannot remain as detached with a family as one can with an individual patient; it is almost impossible not to get caught up in the drama of the family interaction. There is also something about working with a family as opposed to working with individuals which tempts one to pass judgment under the guise of being objective. When a child is being cruelly exploited or when someone is help- lessly squirming under the impact of a devastating "damned if they do and damned if they don't" bind, the therapists find it difficult to maintain clinical detachment. With a family there is a great temptation to circumvent defenses, to get to the heart of the matter, to do less structuring and less preparation for an interpretation, to disregard all the do's and don't's which had been learned while training to be psychotherapists. This does not mean that this reactive procedure is wrong; however, with a family a different set of rules of therapy seem to apply, and this attitude seems to be a natural outgrowth of seeing an entire family together and having to deal with the raw materials of life, so to speak. Family therapy can be heady stuff for therapists; there is a magnetic compulsion to re- fashion our own parents and make a better mother and father out of the parents under observation. What an ideal opportunity to reconstruct one's own family struggles so that in *this* family they can be worked through and mastered!

The safeguard usually recommended for minimizing countertrans- ference distortions is one's own personal analysis or psychotherapy, but no amount of analysis really frees anyone from all neurotic proclivities, and besides psychoanalysis cannot directly deal with transactional family elements. In our organizational set-up, through direct observation of sessions by the entire therapy group and by tape recordings, there does exist the opportunity for staff members who are not involved in the therapy to comment on countertrans- ference falsifications as well as sticky reality problems. (For ex- ample, one therapy team needed considerable help from the staff in handling their feelings about overt, consummated incest which occurred in one family.) Continuous discussion of dynamics, goals, techniques, transference, and countertransference phenomena between co-therapists between therapy sessions has been found to be essential. These goals can be much better accomplished in staff conferences where independent observers can lend their impressions and help clarify team differences. Introduction of a third therapist in the therapy sessions as temporary consultant has been particularly useful when the therapists were in danger of being absorbed into the family system and of following only certain grooves and chan-nels, losing their freedom of action.

Family therapy is emotionally demanding work which creates intense feelings in therapists which must be contained during ses-sions, or at least given therapeutic expression. Behind the observation mirror, however, the staff of therapists frequently vent their frustra-tions by becoming childish with each other, making snide remarks or hostile interpretations about a family, joking and taunting—all from the position of this privileged sanctuary. We have found this sort of release necessary and have even wondered whether family therapy can ever be done in isolation from one's colleagues.

CO-THERAPY TEAM RELATIONSHIP

Ever since we first began treating families it has been routine for us to use therapy teams of two rather than a single therapist, but we do acknowledge the fact that some therapists in other family therapy centers are willing to face a family alone and, by their accounts, are able to work effectively in that manner. We frankly admit, moreover, that the team approach was probably originally created more for the security of the therapists than for the family, for if therapists cannot be secure they will diminish their usefulness to patients. The security of the team relationship is a necessary resource, in our judgment, because family therapy, especially on a long-term basis, can create strong and alien feelings which can be profoundly disturbing. The system of the family is much more powerful and practiced than that of any therapy team.

As we amassed experience through our *modus operandi*, we learned that working as a team, in spite of disadvantages, introduced another dimension which had its own therapeutic value, e.g., giving a family a set of parents. The total therapy process, then, has come to include not only the intrafamilial dynamics, but the dynamics of the team relationship and the impact of the team and the family on each other. The entire process is all one, although for purposes of discussion in this chapter each factor has been artificially abstracted from the interconnected aggregate. A more elaborate report on co-therapy team relationship in our unit is given in a paper by Rubin-stein, Weiner, *et al.* (1964).

The dynamics of the relationship between co-therapists is involved and exists on a number of levels. The therapists choose to work with each other partly on the basis of extremely subtle, unconscious cues which are probably related to having had, in their own families of origin, similar experiences, style of expression, quality of affect, etc.—all of which draw them to each other and enable them to work out their differences in relatively congruent manner. The co-therapists may seem to be quite different kinds of people working in complementary fashion, yet they probably share similar introject experiences. Their basic personality affinity supersedes differences in sex, profession, culture, religion, or theoretical orientation and, in all likelihood, accounts for the fulfillment of deep needs in the relationship as well as for transference distortions. The trust, confidence, and sensitivity which the therapists have toward each other is a prerequisite in their ability to work with families; this primary concordance can tolerate divergence between them as well as allow them to handle family anxiety. As in a marriage, a team relationship has its own evolution and phases, and the ambivalences between therapists, often exploited by the family, have to be worked through. If the foundation of the relationship is solid enough, the two therapists can alternate being child and parent for each other, even while being two parents or husband and wife for the family. If there is not a good team relationship good family therapy cannot be done.

We have learned that when the family therapy has bogged down or is floundering, the first effort to diagnose the difficulty should be directed toward the team relationship rather than the family. If one therapists gets disturbed by something going on in the family he should first look for some difficulty in the team relationship. In our unit if the team is unable to resolve the problems on its own, the entire staff observes a family session or listens to tape recordings of the sessions. When the team members can overcome their individual and collective defensiveness they can examine the source of their difficulties with each other. For example, one therapist may feel excluded because the other therapist has established proprietary rights over a family member; when a therapist gets more from a family member than he does from his team-mate he is behaving like the parent in the schizophrenic family who turns more to his child than to his mate. Part of the process which occurs between the co-therapists is a function of the group process of the entire staff; the total family of therapists, of course, has its own system, rules, and myths. Sometimes the behavior of the therapists is monitored more by the impression they are trying to make on their colleagues behind the one-way mirror than it is by the team strategy or the needs of the family.

The bond of the team relationship enables the therapists to tolerate wide deviance in style as well as tests which the family will make upon the relationship. One therapist may deal with primary process material and one with secondary process material. One therapist can stay relatively free of the family entanglement and rescue his co-therapist when the latter loses objectivity. Even a smoothly functioning team with long experience in working with each other can be ruffled by certain family maneuvers. One of the severest tests occurs when the family attempts to split the therapists into good and bad objects, isolating the bad one. This omnipresent human phenomenon has a variety of motives behind it: it may be seen as a remnant of former attempts to divide and conquer between parents, the testing out of parents; it may serve resistance purposes, or may lead to the arousal of jealousy or competition between therapists. The maneuver can be especially effective if there are latent rivalries between the therapists or if it fits in with the unconscious need of one therapist to be seen as the giving, over-responsible one, or the unconscious need of the other therapist to be seen as the "baddy." If one therapist has a strong need to be liked by a family, the other team member can be regarded as being in the way or perhaps even used as an avenue to gratification from the family. There is a sibling paradigm in this team problem: it feels better to outdo a sibling for parental love than to be an only child with no one to compete with. Another problem arises when one team member is regarded as the senior therapist and the other as the junior therapist. Frequently the family will impose their structure on the therapy team (e.g., a Jewish doctor regarded as the senior therapist by a Jewish family, or, if one of the therapists has been the individual therapist for the designated patient he will be regarded as "the doctor" by the family). The preferred therapist cannot help but respond to the family's view of himself. Some of these problems should be brought out into the open and discussed with the family; if the therapists do not communicate with each other, the family will not. The emergencies and trials which the family goes through in therapy frequently bring the team members closer together, and thereby unite the team and the family.

There are some families who will not allow the therapists to enter their system because they utilize passive techniques of non-involvement. These kinds of families, which usually contain an acting-out member, are shallow and superficial once the immediate crisis is past (e.g., when the police arrest the child). They come to the sessions, but their silent behavior says, "Do me," as if to say, "Okay, we're here; now do something for us, without our having to ask for it." The security in the team relationship is very important on these occasions because of the anger and anxiety aroused in the therapists. The co-therapists, after making efforts to provoke feelings and interaction between family members, frequently have to rely on each other for contact or have to learn to use each other to maintain silence. The families who let the therapists into the system too quickly can be deceptive, and it is occasionally necessary for the therapists to save each other from engulfment.

In conclusion, we have found that there is a quality about the relationship of a good therapy team which helps allay family anxiety so that the members can more freely explore the depths of their relationships. The team relationship itself helps create hope for the family that something better can come out of their misery.

Terminal Phases of Family Therapy

Among the vast unexplored areas of family therapy lies the question of the dynamics and handling of the final stages of treatment and its termination. There is not a great deal of information on this area, not only because there are so few places in the country where long-term family therapy is done, but also because there are not many families who reach the phase of natural termination (i.e., a termination mutually agreed upon by the therapists and the family with the unanimous conviction that growth has taken place). We have not been operating long enough to see enough families reach the final phases; also, the dynamics of the termination process are difficult to understand.

Family resistance of all types characterizes the final as well as the middle phases of family therapy, but they assume a somewhat different form. For a long time there is much monotony as each member of the family reports the same material over and over again, eternally adding two and two and getting five. There is certainly no undeviating progression; a new connection is made here, a bit of backsliding there; several members are ready to move ahead to new definitions of relationships, but one member keeps obstructing the process; or a combination of two retards a third. The same old family patterns and habits constantly pull the family backwards at the same time that these desperate people are looking for a way out of their wretchedness. Interpretations that had been repeated many times are reacted to as if heard for the first time.

When the family system begins to crack, intense turmoil is precipitated; there may be threats of suicide, murder, and divorce. Rupture of the system also creates anxiety in the therapists who may react by going in one of two directions: by offering more support, more frequent sessions, or offers of individual therapy. Or, the therapists may begin to withdraw from the family; later reflection may make them realize that they have been giving clues that the family should terminate—by coming late to sessions, getting more impatient, increasing the amount of interpretations, insisting on conditions they know the family will not meet, or attending to the manifest, negative side of the family's ambivalence about coming to the sessions. We have found the threat of termination to be a powerful mobilizer for inducing motivation for change and loosening things up. When we ask some families why they come week after week without essentially changing, they rarely can verbalize their goals except to reply, "We want our daughter or son to get well," or "We need a happier family." When we point out the futility of continuing without some evidence of a desire for change, great apprehension arises, even in parents who have never accepted the idea that they are patients or have paid only lip service to the idea. One mother hinted darkly that if we dropped them she'd make her child sick again. The family members are in great conflict between the over-powering urge to maintain the status quo, the previous homeostatic balance on the one hand, and the dependent desire to please the therapists, to be liked and accepted by them on the other hand. Yet they are often honestly confused as to what "change" means. One of the mothers, who had controlled all the family money and had the house in her name, interpreted change as doing more, rather than less, of what she was already doing; she said, "I've already done enough; I can't possibly do more!" Her husband started off one of the meetings saying, "Well, I suppose it's required that I be a stronger, more dominant man," and then he checked with his wife and asked, "Don't you think so, dear?"

The family then enters a frozen state of suspended animation where the old ways are no longer effective and the new ways are not yet available. This state may last a considerable time, and families may be fixated there and never move ahead. It is a painful period for everyone. Ever so slowly, with the families who do make progress, the family members begin really to listen to each other and to the therapists. Gradually they find that the old gratifications no longer seem to work. There just doesn't seem to be much point, somehow, in continuing the relentless alienation or ruthless accusations. They are the same people, and yet there is something different in the family atmosphere; perhaps that nameless dread no longer seems to be hovering over the family. The parents may be able to be less fearful that their daughter will be raped if she goes out on a date, and the children may be less concerned with what goes on in that bedroom which has come to be occupied by both parents. The husband may see the essential unhappiness behind his wife's shrewish ways and may use her less as a censuring mother. The wife may be able to feel more like a woman since she doesn't feel so compelled to see the husband as a tormentor or serf. Unlike other forms of psychotherapy, there is not much verbalized insight; the family members seem to get along better, but have great difficulty understanding why they do. One could draw a parallel with some forms of child therapy, where a child may benefit by the experience without even knowing he was undergoing treatment.

The dynamics involved in terminations which occur precipitously, either in the early, middle, or later phases, can be most instructive. One of the major reasons why families terminate suddenly is based on an awareness of what the therapists are doing to the system, as well as on an unwillingness to change. Counterpoint to this theme is the transference-countertransference gambit whereby the family's needs and the therapists' needs are tested out against each other. That is, a struggle ensues between therapists and families as to "who wants who." When the family senses that they are going to be abandoned, they want to quit, giving the message, "I'll reject you before you can reject me." Although families feel libidinally rejected when therapists threaten termination, they often learn, too, that they can hurt the therapists by rejecting them. If the therapists have greater need for the family than the family has for them, then the family is stronger, and vice versa. We have learned from this realization and the fact that the families' involvement with the therapists often increases when the therapists become less interested in changing them that therapy teams often need help from the rest of the staff to "play it cool" or to let a family go. Greater experience has led our therapists not to show eagerness to possess or retain families; when the families sense this, they put more serious effort into their therapy work. The relationship with the team member, we have learned, will remain long after the family has departed.

Hiatuses in family therapy have their usefulness, as they do in individual therapy. Some families have interrupted treatment and returned as new families, with new attitudes and motivations. For some of these families, we later realized, the rejection of the therapists represented a step toward individuation and growth; the separation was a trial action. When they rebuffed the therapists they did not truly look upon the therapists as the bad parents; in the unconscious the only really bad parents are those who get sick, leave, or die. These families needed to test whether the therapists would be available when needed, would be *there*. During the course of therapy this testing out may assume the form of missing appointments or behaving irresponsibly, to see whether the therapists would go after them or rescue them, to see how much the therapists wanted them.

One of the most important observations we have made on the question of termination is how dependent these families become on the whole treatment process. The new, artificial family created by the treatment situation acts as a crutch for the family, and its withdrawal is frightening to the family members. Implicit in many of the statements during the sessions is the plea that the therapists accept an enduring consignment to take care of them. As a matter of fact, when the family members are asked to define their own goals of treatment they behave as though they cannot commit themselves to treatment unless they feel that the therapists are making the first commitment to them; they seem much more concerned with whether *we want them* (to continue with the treatment) than they are with their own personal aspirations.

The dynamics of termination are central and are suffused throughout all other problems of family therapy. As more experience is gained in the area of termination we may come to understand more about how to anticipate and handle resistances in all phases.

A Subjective Evaluation of Family Therapy

The question we have seriously asked ourselves is: If family therapy "works," how could it? Though it may not be fair to compare family therapy to individual psychoanalysis, the major surgery of psychotherapy, one must consider what is involved in changing the human personality. Even under the ideal conditions of analysis, five times a week, the patient must go through the long, painstaking process of enervation of defenses, surmounting resistances, deep regression, transference neurosis, working-through, and finally, if analysis is relatively successful, there is abandonment of fixations, diminishing of primary-process phenomena; the patient ends up doing things for himself rather than for the analyst and seeks gratification of needs through the reality principle. Analysts can state with conviction that in order to effect really meaningful change and achieve resolution of deep-seated personality problems, no part of this process can be skipped or aborted, and even under these ideal conditions the clinical outcome is uncertain. Then, it might legitimately be asked, how can you possibly hope to bring about real change under the unmanageable conditions of seeing four or five people together once a week? In the analytic situation, when an interpretation is made, the patient usually responds with self-justifying statements and a variety of resistance maneuvers while the analyst patiently listens; at a certain point there is a long pause, and then the patient usually considers the interpretation, sometimes grabs hold of it, and then begins to speculate on its implications in his life and possibly goes back to its earlier antecedents. In family therapy, where the lines of inquiry cannot be pursued without interruption, where each person, in the early phases at least, stops at the point of blaming the other and is intent on saving face in front of the family, is it possible even to approximate the working-through of resistances? Are not the most heavily charged events and fantasies of a person's life deeply buried under so many layers that they require special techniques of individual therapy to be revealed? Are not very early conflicts in each person too far removed from the immediate situation for them to be traced back from derivatives to their past connections? How can a severely regressed family possibly abandon infantile needs?

Despite every theoretical reason why family therapy should not work, we who have been doing it have developed an inner conviction that it does work for most families and that it has even greater potential for becoming more effective as more is learned. But what do we mean by the treatment "working"? First, it is necessary to use criteria of change different from those applied to individual therapy. The criteria of interpersonal and transactional processes are pertinent, even though our conceptual standards for evaluating these kinds of changes are in a primitive stage. On what level should we look for change? Do we seek changes in attitudes, in behavior, on the level of deep needs, homeostatic balance, shifts in alliances? Do we seek freedom from symptoms for the designated patient? Do we find, instead, exchange of symptoms among family members? Do we look for differentiation from each other in the family members, less family distress, more togetherness, less togetherness, more unqualified communication messages in the family? Do we try to help the family members get more meaning our of life, or, in the last analysis, as in all forms of therapy, do the patients set their own goals? This criterion, too, is not dependable, inasmuch as the goals, based on accumulated insight as the treatment progresses, are often quite different at the end of treatment than they were at the beginning. Besides, are not estimates of health needed from therapists and society? But what constitutes a healthy family? What right do the therapists have to decide what the good family life is? Should family therapists not avoid being agents of society in making families conform to some idealistic standard? And so on.

Rather than attempting to deal with the foregoing questions, we can specify some concrete, operational ways of estimating family improvement. Intrapsychic changes lead to interpersonal ones, but interpersonal changes in turn lead to intrapsychic alterations, especially when the changes are shared jointly within the most basic living unit, the family. We know families have improved when we notice continuity in the sessions and when the family is able to resolve conflicts at home instead of bringing them to the therapists to solve. We know there is growth when the family members use each other less as transference figures and seem more like real people to the therapists and to each other. When the family pathology is lessened the family members can enjoy each other and life better. Without attempting to specify precisely what is meant by our language, we do find that greater individuation occurs, so that the shared ego of the family slackens and separation of the members from the system can be tolerated. Each individual becomes more free to explore an individual definition of self, which may be quite different from his role as formerly viewed by the family. The affect which was discharged into the family arena becomes more dispersed and less primitive gratification value is attached to it; the old "kick" out of the family craziness is gone. Emotional forces tend to become less family-adhering so that, for example, the sexual energies of the children can begin to turn toward extrafamilial figures. Communication tends to open up between parents and, despite the initial confusion, futility, and disappointment when they really open their eyes to each other, the marriage partners usually end up with more sympathetic views of each other and, consequently, increase their chance of a meaningful relationship. Improvement in the marriage, as we have said, is almost invariably followed by emotional growth in the children. As the parents were "fed" by the therapists they came to feed less on their children. Perhaps most important of all, the families discover that there are other ways of behaving toward each other and still remain a family.

Family therapists are hopeful about their work because they have seen improvement in families where a great deal of prior individual therapy for the various members did not materially change anything.

The family as an institution has survived many thousands of years as the most workable living unit for human beings because, as the mediator of the culture in preparing the young for the next generation, it has served to digest social change as well as act as a flexible bulwark against upheavals which have occurred through time. It is perhaps not accidental that, despite a century of enlightened psychiatric endeavor, it has taken so long to get around to treating the family unit as the patient. Most people rather instinctively regard the family as sacrosanct, as perhaps the last bastion of freedom left to man. (Note, for example, the recent protests against psychological tests in schools which inquire into personal aspects of family life.) Where else but in his own castle, with his own family, can a person pick his nose, flatulate, lose his temper with impunity, whine, let the child in him emerge—in short, regress and "be himself"? Although the reader may have gained the impression that we have focused heretofore only on the pathologic and the bizarre in family life, we fully recognize the emotional refuge and deep satisfactions in family living. Even in the most alienated families the blood ties and continued associations create loyalty and a kind of caring—the family jokes, holiday celebrations, the smell of cooking, etc. Nonetheless, family gratifications can sometimes paradoxically provide the background for human tragedy and emotional disturbance of endless variety—the cruel rejections, the discriminations, the child unloved as a person, the humiliations, the parentification of the child, the lack of intimacy, the overindulged, the unrealized fulfillments and thwarted potentials, and the outrages against the human spirit.

People are often misled about the degree of pathology in those they think they know well because most people, in customary social relationships, manage to conceal not only their fantasy life but many aspects of their overt infantile behavior which is acted out only with certain special people (e.g., a mate, child, sibling, parent, friend). The individual psychotherapist or analyst does become acquainted with the fantasy life, but even they can misjudge the full impact of a person's pathology because they get only second-hand reports about the quality of the social interaction and, except for transference, rarely see it unfold before them. The distorted behavior may not even appear in full force in the transference if it is being acted out in especially intense fashion with someone outside the sessions. Family therapy is the only kind of therapy which can witness the "sick" behavior with the key figures as it actually occurs *in vivo*. Therefore, no matter how mature some people seem to be in ordinary social relationships, certain childish features of their personality emerge only when they are in the presence of members of their family. The layman knows this when he says, "You have to live with a person to know what he's really like." As one woman put it, "In the outside world my husband is the essence of goodness. He is capable and admired; he goes out of his way to do things for everyone. Everywhere I go people tell me what a lucky person I am to be married to him. Yet the minute he walks in the front door something happens, because to his family he can give nothing and he acts like a little boy!" The private "back-room" of the family is rarely exposed to outsiders, in contradistinction to the "front-room" exhibited to the public (Goffman, 1956). Even close friends can "know" a family for years and not be aware of not only the family skeletons and scandals consciously concealed, but of the sometimes weird underground of the family.[4] The footnotes in the biographies of famous people only

---

[4] Perhaps this is what the author of the play *Five Finger Exercise* (Shaffer, 1959) was getting at when the tutor comes to live with the family and the son tells him upon their meeting, ". . . Well, let me give you a warning. This isn't a family. It's a tribe of cannibals. Between us we eat everything we can . . . You think I'm joking?" The tutor, feeling uncomfortable, replies, "I think you're lucky to have a family." And the son says, "And I think you're lucky to be without one . . . I'm sorry. I'm making tasteless jokes. Actually we're very choosey in our victims. We only eat other members of the family."

hint at the deeply personal but extravagant and strange practices which occur in every family in some form and degree, even in those families known to the community as ideal.

To expose the subterranean currents of family life occasionally makes the therapists uneasy. Some of the disclosures in the family meetings have the disturbing and embarrassing quality of an obscenity uttered in church. In individual therapy we have become used to the patient's relating intimate events with great guilt or shame, reliving with acute suffering the death of a child or a parent, re-experiencing the feelings that a brother or sister was preferred, describing masturbation fantasies, etc. One sees in the privacy of the office all the beauty and ugliness of the human character. But it is quite another sort of discomfort when these things are disclosed semi-publicly, e.g., when the son comes increasingly to have poorly disguised contempt for his soft, ineffectual father who always abdicates on making decisions, or when the simmering, spiteful battle between mother and grandmother culminates in the scathing denunciation, "You should never have had children!" or to witness the horror in the mother who has become aware of how she has hurt her child, or to hear a "well" sibling say to her sanctimonious mother, "You know, mother, you really do rotten little things." Though the children are used to seeing their parents' childish behavior in the home, to see it openly displayed in front of outsiders, the doctors, is humiliating for them.

It must be remembered that we often see these families at their worst; the father whom we see as a "passive-dependent character with depressive features" may be, to his children, a warm, lovable person with other sides to his personality. The alcoholic mother is sometimes more affectionate with her children than other, more proper mothers. No matter how bad, unsuccessful, or unlovable a parent may seem to others, the children may "love" him or her unreservedly and fiercely, and it's difficult for parents to give this up. Every therapist has seen that no matter how repugnant or peculiar a patient or family may seem on first contact, after they have been worked with for a while they seem more like persons and one can understand a little more why they do what they do, that given their particular background and present circumstances, they do what they *have* to do. On the subjective side, the therapists have a mélange of feelings as they sit with these families: empathy, hate, bafflement, isolation, love, disgust, sympathy, etc. Cognitively, they evaluate, judge, sense, combine strategy with the co-therapist, maneuver, self-observe, etc.

We have occasionally wondered about how families were being disturbed by the therapy. It is not unusual to hear patients in individual therapy complain that they're worse off than when treatment started. Families, too, often report that they are more disrupted; there are threats of divorce and murder (none of which have actually been carried out), complaints that we are "ruining" the family, reports of more contention in the home, etc. As we have examined this question more closely, however, we ask: What was the state of affairs with the family before we came into the picture? Was their relative serenity achieved by sacrificing one member of the family as the patient? Had there not been deep but unrecognized dissatisfaction for years? Any investigative procedure is bound to disturb rigid patterns, cause more distress, frustrate intrafamilial vested interests, and make things temporarily appear much worse. It is interesting that as we have become more experienced in family therapy we have heard fewer complaints of his sort. As in all forms of psychotherapy, family therapy undoubtedly has its spreading side-effects. Families occasionally over-analyze at home and interpret to each other; they may even use therapists' statements made during sessions to bolster an argument at home (e.g., "See, the doctor said you have hostile feelings toward your mother and you take it out on me"). Extended family members may find changes in the family members most upsetting.

It is interesting to speculate why Freud, with all his genius for apprehending so many fundamentals truths about the nature of man, stopped short of fully recognizing and therapeutically handling the interpersonal, interlocking pathology *among* people intimately involved with one another. Though, in one sense, no one understood intrafamilial struggles better than Freud, his emphasis on the reconstruction and elaboration of the family dynamics within one mind, and his discouragement of involvement of family members in the treatment process of individuals established the practice of the exclusion of the family in most forms of psychotherapy. Heretofore science has always had to rely on information *about* the family second-hand, from reports given by patients, from questionnaires, or from individual members of the family seen separately. By observing the family interacting together phenomena began to be discovered which had never before been known to exist because the special conditions for their disclosure had never been present. It is likely that this generation of family therapists have made their contribution by identifying the family concept and recognizing some of its profound implications; perhaps it will take another generation of clinician-theoreticians to further integrate the intrapsychic and transactional spheres before family therapy will be a refined, specific form of treatment with known limits. Practical considerations of the treatment aspect aside, in the long run the significance of the family transactional approach is that it represents a major conceptual challenge to contemporary psychopathology and personality theory as a whole.

We are only now beginning to realize some of the wider connotations and consequences of the family approach. Family therapy, which originally focused on schizophrenic patients and their families, has come to be applied to a wide variety of clinical conditions in the designated patient, including the neuroses, acting out character disorders, resistant psychosomatic conditions, learning problems, problems of ego-restriction and inhibition, alcoholism, problems of the aged, sexual deviation, etc. Suicide prevention centers are learning that suicides have a better change of being thwarted when the whole family is seen and the meaning of the suicide attempt or threat can be better discerned. The traditional child guidance approach is gradually giving way to the family approach in a number of states, and the community mental health centers of the future may well become family mental health centers. Even in those clinic situations where family therapy cannot be undertaken, clinicians are beginning to discover the value of the intake family diagnostic interview as a routine work-up since it has been realized that this approach represents the best method of ascertaining the meaning of the illness and what went on in the family to help create it. Family therapy is here to stay, but because there are so few trained family therapists, because it is such a time-consuming endeavor, and because knowledge in the field is still in its prodromal stages, family therapy will remain a highly selective, limited procedure for some time to come, although adaptations of some of its tenets may someday be applied to some of the social ills of our day. The ultimate value of family therapy probably lies in the area of prevention; the children in the treated family who will marry and form families of their own will have a greater capacity to create healthy family living.

References

ACKERMAN, N. W. (1960). Family-focused therapy of schizophrenia. In S. C. Scher and H. R. Davis (Eds.) *The out-patient treatment of schizophrenia*. New York: Grune & Stratton.

BELL, J. E. (1961). *Family group therapy*. Washington, D.C.: Public Health Monograph No. 64, Dept. of Health, Education and Welfare.

BELL, N. W. (1962). Extended family relations of disturbed and well families. *Family Process 1*, 175–193.

BOSZORMENYI-NAGY, I., AND FRAMO, J. L. (1961). Hospital organization and family oriented psychotherapy of schizophrenia. Montreal: *Proceedings of the 3rd World Congress of Psychiatry*.

BOSZORMENYI-NAGY, I., AND FRAMO, J. L. (1962). Family concept of hospital treatment of schizophrenia. In J. H. Masserman (Ed.) *Current psychiatric therapies*, vol. II. New York: Grune & Stratton.

BOWEN, M. (1961). Family psychotherapy. *Amer. J. Orthopsychiat. 31*, 42–60.

CARROLL, E. J. (1960). Treatment of the family as a unit. *Penna. Med. J. 63*, 57–62.

DICKS, H. V. (1964). Concepts of marital diagnosis and therapy as developed at the Tavistock Family Psychiatric Units, London, England. In Nash, E. M., Jessner, L., and Abse, D. W. (Eds.) *Marriage counseling in medical practice*. Chapel Hill: Univer. No. Carolina Press, Ch. 15.

ERIKSON, E. (1950). *Childhood and society*. New York: Norton.

FAIRBAIRN, W. R. D. (1952). *An object-relations theory of the personality*. New York: Basic Books.

FRAMO, J. L. (1962). The theory of the technique of family treatment of schizophrenia. *Family Process 1*, 119–131.

GOFFMAN, E. (1956). *The presentation of self in everyday life*. Edinburgh: Univer. of Edinburgh, Social Sciences Research Centre.

GUNTRIP, H. (1953). The therapeutic factor in psychotherapy. *Brit. J. med. Psychol. 26*, 115–131.

HALEY, J. (1959). Family of the schizophrenic: a model system. *J. nerv. ment. Dis. 129*, 357–374.

HALEY, J. (1963). Marriage therapy. *Arch. gen. Psychiat. 8*, 213–234.

HANDLON, J. H., AND PARLOFF, M. B. (1962). The treatment of patient and family as a group: is it group psychotherapy? *Int. J. grp. Psychother. 12*, 132–141.

HILL, L. (1955). *Psychotherapeutic intervention in schizophrenia*. Univer. Chicago Press.

JACKSON, D. D. (1959). Family interaction, family homeostasis and some implications for conjoint family psychotherapy. In J. H. Masserman (Ed.) *Science and psychoanalysis, II Individual and familial dynamics*. New York: Grune & Stratton.

JACKSON, D. D., AND WEAKLAND, J. H. (1961). Conjoint family therapy: some considerations on theory, technique, and results. *Psychiatry 24*, 30–45.

KUBIE, L. S. (1956). Psychoanalysis and marriage: practical and theoretical issues. In V. W. Eisenstein (Ed.) *Neurotic interaction in marriage*. New York: Basic Books, Ch. 2.

LIDZ, T., FLECK, S., ALANEN, Y. O., AND CORNELISON, A. (1963). Schizophrenic patients and their siblings, *Psychiatry. 26*, 1–18.

MENNINGER, K. (1958). *The theory of psychoanalytic technique*. New York: Basic Books.

MIDELFORT, C. F. (1957). *The family in psychotherapy*. New York: Blakiston.

NIZER, L. (1961). *My life in court*. New York: Doubleday.

PROUT, C. T., AND WHITE, M. A. (1956). The schizophrenic's sibling. *J. nerv. ment. Dis. 123*, 162–170.

REDL, F. (1948). Resistance in therapy groups. *Hum. Relat. 1*, 307–313.

RUBINSTEIN, D., AND WEINER, O. R. (1964). Co-therapy teamwork relationships in family psychotherapy. (With collaboration of Boszormenyi-Nagy, I., Dealy, M., Framo, J. L., Lincoln, G., Robinson, L., and Zuk, G.) Paper read at Conference on Family Process and Psychopathology: Perspectives of the Clinician and Social Scientist. Eastern Pennsylvania Psychiatric Institute, Philadelphia, October.

RYCKOFF, I., DAY, J., AND WYNNE, L. C. (1959). Maintenance of stereotyped roles in the families of schizophrenics. *A.M.A. Arch. gen. Psychiat. 1*, 93–98.

SCHAFFER, L., WYNNE, L. C., DAY, J., RYCKOFF, I. M., AND HALPERIN, A. (1962). On the nature and sources of the psychiatrists' experience with the family of the schizophrenic. *Psychiatry 25*, 32–45.

SEARLES, H. F. (1958). Positive feelings in the relationship between the schizophrenic and his mother. *Int. J. Psychoanal. 39*, 569–586.

SEARLES, H. F. (1959a). Integration and differentiation in schizophrenia. *J. nerv. ment. Dis. 129*, 542–550.

SEARLES, H. F. (1959b). The effort to drive the other person crazy—an element in the aetiology and psychotherapy of schizophrenia. *Brit. J. med. Psychol. 32*, 1–18.

SEARLES, H. F. (1961). Anxiety concerning change, as seen in the psychotherapy of schizophrenic patients, with particular reference to the sense of personal identity. *Int. J. Psychoanal. 42*, 74–85.

SHAFFER, P. (1959). *Five finger exercise.* New York: Harcourt Brace.

SONNE, J. C., SPECK, R. V., AND JUNGREIS, J. E. (1962). The absent-member maneuver as a resistance in family therapy of schizophrenia. *Family Process 1*, 44–62.

SZASZ, T. S. (1957). A contribution to the psychology of schizophrenia. *A.M.A. Arch. Neurol. Psychiat. 77*, 420–436.

VARON, E. (1958). Defenses inherent in the group situation. Jewish Family & Children's Bureau, Baltimore (mimeo).

WHITAKER, C. A. AND MALONE, T. P. (1953). *The roots of psychotherapy.* New York: Blakiston.

WHITAKER, C. A., MALONE, T. P., AND WARKENTIN, J. (1956). Multiple therapy and psychotherapy. In F. Fromm-Reichman and J. L. Moreno (Eds.) *Progress in psychotherapy.* New York: Grune & Stratton, 210–216.

WHITAKER, C. A. (1958). Psychotherapy with couples. *Amer. J. Psychother. 12*, 18–23.

WYNNE, L. C., DAY, J., HIRSCH, S., AND RYCKOFF, I. (1957). The family relations of a set of monozygotic quadruplet schizophrenics. Zurich: *Congress Report of the 2nd Internat. Congress for Psychiatry, 2*, 43–49.

YI-CHUANG LU. (1961). Mother-child role relations in schizophrenia: a comparison of schizophrenic patients with nonschizophrenic siblings, *Psychiatry 24*, 133–142.

5

MURRAY BOWEN

Family Psychotherapy with Schizophrenia in the Hospital and in Private Practice

The specific method of family psychotherapy in the treatment of schizophrenia which will be described here was developed as an integral part of a theoretical premise about the nature and origin of schizophrenia. The theoretical premise was later extended to "a family concept of schizophrenia," and more recently to "a family theory of emotional illness." Much of the theoretical and background material has been reported in Bowen, Dysinger, Brodey and Basamania (1957); Bowen (1959); and Bowen, Dysinger and Basamania (1959). The family concept of schizophrenia is discussed in Bowen (1960) and family psychotherapy with schizophrenia in Bowen (1961).

Presented here is a series of sections beginning with broad theoretical concepts and proceeding through more specific theory and clinical application of the theory to a clinical description of family psychotherapy. Considerable emphasis is placed on the theoretical orientation. The psychotherapist establishes and controls the milieu in which the psychotherapy takes place, and his theoretical thinking about the nature of the problem to be treated determines his approach to the problem, the procedures he will use, the observations he

213

214 INTENSIVE FAMILY THERAPY

will make and the way he will respond and react as the therapy proceeds. Thus, it is profitable to know the therapist's specific theoretical emphasis in any description of a method of psychotherapy.

The specific order of this presentation is as follows: The first section is a brief review of important steps in the development of the family theory. This is presented to clarify differences between family theory and individual theory which conceives of emotional illness as a psychopathology confined within the person of the patient. It is difficult to communicate a family orientation to those whose thinking and perceptual systems operate in terms of individual theory. Differences between individual and family theory are repeated in a different context in each section of this chapter. The second section is a specific consideration of important points in the theoretical orientation. The third section is a brief summary of the family theory of emotional illness. Schizophrenia is seen as a part of the total spectrum of human adaptation. An understanding of less severe types of emotional illness has much to contribute to the understanding of schizophrenia. The fourth section is a description of the family projection process by which a parental problem is transmitted to a child, a process especially important in schizophrenia. The fifth section is a description of a clinical program designed to modify the family projection process in the hospital and in private practice. The sixth section deals with specific principles and techniques in the use of this method of family psychotherapy. The last section is an estimation of the current status of the method of family psychotherapy being presented.

Background Information

In the development of the family theory of emotional illness, the initial work was based on previous experience with individual psychotherapy in schizophrenia. It began with a five-year clinical study[1] in which various members of patients' families, as well as the patients, were treated in individual psychotherapy. As the emphasis shifted to include family members, the relationship system between family members came into prominence. Attention was focused on the symbiotic attachment between mothers and patients. Of particular interest was the cyclical nature of the symbiotic relationship in which each pair of mothers and patients could at times be so close that they were "emotional Siamese twins" or, at other times, so distant and hostile they repelled each other. Charac-

---

[1] Conducted at the Menninger Clinic and Shawnee Guidance Center, Topeka, Kansas, 1949–1954.

teristics of the symbiotic relationship were incorporated into a detailed hypothesis concerning the etiology of schizophrenia.

The most important steps in the development of the family theory were made during a formal family research study[2] in which schizophrenic patients and their families lived in residence on a psychiatric ward. At the beginning of the research the hypothesis from the previous work was incorporated into a research plan for mothers to live on the ward with the schizophrenic patients. The research revealed striking "new" characteristics of the mother-patient relationship not clearly "seen" in the previous work. These characteristics will be described in the next section. Why had these observations been obscured in the previous work? The hypothesis was the same and the families had the same kinds of clinical problems. Two factors seemed to account for the change. One factor was the close living situation in which the relationship actions and responses were more intense, but the most important factor seemed to be "observational blindness" in the investigators. Man can fail to see what is before his eyes unless it fits into his theoretical frame of reference. For instance, man had been looking at the bones of prehistoric animals for centuries without really "seeing them"; he believed the earth had been created exactly as it is now, and he could not "see" the bones until there was a theory of evolution. The initial work with families was based on individual theory, which is so focused on the patient that it was not possible to really "see" the family. The shift to the hypothesis about the symbiotic relationship was a move toward a family orientation. I believe the specific shift was determined more by limitations in theoretical thinking than by the accuracy of the concept in describing the family phenomenon. The symbiotic relationship had been described in the literature; it was a compatible extension of individual theory, and it accurately described one area of the family phenomenon. Only the mother-patient relationship came into focus because the remainder of the phenomenon was obscured by "observational blindness." The "living together" research was another move toward a family orientation. Although the hypothesis was still stated exactly as in the informal study, the attitude behind the living together situation helped set the stage to "see" the family better. Increasing ability to "see" the family, plus the increased intensity of the relationship characteristics, were sufficient for the new observations to break through. Once seen, the new relationship phenomenon was so forcefully present that it pervaded the entire operation. It was then possible to see the phe-

---

[2] Conducted at the Clinical Center, National Institute of Mental Health, Bethesda, Maryland, 1954–1959.

nomenon clearly in concurrent work with outpatient families in which the phenomenon was less intense in its manifestations.

The most important step in the development of the family theory was based on the "new" observations and was made late in the first year of the research study. The hypothesis was extended to include the entire family in the theoretical premise, the research design was modified to permit both parents and other family members to live on the ward with the patient, and the psychotherapy was changed from individual to family psychotherapy. During the last four years of the research study, the theoretical premise was further defined and extended into a family concept of schizophrenia, and the family psychotherapy was developed as an integrated part of the family concept. Concurrently with the live-in research study, an increasing number of outpatient families were treated in outpatient family psychotherapy. Since 1959, the author's work in family psychotherapy has been confined to outpatient work and to private practice.

The most recent steps in the development of the family theory were based on experience with family psychotherapy for families with problems less severe than schizophrenia. This includes some 250 families with problems ranging from simple neuroses to those of near psychotic degree. It was surprising to find that all the family dynamisms so striking in schizophrenia were also present in families with the least severe problems and even in "normal" or asymptomatic families. Experience supports the view that the difference between schizophrenia and less severe psychopathology is one of degree. Changes during family psychotherapy are important in understanding the family phenomenon, and the rapid changes in families with neurotic problems provided a range of observations not possible with the slow indefinite changes in schizophrenia. Experience with less severe problems provided the observations for expansion of the family concept of schizophrenia into the family theory of emotional illness. The present theory conceives the entire range of human adjustment to be on a single scale, with the highest levels of maturity at one end of the scale and the lowest forms of maladaptation and emotional illness at the other end of the scale.

THEORETICAL BACKGROUND

Important differences between individual and family theory were brought into sharp focus at the end of the first year of the research by the decision to change from an individual to a family orientation. The first year the theoretical orientation was based on *individual* theory; each patient and each mother had *individual* psychotherapy, and the research was directed at defining the interlocking of *individual* pathologies. The change was based on the newly observed characteristics of the mother-patient relationship. The mother-patient symbiosis was much more intense and extensive in actuality than had been postulated in the hypothesis. The symbiotic "emotional oneness" was not an entity in itself but a fragment of a larger family "emotional oneness." Concurrent observations of outpatient families suggested that fathers were as involved as the mothers in the emotional oneness and that other family members were also involved. Family relationships alternated between overcloseness and overdistance. In the emotional closeness phases, the intrapsychic systems of involved family members were so intimately fused that differentiation of one from the other was impossible. The fusion involved the entire range of ego functioning. One ego could function for that of another. One family member could accurately know the thoughts, fantasies, feelings, and dreams of the other. One family member could become physically ill in response to an emotional stress in another. Every detail of a patient's psychosis could have its mirror image in the mother. There were examples in which the patient's psychosis acted out the mother's unconscious. In the angry distance phases, family members could "fuse" with other family members, or certain nonrelatives, such as members of the hospital staff, and the other person would also "fuse" into the family problem. Another manifestation of the family oneness was the spontaneous, fluid shifting of ego strengths and weaknesses from one family member to another. Part of a "pathology" could be in one family member and other parts in other family members. It suggested a family jigsaw puzzle of strengths and weaknesses, with each family member holding pieces of the same puzzle and with considerable trading of pieces. These observations suggested the concept, "the family as the unit of illness." A part of the total problem was in each family member, and perception of the total problem was not possible from examination of the parts separately. In some families, individual psychotherapy with a single family member would tone down the emotional process in the entire family for varying periods of time. Research observations suggested that the larger family emotional oneness had the same basic characteristics as the mother-patient symbiosis. Terms such as "emotional fusion," "emotional connectedness," "emotional stuck-togetherness," and "ego fusion" all accurately describe the phenomenon. The "symbiotic" hypothesis was discarded and thinking was directed to a larger family phenomenon.

There were critical practical and theoretical issues in the decision to change to a family orientation. Practical considerations favored individual theory and individual psychotherapy, both within "known" areas of theory and practice, but the observations suggested the family phenomenon was more complex than the interlocking of individual pathologies. Strict theoretical thinking favored a complete change to a family orientation but the initial "family" hypothesis was poorly developed and family psychotherapy seemed incomprehensible. Various combinations of individual and family orientation were considered but any combination plan contained drawbacks. For instance, experience suggested that any individual psychotherapy might obscure "family" observations. After much deliberation, and in spite of doubts that it could be successful, a decision was made to put the entire effort into family research observations, into extension of the family hypothesis, and into an attempt to develop a method of family psychotherapy and give it a fair trial "before returning to the individual orientation." Clinically, the idea was to include sufficient family members in the study to have the essential parts of the "family jigsaw puzzle" together at the same time and to attempt psychotherapy with all the "puzzle parts" present. The most serious doubts concerned the family psychotherapy. Because of orientation in psychoanalysis and individual psychotherapy, I believed the only way toward emotional maturity was careful analysis of the transference relationship between patient and therapist, and I assumed that the proposed "family psychotherapy" could be no more than preparation for eventual individual psychotherapy for each family member. Nevertheless, it was decided to discontinue all individual psychotherapy, and a method of family psychotherapy was devised to fit the clinical problem as defined by the theoretical premise.

The shift to the family orientation constituted a turning point that might not have been possible without the "total commitment" to the family. The family theoretical premise made it possible to "see" an exciting new dimension of clinical observations that had been obscured by individual theory. After a brief time it became evident that family psychotherapy had promising possibilities for the future. Some of the difficulties in the operation of a family orientation in an "individual" environment will be discussed later. This method of family psychotherapy has now been used for eight years with over 300 families. There have been 63 families with a schizophrenic family member in family psychotherapy for periods ranging from seven weeks to over seven years. This includes 51 families with one severely impaired adult schizophrenic offspring, ten families with a psychotic spouse, and two families with severely impaired young children diagnosed as suffering from autism or childhood schizophrenia.

Family Theory of Emotional Illness

It is difficult to conceptualize a family emotional oneness and even more difficult to communicate the idea to those whose focus on the individual makes it difficult for them really to "see" the family. I have used the term "undifferentiated family ego mass" to refer to the family emotional oneness. The term has certain inaccuracies but it aptly describes the over-all family dynamics, and no other term has been as effective in communicating the concept to others. I conceive of a fused cluster of egos of individual family members with a common ego boundary. Some egos are more completely fused into the mass than others. Certain egos are intensely involved in the family mass during emotional stress and are relatively detached at other times. The father and mother are always maximally involved. At times the ego mass may include only a small group of the most involved family members. At other times the active fusion may include members of the extended family network and even nonrelatives and pets. Live-in servants are often more "fused" into the family ego mass than certain blood relatives who are more differentiated. Sonne and Speck (1961) have included pets in family psychotherapy. The ego fusion is most intense in the least mature families. In a family with a schizophrenic family member, the fusion between father, mother, and child approaches maximum intensity. Theoretically, the fusion is present to some degree in all families except those in which family members have attained complete emotional maturity. In mature families, individual family members are contained emotional units who do not become involved in emotional fusions with others.

Clinically, the undifferentiated family ego mass is considered equivalent to a single ego. The family psychotherapy is directed to the family ego mass, without specific regard for the individuals involved in it at the time. The psychotherapist relates himself to the family ego mass in the same way that he relates himself to an individual ego in individual psychotherapy. The family members who are included in the family psychotherapy at any one time depend on the dynamics in the family ego mass and the immediate therapeutic goal. The therapist may approach the family ego mass with all involved family members present, with any combination of family members present, or with only one family member present. Family psychotherapy with a single family member is difficult to explain to those who use a different theoretical orientation. The family psychotherapist who relates to the family ego mass *through* a single family member employs a psychotherapeutic principle similar to that used in individual psychotherapy when the therapist relates himself to the "intact portion of the patient's ego" or to the "mature side of the ego." Since the two spouses (or parents) are the two family members most involved in the family ego mass, the most rapid family change occurs when the spouses are able to work as a team in family psychotherapy. The final stage of successful family psychotherapy includes the two spouses working together on their individual and joint problems.

According to the family theory of emotional illness, children grow up to achieve varying levels of differentiation of "self" from the undifferentiated family ego mass. Some achieve almost complete differentiation to become clearly defined individuals with well-defined ego boundaries. This is equivalent to our familiar concept of a mature person. These individuals are contained emotional units. Once differentiated, they can be emotionally close to their own family members, or to any other person, without fusing into new emotional onenesses: People tend to marry spouses who have identical levels of differentiation of self. When the well-differentiated person marries a spouse with an equally high level of identity, the spouses are able to maintain clear individuality and at the same time to have an intense, mature, nonthreatening emotional closeness. These spouses do not become involved in the fusion of "selfs" that occur in marriages of less differentiated spouses.

If the entire range of differentiation of self is considered on a single scale, with the highest level of differentiation of self and theoretical complete emotional maturity at the top and the lowest level of maladaptation and the severest forms of emotional illness at the bottom, the following would be the relative scale positions of the diagnostic categories that are pertinent to this presentation. The person who later develops a neurosis belongs somewhere in the middle of the scale, the person who later becomes the parent of a schizophrenic offspring belongs toward the lower end of the scale, and the person who later becomes schizophrenic belongs at the lower end as a "no self" who functions on a "self" borrowed from others.

People who become parents of a schizophrenic offspring illustrate an important facet of the theory. These are people with very low levels of differentiation of self who somehow manage to function fairly well in their life adjustments. As children, they do not begin the steady process of "growing away from their parents" as do their more differentiated siblings. Instead, they remain emotionally undifferentiated in the ego mass with their parents. After adolescence, in an effort to function without their parents, they "tear themselves away" to establish "pseudo selfs" with a "pseudo separation" from the parental ego mass. This may be achieved by denial while still living at home or it may be reinforced by physical distance. The young adult who runs away never to see his parents again may have more basic attachment to his parents than siblings who continue to live with the parents. The Achilles heel of these people is a close emotional relationship. They may function successfully in business or a profession as long as they keep relationships casual and brief, but in a marriage to a spouse with equally poor differentiation of self, they become overly involved emotionally. The new spouses fuse together into a new family ego mass in which the tenuous ego boundaries are obliterated. This is a replica of their former emotional fusions with their parents. This same process, on a less intense level, occurs in spouses with higher levels of differentiation of self, but the process is most striking in people who become parents of a schizophrenic offspring.

People who later become schizophrenic will illustrate one of the lowest levels of differentiation of self. The main difference here is that these people are never able to "tear themselves away" to achieve an adequate level of "pseudo self." They continue to function as dependent appendages of the family ego mass. Some achieve so little self that they collapse into psychosis during their first efforts to function independently of the parents. Some achieve sufficient "pseudo self" to function for brief periods alone, but any long-term separation from parents is accomplished only by finding a new family ego mass to which they can append themselves. Their life adjustment depends on the all-important attachment to others who will guide and advise them and from whom they can borrow enough self to function. They may make it through life without serious trouble but they are extremely vulnerable to the loss of the important other, and they can collapse into psychotic nothingness in the face of life events that threaten or disrupt their dependent attachments.

An important point in family theory is the fusion that takes places in a newly married husband and wife into a new family ego mass. This is most intense in spouses with low levels of differentiation of self. Both spouses long for closeness but closeness results in fusion of the two "pseudo selfs" into a "common self," with obliteration of ego boundaries between them and loss of individuality to the "common self." To avoid the anxiety of fusion, they keep sufficient emotional distance, called the "emotional divorce," for each to maintain as much "pseudo self" as possible. In general, the course of the new family ego mass is determined by (1) the pattern of dynamics within the ego mass and by (2) relationships to those outside the ego mass. Dynamics *within the ego mass* are determined by the way the spouses fight for, or share, the ego strength available to them. One spouse usually functions with a dominant share of the ego strength. At one end of the scale are marriages in which both spouses "fight for their rights." A conflictual marriage results. The conflict subsides when either "gives in." In the middle group are the marriages in which differences are resolved by one spouse who reluctantly "gives in." The spouse who gives in "loses strength" to the other who "gains strength." At the other end of the scale are the marriages in which one spouse works actively to be the dependent one who gives in, becoming a "no self" who supports the strengthened self of the other. A spouse who habitually "gives in" can reach a state of sufficient "no self" to become incapacitated with (a) physical illness, (b) emotional illness or (c) social dysfunction, such as work inefficiency, drinking, or social irresponsibility. A marriage might become permanently stabilized with the "no self" spouse disabled with a chronic illness.

Relationships to those outside the family ego mass determine the intensity and extensiveness of the emotional phenomenon within the family ego mass. The important outside relationships are usually to relatives in the extended family network, but nonrelatives can serve the same function. When outside relationships are not too intense, the emotional intensity within the ego mass is toned down. When outside relationships become intense, the problems within the ego mass are "transmitted" to the outside person who then becomes fused into the family ego mass. Spouses may maintain their most important relationships to the past generation, their parents; to the present generation, their siblings; or to the future generation, their children. A small percentage of spouses keep their problems almost completely contained within a small area. For example, there are marriages with intense problems almost completely contained between the spouses, with intense marital conflict or one chronically ill spouse, and with little or no involvement of their children. There are also marriages in which the full weight of the parental problem is transmitted to a single, maximally impaired child, leaving the parental relationship calm and harmonious. In the average family the spouses maintain important outside relationships in more than one area and the problem is "spread" over a larger area of the family relationship system.

Schizophrenia develops in a family in which the parents have a low level of differentiation of self and in which a high level of the parental impairment is transmitted to one or more of their children. The important variables in the process are (1) the severity of the problem in the parental ego mass and (2) the degree to which the parental impairment is transmitted to a single child or is "spread" to multiple children or to other relationships in the extended family. For instance, a less severe parental problem transmitted to a single child would produce more severe schizophrenia than a very severe parental problem "spread" to multiple children. Schizophrenia is viewed as the product of a family process in which a child in each generation is more impaired than the parents (children less involved in the process may have higher levels of differentiation of self than the parents). The process repeats for several generations until there is an offspring with a low level of differentiation of self, who, in a marriage, will have sufficient impairment in the parental ego mass to produce schizophrenia in a child. In a previous paper (Bowen, 1960), I hypothesized that it requires three or more generations for schizophrenia to develop. That hypothesis, based on the family concept of schizophrenia, considered that the three-generation process can proceed from fairly well-adjusted parents in the first generation to schizophrenia in the third generation if the parents transmit a major part of the parental problem to a single child in each generation. In most situations there are varying degrees of "spread" in the transmission process, which requires more than three generations for the development of schizophrenia. In this presentation it is not possible to consider variables in families with multiple psychotic offspring, nor the variables operative in divorce, death, and other serious family disruptions.

The Family Projection Process in Schizophrenia

This section will be devoted to the predominant mechanism in schizophrenia, the mechanism through which the parental problem is transmitted to the child. The process can begin long before the child is conceived, when the mother's thoughts, feelings, and fantasies first begin to prepare a place in her life for the child. We can wonder if the pattern of the mother's thinking and fantasies came from her own mother! The process takes a definite form during the mother's pregnancy and it continues through the years with different manifestations in different life stages. The child functions as a stabilizer for the parents, converting the unstable father-mother ego mass into a more stable triad. Parental stability depends on the child functioning as the "triadic one."[3] The child needs parents as stable as possible. His existence is so involved in "being for the parents" that he has no "self" of his own. The parents are made anxious by events that threaten to remove the child from his stabilizing function in the triad, such as "growing away" or "moving away."

---

[3] The one who develops schizophrenia is conventionally referred to as "the psychotic one," "the schizophrenic one," or "the patient." I prefer to use the term "triadic one" because it designates one component part of the family ego mass.

The triadic emotional process is adaptive and it can re-establish itself after most threats. One of the greatest threats is the psychotic collapse which prevents the usual functioning of the triadic one, but the process can even survive this threat and continue with the parents living at home and the triadic one institutionalized as a permanent ward of the state.

The term "family projection process" refers to the mechanisms that operate as the parents and the child play active parts in the transmission of the parental problem to the child. To account for the process with individual theory, it would be necessary to postulate "projection" by the parents and "introjection" by the child. The parents may force the projection against resistance until the child finally accepts the projection, but most often the parents initiate the projection and the child accepts it. Or the child may initiate the projection and coerce the parents to agree that he is the cause of the family problem. The terms "blamer" and "self-blamer" describe one aspect of the projection process. On one axis of functioning, people divide themselves into "blamers" and "self-blamers." In a tension situation, both look for causes to explain the situation. The blamer looks outside of self; his perceptual system is attuned to finding the causes in the other or in the environment, and he is incapable of looking inside of self. The self-blamer accurately perceives causes in self but he is as impaired at looking outside himself as the blamer is at looking inside of self.

The *real* cause of any situation is probably a combination of internal and external factors. Theoretically, a mature person can objectively evaluate both the internal and external factors and *be responsible for the part self plays*. The more immature the people, the more intense the blaming and self-blaming. The following example illustrates one aspect of the projection process. Persons A and B are equally responsible for an embarrassing situation. Person A begins thinking, "If I had not been so awkward, this would not have happened." At the very same moment, B is thinking, "Look at the mess caused by A's awkwardness." The process is completed without a word being exchanged. Both blame A, both are blind to the part played by B, and both act as if their diagnosis is accurate. Under certain circumstances the blamer can become self-blamer and the self-blamer a vehement blamer. The schizophrenic person is predominantly a self-blamer. He can even feel himself to be the cause of floods, storms, and earthquakes. When he reaches an overload of self-blaming he can erupt into blaming. The self-blamer is as irresponsible as the blamer in assuming responsibility for self.

The parental problem is most often projected to the child by the mother, with the father supporting her viewpoint. She is an immature person with deep feelings of inadequacy who looks outside herself for the cause of her anxiety. The projection goes into fears and worries about the health and adequacy of the child. The projection searches out small inadequacies, defects, and functional failures in the child, focuses on them, and enlarges and exaggerates them into major deficiencies. There are three main steps in each episode in the projection process. These steps are important in the later treatment of schizophrenia. The first is a *feeling-thinking* step. It begins with a *feeling* in the mother which merges into *thinking* about defects in the child. The second is the *examining-labeling* step in which she searches for and diagnoses a defect in the child that best fits her feeling state. This is the "clinical examination-diagnosis" step. The third step is the *treating* step in which she acts toward and treats the child as though her diagnosis is accurate. The projection system can create its own defects. For instance, the mother *feels* and *thinks* about the child as a baby (there is an infantile self in the most mature of us), she *calls* him a baby and she *treats* him as though he is a baby. When the child accepts the projection, he *becomes* more infantile. The projection is fed by the mother's anxiety. When the cause for her anxiety is located outside of the mother, the anxiety subsides. For the child, accepting the projection as a reality is a small price to pay for a calmer mother. Now the child *is* a little more inadequate. Each time he accepts another projection, he adds to his increasing state of functional inadequacy.

The projection system can also utilize existing minor defects. Some of these require an examination and diagnosis by an expert to confirm the presence of the defect. Parents can go from one physician to another until the "feared" defect is finally confirmed by diagnosis. Any defect discovered in physical examinations, laboratory tests, and psychological tests can also facilitate the projection process. The family projection can pour into a newly discovered innocuous congenital anomaly and convert it to a disability. The important function of the process is to locate and confirm that the "cause" is outside the mother. One need listen to such a mother only a few minutes to hear her invoke outside opinions, diagnoses, and tests to validate the projection.

The projection process reaches a critical stage when the triadic one collapses into psychosis and can no longer function as the absorber of the family projection. Family anxiety is usually high. It is not the psychosis itself that causes the family anxiety but the inability of this triadic one to continue his usual function in the triad. Family anxiety is less intense when the psychosis develops slowly or the psychotic one is quiet and cooperative and continues to serve the purposes of parental projection. Parents may not even seek help for the quiet psychotic one unless urged by some outside person or agency. The intense anxiety occurs when the psychotic collapse is sudden and the psychotic one not only rebels against accepting the projection but turns into a vehement "blamer" who denies the existence of a problem, while, in addition, causing problems with irresponsible behavior.

The three steps of the family projection process come into prominence when the family seeks psychiatric help for the psychotic collapse. Parental anxiety motivates an increased drive to call the triadic one "sick," to confirm the sickness with a diagnosis, and to start a treatment program. When the diagnosis is confirmed and the triadic one becomes a "patient," another family projection is completed and parental anxiety subsides. *The step into mental illness is probably the most critical in the long series of family projection crises.* One of the important theoretical and psychotherapeutic propositions of the family theory revolves around this point. The usual psychiatric approach is to examine the patient, confirm the presence of the pathology with a diagnosis, and recommend appropriate treatment. The psychiatric consultation fits, step by step, with the family projection process. Thus, a time-proven principle of good medical practice serves to support the parental projection process in the family, to crystallize and fix emotional illness in the patient, and to help make the illness chronic and irreversible. A therapeutic approach to this dilemma, based on the family theory of emotional illness, is described in the next section of this chapter.

Many years of successful parental projection precede the step into mental illness. In some families the groundwork is so complete and the family members are so fixed in their functioning positions[4] that "the step" does little more than officially note what has already come to be. In these families the triadic one readily accepts the projection and the new designation "patient" and the working contract between family and psychiatrist is one in which the psychiatrist assumes responsibility for the end product of the long family projection process. The chances of modifying the family process are remote. In other families "the step" is bigger, the triadic one opposes the diagnosis and the designation "patient," and, if the psychiatrist avoids supporting the parental side of the projection, the prognosis for modifying the family process is better. Functionally, "the step" is one in which the family problem is projected into the triadic

[4] The term "role" as defined by Spiegel (1960) might be more accurate than "functioning positions" but I have not been able consistently to adapt role concepts to this work. Rather than permit loose and inconsistent use of role theory, other descriptive terms have been used.

one and fixed there with a diagnosis. When the psychiatrist accepts the responsibility for treating the illness in "the patient," he condones the externalization of the parental problem to the patient, assumes responsibility for the patient (the family problem separated from the family), and permits the parents to continue projecting onto the patient, without holding the parents responsible and accountable for the consequences of their projection. The parents often become students of emotional illness and use psychiatric terms and concepts to better facilitate the projection to the patient. Thus, our usual psychiatric approach to the treatment of the psychoses is one in which the family, the patient, the psychiatrist, and society all play a part in "acting out" and perpetuating the family projection, in turning the problem in the patient into a chronic one, and in creating a situation which permits the family projection to continue long after the patient has become the permanent responsibility of the state. There are outpatient situations in which the psychiatrist is even more effective in facilitating the family projection process. For instance, individual psychotherapy with a "patient" still living with his parents may support the patient sufficiently for him to continue as an unusually effective absorber of the parental projection.

A final clinical characteristic of the family projection process that is important to this presentation is the lack of responsibility for "self" in those who participate in the projection process. A "blamer" who projects his problem to others is not responsible for self. The "self-blamer" is equally irresponsible. He blames himself to relieve anxiety and not to assume responsibility for himself. Our concept "disease" and "illness" conceives of the problem as a dysfunction determined by forces beyond the control or the responsibility of the family.

Clinical Efforts to Modify the Family Projection Process in the Hospital and in Private Practice

The ward milieu program and the family psychotherapy were both designed to modify the family projection process. This section is devoted to clinical management of the three steps in the family projection process: (1) *thinking* of the triadic one as sick, (2) *diagnosing* the triadic one and designating him "patient," and (3) *treating* the "patient" as a sick person. Also included in this section will be a clinical discussion of *responsibility*. The clinical effort was to *think* and *act* toward the families according to the family orientation. This meant avoiding the concepts "sick," "illness," and "patient" and avoiding the use of diagnoses and treating the triadic one (or any other family member) as a sick person. It was not possible to achieve more than partial success with the live-in families, but the effort provided much knowledge about schizophrenia and the experience has been invaluable in subsequent family psychotherapy. A review of the clinical effort with the live-in families will provide another view of the differences between individual and family theory and a glimpse of the depth of change involved in a shift to family theory and family psychotherapy.

Social custom, laws governing sickness and mental illness, and our most basic, time-proven principles of medical practice are all oriented around the individual theory of disease. Medical practice and hospital structure adhere strictly to "sickness-patient-diagnosis-treatment" principles. Any small deviation from standard procedure can cause a reaction within a medical or hospital organization. In this study, which was carried out in a research hospital, permitting some flexibility in operation not possible in a strict medical service institution, an effort was made to anticipate the issues that would arise in the research and to arrange as much "research freedom" as possible from the enforced use of individual principles and procedures. The hospital administration was interested in helping to facilitate the research, but when issues were better defined, it became clear that a medical administrator can "interpret" but not change medical structure. Other than the flexibility permitted for any research, and certain favorable interpretations by the hospital administration, the research operated according to routine medical structure. I, as project administrator, was responsible and accountable to the hospital for every item of individual procedure. Within the confines of the ward, a different milieu was established. Numerous people have said that this research should not have been done in a hospital because of the traditional attitudes of hospitals about sickness. On the other hand, the very same issues are involved even in the private practice of family psychotherapy through a similar attitude to illness on the part of the legal and medical institutions of society. For example, dangerous acting out by one psychotic family member can threaten the therapist with medical-legal breach of responsibility; the charge may be made that the psychotic should have been considered a patient requiring hospitalization.

Some problems were encountered during the first year before the family orientation was started. Three mothers and three patients participated in the study. The mothers were permitted either to room with the patient, or to live outside and spend daytime hours with the patient. One mother chose to room with her daughter; the other two chose to live outside. Emphasis was placed on the "presence" of the mothers. They were not required to function as mothers. The live-in mother was required to fulfill the administrative requirements for "patients," and though she was diagnosed "Normal Control" and her patient status was toned down, she was still a "patient." The other mothers had privileges to eat on the ward and to participate in hospital activities. They were expected to assume some responsibility for the care of the patient but these mothers were never responsibly involved in the study. The staff was responsible for the patients and the mothers were privileged "visitors." The system actually permitted the mothers an ideal situation for carefree projection of their problems to the patients; they could be irresponsible in upsetting the patient and return home, telling the nurse, "*Your* patient is upset." The treatment results were rather good by usual individual standards but individual psychotherapy kept the family problems divided. Critical issues could be avoided by each expecting the other to deal with the issue, and no family went beyond the passive attitude of cooperating while waiting to be changed.

With the shift to the family orientation, all family members were required to live in. The parents and normal siblings were diagnosed "Normal Control" and the psychotic family members "Schizophrenia." Family members had all the records and routine procedures required for "patients." Freedom for fathers to continue their regular work and for other family members to participate in outside activity was permitted by routine 72-hour "patient" passes. Absences over 72 hours required a discharge and a new admission. The maintenance of the project in a hospital required innumerable admissions, discharges, physical examinations, and routine laboratory studies to meet the requirements of good medical care for patients. The administrative structure permitted short cuts in administrative steps but it did not permit elimination of steps.

An important part of the clinical program to deal with the family projection process was the requirement that the parents be responsible for the psychotic family member. The doctors and nursing staff would be available to help the parents but not to assume direct responsibility for the "patients." One parent was required to be with the "patient" at all times. When both parents were away from the ward at the same time they would ask the nurses to be responsible for the "patients." It was almost two years before the staff achieved a reasonable working version of the clinical program. There were three main areas of difficulty in implementing the plan.

The first area of difficulty had to do with the individual medical orientation of the staff. It was second nature for staff members to think in terms of the individual, to "assume responsibility for the patient," and to "feel with" the patient and be angry at the parents. It required time and intimate exposure to the families for the staff to *know* the family orientation. Early efforts to change concepts and terms were no more than "play acting." Shortly after the staff began to avoid the use of the word "patient," the head nurse protested the emptiness of changing words; three years later she wrote a paper, "The Patient Is the Family" (Kvarnes, 1959). Among the terms that replaced "sick," "illness," and "schizophrenia" were "dysfunction," "incapacity," and "functional collapse." Among the terms that replaced "patient" were "impaired one," "disabled one," "collapsed one," and "triadic one." In due time, the family orientation became almost as comfortable as the old, especially when families began to respond favorably to the family approach.

The second area of difficulty was intimately connected with the first. The hospital administration required an individual orientation, in conflict with the policy of the research ward administration. The staff complied with the minimal individual requirements of the hospital, but within the ward the staff attempted to think and act the family orientation. The hospital designated each family member a "patient" and required the physicians to be responsible for "patients" under their care. Within the ward there were "family members" instead of "patients" and parents were required to be responsible for all members of their families. The families understood the two orientations and they became students of the fine points of difference between them.

The third area of difficulty was within the families. The family projection process is forceful. It has an amazing capacity to utilize existing structure to project the problem to the triadic one and to make the environment responsible for the externalized problem. When the staff no longer accepted as much responsibility for emotional functioning in the families, the family process found new ways to make the staff responsible. Since the physician was responsible for the physical health of his "patients," an increasing number of family problems became manifested as physical illness, and families overused the ward physician and medical structure to make the staff responsible. Finally the staff developed a system equivalent to a physician in private practice. A "clinic" with regular office hours was established on the ward, and for routine problems, the families made clinic appointments. The family living quarters (twin bedrooms on the ward) were equivalent to private homes. Family members went to the "clinic" for consultation and returned to the "home" where they were responsible for following the recommended treatment. Families were provided with supplies of most drugs to be kept in their "homes." This kind of an arrangement would not have been possible in any but a research setting.

One series of events will convey much about the "responsibility" problem. Parents were free to take the "patients" into the community "when they were capable of controlling the psychotic behavior." They could ask a staff person to accompany them if they doubted their ability to manage the situation. There were frequent complaints from merchants, local citizens, and from other departments in the hospital reporting disturbing behavior. Each incident was discussed with the families. The families would "explain away" the incidents by calling them fusses or disagreements; by blaming the public's lack of understanding about emotional illness; by diagnosing the complainant as an upset, touchy, neurotic person; or by a discussion of whether or not the complaint was justified. The families would promise to try harder. The staff went through a period of being overhelpful to the families in specifying off-limits areas and in helping them to understand and deal with disturbed behavior. The frequency of incidents remained the same except that they occurred in unusual places or in circumstances that "you did not tell us about." Finally came the awareness that the staff attitude played a part in the problem. In providing help and instruction, the staff doubted the parents' ability to find their own solutions. The families had been scolded for their mistakes but they had not been told exactly what was required.

When we became aware of this, the families were told that the research project required the parents to assume responsibility for the disturbed family members and that they had considerable freedom to go and come in the community as long as they could control the behavior of disturbed family members. They were reminded that we lived in a community where people had the same fears and concerns about mental illness as people everywhere, that we had a responsibility to the community, and that the goal was the prevention of complaints, whether justified or unjustified. The families were told that they were held responsible for learning the rules of the community and the hospital and that a condition for continued participation in the research project was that there be no complaints about disturbed behavior off the ward. Complaints from the hospital and the community stopped. The formerly irresponsible parents became overly responsible. When the disturbed family members became upset, the parents initiated their own systems of control. When an upset became too great, the family might ask permission of the other families to lock the ward for a few days until the upset subsided. This experience, now confirmed by other subsequent experiences, provided evidence that the parents of a schizophrenic offspring, who commonly function as helpless and irresponsible people, have the capacity to function responsibly when it is required. My own functioning as project director played an important part. I had assumed responsibility, with the hospital administration, for stopping the incidents, and when I functioned more responsibly, it was possible to require families to be responsible. Interestingly, it was during the periods when the parents were functioning responsibly that families made the most progress in the daily family psychotherapy meetings.

The live-in families provided a unique and rewarding research experience but a live-in environment is not the most favorable for change in family psychotherapy. It was possible for families to assume a fairly good level of responsibility for the psychotic family member but the parents became overdependent on the hospital resources available to them, which precluded development of their own resources. Family psychotherapy has been more successful with families responsible for the care of the psychotic one in the home.

Clinical results in dealing with the family projection process have been best in outpatient work and private practice. The process that drives toward "sickness-patient-diagnosis-treatment" issues is fed by anxiety. In the early clinical efforts I too often found myself opposing the projection process. The most profitable approach has been to avoid becoming entangled in the issues of the family projection process and to direct attention to the parental anxiety that feeds the projection. A few hours spent with one or both parents is often enough to relieve the immediate anxiety and convert the situation into a calm, productive, family psychotherapeutic effort. When family anxiety is very high and it is not possible to avoid the sickness-diagnosis issues of the projection process, I state my theoretical position as clearly as possible and quietly refuse to participate in action designed to fix the problem in the patient, or I refuse to continue working with the family unless parents are willing to assume some responsibility for their part in the problem.

The issues in the family projection process come into clear focus with the proposed first hospitalization for an acute psychotic disturbance, especially when the psychotic person is protesting that he is not sick and the projection process is insisting on a diagnosis and hospitalization. Much is gained if a diagnosis and hospitalization can be avoided and the projection process can be modified before the family takes this additional major step in confirming emotional illness. If hospitalization is necessary, I prefer that it be for reasons other than "sickness." The following describes my current approach to the situation in outpatient work and private practice. There are three main reasons for hospitalization: (1) The family demands it because the family has reached a tolerance for the disturbance in the home. (2) The community demands it because of offenses to the community. (3) The disturbed person requests it for himself. The first reason is the important one for this presentation. When hospitalization is the issue, the family expects the psychiatrist to use illness as the reason for hospitalization. With this approach, the patient is told that he is sick and he must be hospitalized for treatment. With the psychiatrist responsible for the hospitalization, the family tells the patient, "We are sorry you are sick and have to go to the hospital. You will get good treatment there. When you are well, we want you home." According to a family approach, this sequence contains reality distortions. The first is the concept "sick" and "hospital." The degree of "sickness" is not the real reason for hospitalization. Families keep severe degrees of "sickness" at home as long as the person behaves himself. The real reason is that the family wants the disturbing behavior removed from the home. Hospitalization is more for the family than the patient. Another distortion is, "When you are *well.*" This really means, "When you no longer disturb the family."

An impaired ego can deal with hard facts of misbehavior, but it has more difficulty with the reality distortions in "sickness" reasons. A resisting person's ego does not perceive "sickness" with his own perceptual system, and he is at a disadvantage when hospitalized for a reason he cannot perceive within himself. If he insists on his own perception that he is not "sick," he is uncooperative and in conflict with his environment. If he accepts the "sickness" reason, he agrees to something he cannot perceive within himself and he becomes dependent on the environment to teach him about "sickness." There have been amazing benefits when the family assumes responsibility for hospitalization and uses "behavior" as the reason. If the situation permits, I will spend days or weeks on this one point before I will hospitalize a person for "sickness." To illustrate, one psychotic son had been resisting hospitalization for several weeks. The effort was directed at helping the parents use "the family" as the reason. When the mother finally said, "Will you go for us, to give us some relief?" the son calmly replied, "That's the first fair proposition I've heard. I am ready to sign myself in any time." The family can use force, such as, "We are sending you to the hospital because we are fed up with your behavior and the problems you create at home," without the complications and penalties that can come from using "sickness" as the reason. In these circumstances the patients approach the hospital differently, their progress is usually rapid, and hospital stays are brief. A clinical case illustrating some of these points is presented in the next section.

The principles that apply to the "sickness" concept are applicable in many areas not specifically related to the family projection process. The following example is from a situation that did not involve a family. A recovering hospitalized patient was permitted his first pass into town. As he started to step into the bus to return to the hospital, he became immobilized, for voices threatened dire consequences if he stepped on the bus. He was delaying the bus in heavy traffic, and the bus company complained to the hospital about "patients too sick to go to town." His doctor restricted him to the hospital because of "behavior" instead of "sickness." He was told that he was restricted because of his "behavior" at the bus stop, and when he was able to behave in a way that did not call attention to himself or interfere with others, he could try again. Within a week he had another town pass and shortly thereafter he was discharged to return to his job. Later in his psychotherapy he reconstructed the series of events. After his restriction, he spent days practicing ways to behave normally in spite of the voices. He became so successful at this that he returned to work while the voices were still present. The restriction for behavior provided him with something he could understand, that he could work on, and that he could change. If restricted for "sickness," over which he had no control, he might have had no choice but to wait and hope the sickness would go away.

Much effort has gone into avoiding the concepts of "sick" and "patient" and the use of "diagnoses," although this effort may seem unrealistic when the triadic one is so disabled and impaired. How valid is the effort and what are the results? I have not yet seen a family projection process completely resolved in a family with severe schizophrenia. When the family is calm, the process can disappear from view, but if anxiety builds up again, the process appears again. Occasionally, parents can be successful in controlling their side of the process, only to have the triadic one begin acting inadequate and impaired in a way that forces them to recognize his "petition for sickness." The schizophrenic person is not oriented to becoming "normal" and he plays an important part in perpetuating the status quo. Mendell (1958) has used a different approach to the dilemma of diagnosing only the patient. He does psychological tests on all key family members which are then used as authoritative evidence to substantiate a diagnosis on all family members. Each "sick" person is then treated in group psychotherapy but with each family member in a different group.

It is with problems less severe than schizophrenia that avoiding "sick-patient-diagnoses" is of direct benefit in helping the family ego mass toward a higher level of differentiation of self. When the family achieves a higher level of differentiation, the projection process disappears permanently. The following is one of innumerable such examples. A husband in his mid-30's had four years of fairly successful psychoanalysis for paralyzing obsessions and phobias that had forced him to give up his work. During his analysis, his wife had a period of psychotherapy. The husband returned to work and became fairly successful but he was a "compensated neurotic" with his sickness under control. The wife was the adequate one who protected him from upsetting situations. In a later period of marital conflict, the wife sought further psychiatric help. The husband refused to participate and the wife began family psychotherapy alone. Her thinking-feeling system was totally occupied with the husband's "neurosis." Early in the family psychotherapy, she was asked if she could stop thinking of him as neurotic, stop calling him neurotic, and stop treating him as an impaired person. She responded, "Okay, but what other term do I use? Do you have a better term?" It was suggested that she "play like" he was not sick, or weak, or neurotic. The suggestion seemed to have missed its mark. About two months later she said, "I have been working on that idea. I no longer call him neurotic or treat him like a neurotic, but for the life of me I cannot stop thinking of him as neurotic." The husband responded to her change with a campaign to act helpless, to call himself neurotic, and to plead with her to mother his helplessness. She refused to give in to his demands. He became angry, accused her of not loving him, and went into a week of individualistic, "I do not need you." Then he joined her in the family psychotherapy and they went on to a good resolution of their problem. From the beginning of their marriage, the husband had been either a potential "patient," an actual "patient," or a compensated "patient," and the wife had been a "mother" to his varying degrees of incapacity. Now for the first time, they were free of the problem and able to be two adult people in their marriage.

Principles and Techniques of Family Psychotherapy

The first structured family psychotherapy was with the live-in families in the research study. Both parents, the schizophrenic offspring, and the normal siblings attended the psychotherapy hours together. This was a nondirective psychotherapy in which the family members "worked together on the family problem." The therapist functioned as a catalyst to facilitate the working together and as a participant observer who was sufficiently detached to observe objectively and interpret the family process. The psychotherapy followed a definite course. The normal siblings soon found reason to separate themselves from the family effort, leaving the father, mother, and psychotic one interlocked in an intense emotional interdependence, which I have called the "interdependent triad." Change within the triad was slow and it appeared to go toward differentiation into three distinct selfs. One parent would pull up to a more confident level of functioning and appear to develop a better defined self with a higher level of identity. Then the other parent would go through the same process, and then the triadic one would appear to "grow up a little." These cycles could take as long as a year. It was hoped the cyclical course would continue until all three emerged as well-differentiated individuals. This did not occur. Some families would continue through a few cycles and stop the psychotherapy during an asymptomatic period or use an angry family incident as a reason to stop. Some families would progress very rapidly for a few months and stop suddenly when symptoms were less troublesome.

A series of experiences led to a modification of the effort to follow the triad through to differentiation. The following is a good example: The daughter, in her late twenties, had spent most of the previous six years in institutions. The father, mother, and daughter attended psychotherapy hours together. Progress was rapid. Within six months the daughter was working and within a year she was on as high a level of confident, adequate functioning as I have ever seen in recovery from schizophrenia. She was free of guilt and defensiveness about the psychotic period. The intensity of the parental relationship pattern (aggressive, anxious mother and compliant father) had receded into the background and the parents were calm and productive. The daughter talked of moving from the parental home to her own apartment and the parents "agreed" with the idea. The daughter asked about "individual" psychotherapy for herself but the plan implied that the parents would stop their participation and the therapist discouraged it. All three continued the psychotherapy together. The day the daughter announced definite plans to move, the formerly calm parents became anxious, pleading, attacking, and helpless, and the old family projection process was back in its full intensity. The daughter decided to "give up her own life goals" for a time "to help her parents." Slowly the daughter's functioning began to fail and within six months she had lost her job and was back in another severe regression. After another ten months she was returned to an institution. This is an example of family reaction when the triadic one attempts to separate self from the parents. Confronted by the parental anxiety, the budding self of the triadic one rushed back into the family ego mass "to save the parents." In recent years, the psychotherapy has been modified to help the family through this separation crisis. As soon as parents and triadic one are aware of the part that each plays in the family process, the parents are seen together with the explicit goal of helping them to separate their lives from the triadic one, and the triadic one is seen alone with the explicit goal of helping him to function without the parents and to resist his automatic emotional "reflex" to "save the parents" (to become the parental projection object) when they are anxious. Results have been better with this approach but it involves a more "supportive" relationship to each side of the family and the basic level of differentiation of self does not change.

The family ego mass in severe schizophrenia is not only an "undifferentiated" family ego mass but in my experience it is "undifferentiatable." I have not yet seen a reasonable resolution of the basic problem in a family with severe schizophrenia. The emotional oneness in schizophrenia is over and beyond other emotional ties. The child is emotionally "welded" into the ego mass with the parents, where he functions as an "ego nothing" which permits the parents to be an "ego something." These three people can be physically separated but it appears impossible for any one to differentiate a "self" from the other two. With the triadic one living away from home in dependent attachments that do not involve the parents, all three members of the triad are more comfortable. The parents function by "borrowing self" from outside themselves and by "projecting their inadequacies" to others. In this situation, the parents perceive no problem within themselves and they have no motivation for family psychotherapy. If the threesome is reunited, the old emotional fusion of the triad is immediately operative again.

The orderly "differentiation of self" from the family ego mass does occur in a wide range of problems less severe than schizophrenia. The differentiation process is most rapid with problems of neurotic degree. The parents can proceed to differentiate selfs from their children (with spontaneous change in the children), from their parents, and from each other; they can attain high levels of identity. The more severe the family problem, the more likely the family to terminate the psychotherapy after symptomatic improvement, as occurs in families with schizophrenia. However, there have been families with transient or borderline psychotic problems in a family member in which family psychotherapy has continued to "differentiation of selfs" from the family ego mass. My goal has been to find a way for complete resolution of the underlying problem in severe schizophrenia. Some families have continued in family psychotherapy for five to seven years with reasonably symptom-free adjustments but no change in the basic problem. In the past three years there has been an effort to involve certain key members of the extended family in the family psychotherapy to add more "strength" to the family ego mass. This effort is too new to report here but initial results appear promising.

Although family psychotherapy has not been successful in resolving the underlying problem in severe schizophrenia, it has been effective in helping families achieve asymptomatic adjustments without changing the underlying problem. The following is an example of a good asymptomatic adjustment with brief family psychotherapy: A 45-year-old mother was in her second acute psychotic episode. For the first episode she had been hospitalized for a year, given electroshock therapy and psychotherapy, and then received two years of outpatient psychotherapy. The second psychotic episode occurred three years later. The husband was anxious and solicitous in relating to the wife's overactive and bizarre thinking and behavior. The wife reacted to his reactions with an increase in psychotic symptoms. The husband agreed to try family psychotherapy with the wife living at home. The husband worked to make the wife's illness the responsibility of the therapist, while he continued to project his anxiety onto her. My effort was to focus on the husband's anxiety, to avoid direct responsibility for the wife's illness, and to hold the husband responsible for the family problem. He did have considerable responsibility with the wife at home, and after two weeks he asked that she be hospitalized because she was "too sick" to remain at home. I maintained the position that home was best for the wife but that he could go toward hospitalization if he had reached his tolerance for the stress at home. He asked a relative to help him supervise the wife's behavior. When the relative became "fed up" with the situation, he asked if I would give the wife "shock treatment." I refused to participate in "shock treatment," and there was an exchange about what kind of "shock" he meant. On his own initiative, he began a very firm management program in which the wife's "privileges" were determined by her ability to control her own behavior. Within ten days the psychotic symptoms had disappeared, and the "perfect result," which the family praises highly, has continued five years. The family had fourteen hours of family psychotherapy over a period of seven weeks.

The following family, who fell within the range of impairment in which complete differentiation of selfs is possible, illustrates several important principles and techniques of family psychotherapy. In this case the family projection process was countered by avoiding hospitalization. Another important principle is illustrated by the technique of conducting family therapy by temporarily seeing only one family member. This was a family with an acutely disturbed 17-year-old son with a problem of borderline psychotic degree who had been an increasing behavior problem since adolescence. His school adjustment had always been poor and the schools had long been involved in diagnosing and understanding the problem, in arranging special programs, and in several recommendations for psychotherapy. The parents attempted to deal with the behavior problems with "discipline," which was really angry retaliation against misbehavior. The son reacted to this with violent, angry outbursts which frightened the parents. The son opposed the parental projection by calling the parents "sick." The psychotherapy efforts had never gone beyond psychiatric consultation because the son insisted he was not "sick" and the parents were immobilized because the son would not cooperate.

In the weeks before the referral, the son's anxiety had increased until he was aloof from the family and was spending afternoons and nights wandering in the community. He was unkempt, his behavior and dress were bizarre, he appeared to be hallucinating, and he was less able to follow simple school routines. He frightened some teachers and certain people in the community. When the school suggested that he be hospitalized, the father sought help in arranging hospitalization. I did not agree with the plan for immediate hospitalization and instead offered family psychotherapy evaluation interviews. The son insisted that his only problem was his parents and he had no need for a psychiatrist. The parents were extremely anxious but they were willing to proceed with family psychotherapy for themselves and to leave the son out of the family effort until he expressed a positive wish for psychotherapy. The son's acting out at school and in the community did not appear too great to risk a family psychotherapy effort. The school agreed to "wait and see" what happened, misinterpreting the therapist's recommendation that the boy not be hospitalized to mean that he should remain in school.

A few days later the school reported that some teachers were frightened by the boy's behavior. The school had long followed the usual steps in the family projection process of *thinking* about, *diagnosing*, and *treating* the son as "sick." The school was reminded that the therapist did not recommend that the boy remain in school and was urged to make decisions on the basis of behavior instead of "sickness," sending the boy home if his behavior did not meet school rules. Some teachers feared it would "hurt" the son to make him deal with reality; they preferred excusing his behavior on the basis that it was "sick." Other teachers, pleased with permission to deal with behavior instead of worrying about "sickness," took firmer reality stands, with considerable benefit to the situation.

The parents made little progress in their first family psychotherapy hours together. Their anxiety was high and thoughts went only to inadequacies in the son. In spite of this, the son's anxiety subsided and within two weeks there were no further complaints from the school or the community. The son expressed pleasure that the parents were finally working on their problem. In the psychotherapy, the parents were in so much basic disagreement about the son that their "selfs" neutralized each other. Their effort ended in the same "selfless" lack of direction that characterized the home environment. It was suggested that one parent try the psychotherapy alone and that they decide which one it should be. During the next six months, the mother was the only family member to attend the family psychotherapy hours. Since the effort in these situations is to help one parent work toward a higher level of identity, the mother was encouraged to define a "self," to become clear about her own beliefs and convictions, and especially to maintain a stand on important family issues without losing "self" in the family emotional field. The mother did well at this, and one fairly definite "self" began to emerge from the "selfless mass" of the family. For the first time the mother began to deal with distraught family situations by controlling her own "self" instead of trying to change the "self" of others.

Within a few months the son's behavior was "almost normal" at school and in the community, but his problem was being acted out within the family. Generally, it is a hopeful sign when acting out in the community shifts back within the family. While the mother was more occupied with her own problem and was less involved in family problems, the father began to "feel with" the son's problems. There was a brief period of closeness between father and son, followed by conflict. The father became a strict "disciplinarian," to which the son reacted with aggressive acting out directed specifically at the father.

The next phase of the psychotherapy began some eight months after the start of the family psychotherapy when the exasperated father demanded the family psychotherapy time for himself. He reported that the family situation was worse than it had ever been, but after a few hours he began to define a "self" and a position for himself in the family. He made more rapid progress than the mother. After a brief period, his thoughts, feelings, and actions were directed more to the mother than the son. About three months after he started, there was a period of overt conflict between the parents. The parents quickly joined forces and began another period of projection of the family problem to the son. The parental conflict subsided and the son went into another period of regression and irresponsible behavior confined within the family. The parents became angry at the son who was still calling them "sick" and who made no effort to help solve the family problem. The son asked for psychotherapy time for himself, the first time he had been seen since the evaluation almost a year before.

The next phase of the family psychotherapy was one in which the son was seen alone in addition to the weekly family appointments which the parents attended together. The son made some progress but soon it became clear that he was "going through the motions" of psychotherapy because the parents insisted. The parents were making little progress on their part of the problem. In these situations, it is common for parental motivation to subside and for parents to depend on the triadic one to solve the entire problem. After two months the son stopped his regular appointments, saying he would return later when he felt the need for psychotherapy. The parents again began projection to the son, who began to act out within the family. The parents, with the tangible problem provided by the son's acting out, were able to focus on a family problem and then to begin the first working together on their own problem.

This family has now had seventy-two hours of family psychotherapy over a period of eighteen months. The son has been able to make passing grades in school for the first time in years, and he was motivated to get a part-time job, but his academic deficit is great and he still has at least another year of high school. The parents continue the focus on their own problem in family psychotherapy but they proceed much more cautiously and slowly at investigation of their own intrapsychic problems than would be characteristic of parents in less impaired families. The family has a higher level of differentiation of self than a family with severe schizophrenia in the triadic one. The ability of the son to oppose the family projection process and the ability of the parents to achieve a reasonable effective level of "self" in acute situations is more "self" than is found with severe schizophrenia. In most families with this level of impairment, the parents find reason to terminate the psychotherapy with some level of symptomatic improvement. The current motivation of the parents to continue suggests that they may be among those to go on to a reasonable resolution of the underlying problem.

Present Status of Family Psychotherapy

It is striking that this method of family psychotherapy, which had its beginnings in the study of schizophrenia, has proven to be effective in resolving the underlying problem in less severe emotional illnesses and ineffective in resolving the underlying family problem in schizophrenia. There are practical and theoretical implications in this. On the practical side, I no longer approach schizophrenia with the expectation that the basic process will be changed by the present techniques of family psychotherapy. In the beginning there was an expectation that the father-mother-patient triad would

242 INTENSIVE FAMILY THERAPY

constitute an autonomous, contained unit within which the problem could be resolved without giving support to each separate individual. But the triad did not prove to be autonomous. I now approach schizophrenia with the expectation that some emotional "support" of the family ego mass by the therapist is necessary, but it makes theoretical and practical sense to direct at least part of the "support" to the parental side of the triad, rather than to the patient alone.

Theoretically, the experience with families adds increasing conviction to the belief that schizophrenia will eventually be explained as an emotional phenomenon if we conceive of an emotional process involving multiple generations. Schizophrenia is as fixed and rigid in the father-mother-patient triad as in the patient, but there is evidence to indicate that the process can be reversed in the family ego mass in which the parents grew up if members of the family of origin are available for therapy.

I view the family projection process as a natural phenomenon that develops as any phenomenon in nature when conditions are favorable for it. At the same time, I believe the "favorable conditions" can be controlled and modified by man if we can be more aware of the way the process operates. Implicit in the family psychotherapy is the assumption that the family projection process does not have to be and that the parents can be responsible for self. The parents in less impaired families can be responsible for self when it is required, but since the parents of a schizophrenic person grew up as triadic recipients of similar but less intense family projection processes in their own families in which responsibility for self was not possible, it is difficult for such parents to assume more than sporadic periods of responsibility for self. Furthermore, on a practical level, it is easier and more expedient for medicine and society to assume responsibility for the projected family problem (the psychotic patient) than to attempt to hold the parents responsible. The family's use of medical structure of "examination-diagnosis and treatment" to further the cause of the family projection process is a monumental problem for which there are no easy answers. If the medical structure did not exist, the families could find other means to make the environment responsible. There is considerable therapeutic advantage when the therapist can deal with the family projection process without diagnosing sickness in the impaired family member.

References

BOWEN, M. (1959). Family relationships in schizophrenia. In A. Auerback (Ed.) *Schizophrenia—An integrated approach.* New York: Ronald Press.

BOWEN, M. (1960). Family concept of schizophrenia. In D. Jackson (Ed.) *Etiology of schizophrenia*. New York: Basic Books.

BOWEN, M. (1961). Family psychotherapy. *Amer. J. Orthopsychiat. 31,* 40–60.

BOWEN, M., DYSINGER, R. H., and BASAMANIA, B. (1959). The role of the father in families with a schizophrenic patient. *Amer. J. Psychiat. 115,* 117–120.

BOWEN, M., DYSINGER, R. H., BRODEY, W. M., and BASAMANIA, B. (1957). Study and treatment of five hospitalized families each with a psychotic family member. Read at annual meeting, Amer. Orthopsychiat. Ass., Chicago, March.

KVARNES, M. J. (1959). The patient is the family. *Nursing Outlook 7,* 142–144.

MENDELL, D., and FISHER, S. (1958). A Multi-generation approach to treatment of psychopathology. *J. nerv. ment. Dis. 126,* 523–529.

SONNE, J., and SPECK, R. (1961). Resistances in family therapy of schizophrenia in the home. Read at Conf. on *Schizophrenia and the Family*, Temple Univ., Phila., March 30.

SPIEGEL, J. P. (1960). Resolution of role conflict within the family. In N. W. Bell and E. F. Vogel (Eds.) *The family*. Glencoe, Ill.: Free Press.

6

NATHAN W. ACKERMAN

PAUL F. FRANKLIN

Family Dynamics and the Reversibility of Delusional Formation: A Case Study in Family Therapy

A family approach to investigation of the schizophrenic phenomenon requires commitment to a point of view. In previous publications (Ackerman, 1960, 1961), we committed ourselves to a theory concerning the schizophrenic illness and also to a theory of family therapy appropriate to this condition. The conceptual frame outlined in these publications assumes a correlation between the schizophrenic process and the homeostatic disorder of the organism. A further assumption is made regarding a basic interdependence between the homeostatic disorder of the schizophrenic individual and the homeostatic imbalance of the family group. The goal of family study is the elucidation of this relationship. In taking this theoretical position, we do not assert an exclusive or an exact one-to-one relation between family and individual homeostasis but only suggest that there may be a significant correlation. We draw this inference from a small but convincing series of empirical experiences in the treatment of the schizophrenic patient within the matrix of the emotional life of his whole family. With this type of intervention, we have been able, to our satisfaction, to alter the homeostatic equilibrium within the family unit and, in parallel fashion, to modify the course of the schizophrenic disorder. In essence, we have been able to bring about a shift in the integrative pattern of family relationships and a concurrent shift in the integrative functioning of the schizophrenic patient in the direction of health.

Let us go one step further in our thinking. In family study and treatment of schizophrenia, we observe circular effects: the influence of family on patient and the influence of patient on family. If, in selected cases, we succeed in reversing some of the central features of psychotic experience by means of family intervention, we are adducing, thereby, evidence of the significant association between family and individual homeostasis. When, by this method, we are able to retard the pathogenic trend and draw the patient back into the real life space of his family group, we infer that the family method of therapy holds the potential power, not only to influence the secondary elaborations, but also to influence the primary manifestations of this disorder. In taking this stand, we do not assert that the social factor is the exclusive etiologic agent; we do not claim a cure. Nor do we say that such improvement can be achieved uniformly with all types of schizophrenia, at any and all stages of the illness, and with every type of family. We contend only that if such a result can be brought about in a few instances, this, by itself, is a significant reflection on the nature of the illness and on the crucial role of family interaction. In present-day controversy, this is an important consideration, since it is often asserted by organically minded investigators that psychotherapy influences the secondary manifestations exclusively, not touching the primary schizophrenic process. We do not agree with this point of view. For us, it is a striking observation that family psychotherapy, under favorable environmental and organismic conditions, seems to affect both the primary and secondary manifestations.

The therapy of the case here described was carried out in the Family Mental Health Clinic of the Jewish Family Service of New York City. This is a research-oriented clinic devoted to the study of the relations of family dynamics and mental health. As is the usual procedure, the family under discussion was first studied in a series of exploratory interviews conducted by the research psychiatrist and observed by the clinic staff. The family was then assigned to a staff psychiatrist for continued study and therapy. Interviews were conducted with the whole family, and also, when indicated, with the patient alone, and the parents alone.

In this family there were individual interviews in the early months with the daughter, and joint interviews with the parents. Later on, the daughter joined in regular family interviews but continued to have some individual contact with the therapist. After a year of therapy, the research psychiatrist had several follow-up interviews with the family, which were filmed for study purposes.

Our purpose in this chapter is to report a study of patient and family in which treatment of the whole family seemed to move toward reversal of the patient's psychotic experience. We present the relevant material in five main sections: (1) the illness situation; (2) the family background and diagnosis; (3) the course of family therapy; (4) verbatim record of a family interview; (5) an interpretive discussion based on the evidence of family study.

The Illness Situation

The patient was a 16-year-old girl brought by her parents for a psychiatric consultation because her mental condition seemed to be deteriorating and the parents were alarmed. For three years the patient had been undergoing psychotherapy in another clinic, with the assumption that she was suffering from a psychoneurosis. Neither this, nor any other diagnosis, had been shared with the parents; they were befogged as to the true nature of the patient's illness and falteringly tried to deny its seriousness. They preferred to view the patient as a child with a "vivid imagination."

The patient was withdrawn, had no associations with her peers, and refused to attend school. At home, she alternated between periods of barricading herself in her room and engaging in belligerent quarrels with her parents and, more particularly, with her grandmother. She made recurrent threats of suicide and exhibited an odd array of mannerisms: a bizarre cough, twirling her hair, averting her gaze, and wormy gestures of her hands and body. At times she used awkward, pretentious phrases that verged on neologism.

Overt signs of illness had appeared at the age of eleven against a background of lifelong shyness and withdrawal. The patient was born while her father was in military service. He met her for the first time when she was three years of age, having been overseas prior to this time. On his return home from the war, he was in poor condition, physically and mentally. He suffered from long debilitating infection and was malnourished, depressed, and irritable. At home, he was accused by his wife and mother-in-law of being overdemanding and of monopolizing his wife's attention, while, at the same time, being critical and irritably rejecting toward the child. When, in the later years, mother and grandmother joined in blaming him for causing the child's mental breakdown, he took sides with the women against himself. He assumed the total burden of guilt and hung his head in shame; he fully believed that he had inflicted severe damage on the child.

But this was not the whole story. The women had made a scapegoat of the father. Clinical study revealed that the child had suffered serious emotional trauma even before the father's return from the war. In these first three years while the father was away, the grandmother governed the family. The mother and grandmother were tightly bound in a dependent, ambivalent relationship. The grandmother was sharply critical of the mother's care of the baby. While resenting the grandmother's carping attack, the mother was unable to fight back. The grandmother accused the mother of neglecting the child, of total ineptness in failing to control the baby's crying, which might waken the grandfather. The grandfather was a shadowy, peripheral figure; he had been a working man and had died six months prior to the first consultation with the family. The grandmother nagged the mother to take the child out into the fresh air and sunshine, on the score that the air in the home was close and foul. In a rationalized, obsessional way, the grandmother pushed the baby out of the home. Though resentful, the mother complied with this coercive pressure. She was split between the need to care for the baby and the need to appease the grandmother. Nonetheless, the tight alliance between the two women continued, and they joined in isolating and scapegoating the father. They set father against daughter, daughter against father. They fortified in the child a barrier of suspicion and fright against the father as a male.

Examination of the patient revealed active hallucinatory experiences. She maintained regular communication with a planet in space called Queendom; she did this by sending and receiving something akin to radar waves. She exchanged messages with the reigning lady in Queendom, "Zena," by means of a "Zenascope." More of this later.

The presenting situation was critical. A prompt decision had to be reached as to the necessity of hospital care because of the danger of violence and/or suicide. Following close study, by means of filmed family interviews, a tentative decision was made to assume a calculated risk in keeping the patient within her own home and undertaking psychotherapy of the whole family.

THE FAMILY BACKGROUND AND DIAGNOSIS

The living unit consisted of the two parents, the maternal grandmother, and the patient, an only child. The grandmother was in her mid-sixties. The father was 47 years old; the mother 45 years old. The parents had been married for twenty years. The father earned a better than average income and the grandmother contributed to the household. Both parents were college graduates, native-born, Jewish.

The parents had been drawn to one another out of their mutual dependent need and their shared ideals of family closeness, security, loyalty, and intellectual striving. In their respective families of origin, they had had certain anxieties in common. The father came from a broken family; the paternal grandfather died in the father's early childhood; the paternal grandmother, domineering and long-suffering, was oversolicitous and intrusive. The mother identifies closely with her own domineering mother, while she viewed her father as temperamental, ineffectual, and yet someone to be feared.

The father is a tall, handsome, distinguished-looking man. He is a rigid, obsessive, perfectionistic individual, with profound feelings of inferiority. He gives the impression of a frightened, guilty, self-doubting boy, rather than a man. He is inclined to be ingratiating and self-apologetic. He is almost womanly in demeanor. He talks in quick spurts or does not talk at all. He is fearful of his emotions and dresses up his thoughts in pretentious, intellectual phrases. He withdraws into scholastic pursuits. All this notwithstanding, he projects a certain childlike appeal and reaches out frantically for approval and support. His main defenses are obsessive obedience, repression of aggression, and emotional detachment. The mother is an attractive woman, but has a bland, vapid, expressionless face. It is difficult to find in her any trace of animation. In a shallow sense, she is an obsessively good person, self-righteous, judgmental, and full of clichés as to what is right and wrong. She shows little spontaneity. She is given to periodic hysterical outbursts and also suffers from migraine. Now and then she bursts into high-pitched, eerie laughter.

The grandmother is a rigid type, a severely dogmatic and aggressive person. She is never wrong and has an immediate answer for every problem. Beneath her hypocritical, self-righteous protests, she is contemptuous of everyone. If she does not get her way, she sulks and makes intimidating threats. She intrudes herself as mother's mouthpiece, harassing father and driving him into an isolated position. Both grandmother and mother have the urge to talk for the father, and also for the daughter. A fragment of symbiosis characterizes the relationship of mother and grandmother. Trying in a futile way to appease the women's fear of masculine aggression, father shrinks from the expression of his male powers.

The patient is an appealing teenager who looks pathetically disorganized and lost. She alternates between panic and explosive, defiant aggression. Her native intelligence, imagination, and perceptiveness show clearly through the curtain of her disturbance. At times her expressions are exquisitely sensitive and seem almost poetic. Mainly, she is in despair; now and again she lashes out in desperation but then withdraws.

On the surface these parents give lip-service to their close partnership, but they have not achieved a satisfying marital union; it is, instead, a parent-child relationship. The father fears the invasive powers of a woman; the mother is suspicious and fearful of male aggression. An undercurrent of competitiveness and hostility aborts the establishment of a firm emotional bond. The parents seem tacitly to collaborate in minimizing the importance of the sexual aspect of their union. When the child was born, it seemed to shatter the tenuous balance of family relationships. She was an intruder and had to be expelled. When she tried frantically to prove that she existed, that she should be given a place, the result was further disruption of the family group. The only alternatives were withdrawal into a psychotic world or suicide. It is on this background that the grandmother insisted that the patient must go to boarding school. This presumably would force her to make friends among her peers.

Casually viewed, this family might appear to be well-integrated, except for the one severely disturbed girl, but this was a deceiving appearance. On deeper examination, it was apparent that this was a profoundly disorganized and split group. In emotional terms, it was a paralyzed family, ridden with guilt and anxiety. The members were severely alienated; they lived in constant dread of the uncontrolled eruption of violence and destruction. In their inner life there was severe prejudice and scapegoating. The one male member of the family was viewed either as a monster or a helpless boy; the one daughter was treated as a disruptive intruder. Both were sentenced by the older women to punishment and exile. On the part of the daughter and father, there was a barely discernible yearning to get together in protective alliance against the older women, but this hardly got off the ground. All three adults united in scapegoating the sick child. They perceived her as a dangerous force and acted as if she must be either controlled or eliminated in order for the family to survive. While in a sly, covert way the patient showed an interest in her father, she mainly avoided him, as he avoided her. Mutually, they shunned direct gaze; they feared to touch one another. Father sensed an erotic element in his daughter's interest, shrank from it as taboo, and feared violence.

A deep rift had grown up between the patient and both parents. When the patient now and then made an abortive thrust to reach out to them, she was rebuffed. She argued with her mother, but her rage was directed mainly against her grandmother. She resisted parental authority, isolated herself in her room, and threatened violence if they invaded her privacy.

Between father and grandmother, there was a smouldering conflict. When originally he failed to oust the grandmother from the family he gave up. But his grudging resentment persisted. Behind his back, the grandmother engaged in a sneaky campaign to tear down his character. At present, the relationship between the father and grandmother is civil, but they hardly communicate. It is a cold war.

The mother, a bland, self-righteous person, slid out from between father and grandmother, as if unconsciously waiting for them to destroy one another. In daily relations with the patient, the adult members of the group were confused, disorganized, defeated, and yet tried to control her by means of threats and bribes.

At the conscious level, mother and father aspired to join in the ideal of a warm, close, loyal family unit. This was a complete fiction, however. In actuality, there was constant fear of the outbreak of open warfare. But the fiction persisted, since the adult members saw themselves as harmonious, peace-loving people. There was, therefore, this sharp, glaring contradiction between the ideal of family closeness and the actual condition, which was one of profound alienation in family relationships. Except for episodic explosions, the emotional climate in the home was static, half-dead; the mood was that of resigned apathy. The members of the group felt trapped. The functions of the family were carried out in a routine, constricted way. The family had little contact with the wider community.

As a family, they were an economic unit, but did not hold together either emotionally or socially. The sexual adjustment of the parents was at a low ebb; child care was disorganized. The family, as family, seemed to move backward, rather than forward; the relationships were severely constricted and lacking in vitality. The emotional atmosphere was pervaded by an attitude of fear and avoidance of life; the growth potential of the family group was almost nil.

The Course of Family Therapy

At the outset, the effort to treat patient and family together proved extremely difficult. The family was confused and fragmented. The grandmother campaigned forcefully for her plan to place the patient in a boarding school. The patient herself requested individual therapy, in complete isolation from her family. For the first four months, the planned procedure of family interviews was obstructed by the split condition of the group. Feeling thwarted, the grandmother aggressively sabotaged the entire proceeding. She competed with the therapist's influence, and she opposed his goal of treating all of them together. This conflict moved rapidly to a climax, after which the grandmother left the home and the therapy sessions.

In this first phase the patient and her family were seen separately. Generally, the patient was interviewed first, and after that her family, including, in the beginning, the grandmother. The early interviews with the parents were monotonous. They showed their bewilderment, fright, and guilt, as well as their deep resentment of the child's behavior. Because of their persistent panic, they continued to deny the severity of the patient's illness. They credited her hallucinatory experiences to her "vivid imagination," and the father minimized her illness by claiming that, like himself, his daughter was interested in science fiction. The therapist challenged this; he categorically asserted the position that the patient was mentally ill.

When they were finally forced to admit the girl's psychosis, the parents came into open conflict with one another. The father displayed a more genuine concern for the child's welfare, while being accused again and again by the older women of rejecting the child. According to both the mother and grandmother, the father rigidly maintained high standards and expectations, especially along intellectual lines. The father was berated for failing to relate to the child, except in terms of scholastic interests, and he submitted to this mortification. He became depressed. But as the therapist gave him increased support by firmly disagreeing that the father was the sole cause of the patient's illness, he felt greatly relieved and his depression lifted. He thanked the therapist volubly.

In the ensuing sessions, the father took a stronger stand against the grandmother's noisy criticisms of the patient. It is noteworthy here, however, that the father, now more openly opposed to the grandmother's aggressiveness, was not directly assertive with his wife. It was self-evident that he was trying to divide mother and grandmother, to free his wife from the grandmother's domination, and to get her for himself once again. In essence, he was reviving his original unsuccessful attempt to join with his wife and eliminate the grandmother from the home.

The conflict between the grandmother and the therapist came to a boil. Talking to her was like conversing with a stone wall, and the therapist expressed his anger to her. The parents were now driven into a corner and forced to choose between grandmother and daughter. It was either one or the other. The therapist pointed out how the grandmother monopolized relations with the mother and competed with the patient. In effect, the grandmother was denying a mother to the sick child. In the choice between grandmother and daughter, the father sided with the therapist. He became outspoken in his desire to separate his family from the grandmother. In contrast, the mother showed conflict and indecision. But, increasingly, she began to ventilate her anger against the grandmother. Finally, the therapist reached an agreement with both parents to "place the grandmother in boarding school," so to speak, rather than the patient. The grandmother was moved to the home of a relative, and after that family therapy moved forward.

In the office, the patient paced up and down agitatedly. She had made several suicidal attempts by swallowing small metallic objects, and she explained that her recurrent cough was an attempt to expel these objects. It was observed, however, that she coughed regularly whenever she darted a glance at her father or at the male therapist. At moments of high tension, when she was in acute conflict over the danger of closeness with her father or with the male therapist, she declared that if she only had the guts, she would jump out of the window.

Bit by bit she revealed the nature of her psychotic experiences. She spoke of hearing voices from another planet, Queendom. The inhabitants of this planet lured her to join them. There, the beings were of another species. They were not human; they were like machines. On this planet no males were allowed; they were all feminine, "not female, but feminine." These creatures were gorgeous beings, with the most exotic coloring of skin and hair. They had hormones, not for sex, but to make them attractive. On this planet there was no reproduction by sexual union, only by fission. The beings in Queendom lived in solar time, not Earthian time. There was no night or day. The inhabitants lived perhaps one hundred and fifty years. They were capable of sleeping for long periods. They were completely self-sufficient and experienced no fatigue. They had the power of clairvoyance. Everything on this planet was factory-made by chemical means. Nutrition was neither personal nor human. The source of food was not Mother Earth, but the factory, where all foodstuffs were chemically produced. In this planet, in outer space, there was no hate, no war, no killing, but also no love. The inhabitants devoted themselves to the cultivation of the arts: music, literature and painting. It was a culture of mind over body. Finally, in this universe there was magic control. There was none of the hate and danger of the Earthian way of life. Yet, some beings in this planet were afflicted with a mysterious disease, which progressively rotted the body while the spirit remained immortal.

Several times the daughter appeared for her session wearing a rubber mask depicting a horribly deformed, diseased person. She stared into a medical book in which there was a photograph of a patient afflicted with ugly, festering, mutilating sores. By implication, this was her fantasy image of her own deteriorating illness.

She explained her urge to be rid of her body: the physical part of her being was an intolerable burden, for it continually had to be fed, nursed, cared for; she wanted only to preserve and enhance her spirit. She sought to eliminate her body and glorify her mind. She was in profound conflict with her bodily needs, especially with her sexual urges. She confided a disturbing encounter with a young man, a waiter at a summer hotel. As she described the incident, in a strange way she had suddenly found herself alone with him, and he took her in his lap and kissed her. She described this young man as a "wolf." He was "not even Caucasian"; he was like "a Formosan monster." When he kissed her, it was as if she felt abruptly transformed from a little girl into a woman. It was a shocking experience. She became panicky and escaped as quickly as she could.

In a peculiar, paradoxical way, despite her fears of sex and men, she showed flurries of intense interest in both her father and the male therapist. In one family session, she dramatized the conflict of allegiance between her psychotic community in Queendom and her real family. She remarked with high animation how perhaps she had made a mistake. She had allowed Zena and the beings in Queendom to talk her into their way of life, where no males were allowed. Maybe she was too obedient. She should have resisted more strongly. She felt tempted to conspire to take a male or two up to Queendom, "just to show them what the male species is like." The male or two were, of course, the father and the male therapist. Since no males were permitted in Queendom, she would have to smuggle them in. But then, "they could only stay a few minutes." She would "keep a sharp eye on them." They would have to behave or right back to Earth they would go.

In the second phase of treatment, when regular family interviews were begun, the patient at first sat as far as possible from her parents. She was hesitant, unsure, frightened. Frequently, as her sense of threat mounted, especially in relation to her apprehension of open hostility, she made a gesture of leaving the room. Each time she did this, the therapist persuaded her to stay. In her mind, he had become her "defender."

Within several weeks, the patient began to touch and even gently to kiss the therapist on the cheek in her parents' presence. The therapist verbalized his wonder that she exhibited this kind of affection toward him but not toward her parents. The father remarked that when he tried to approach her, he was generally met with a belligerent, hostile attitude. When he tried to enter her room, she shut the door in his face and threatened him with a stick. The mother regularly intruded with comments that reinforced the patient's fear of her father, alluding repeatedly to the father's rigid, exacting standards and his rejection of his daughter. It gradually became clear that the main source of hostility toward the patient was the mother, not the father. When the father was critical, he seemed to be acting on cue from the mother. It was the mother who tended to reinforce the barrier between daughter and father.

One incident, in particular, stands out sharply as an example of this trend. The patient brought home from school a failing mark in one of her subjects. The mother warned her against revealing this to the father. When in family interview, however, the therapist, with the patient's permission, brought this failing mark to the father's attention, he reacted not with disappointment and criticism but, rather, with an expression of genuine concern for the way in which the patient felt about this failure.

As these sessions proceeded, one could observe a shift in the alignment of family relationships. The patient's hostility toward the father gradually diminished, and she became perceptively sharper in her attacks on the mother. She alternated these attacks, however, with some recognition, half-apologetic, that perhaps her mother could not really be blamed because she was so dominated by the grandmother. By stages, the patient expressed her anger toward the grandmother with increasing directness and force. On those occasions when the grandmother visited the family, the patient would say to her, "What do you want here? Go home. We don't want you again." But she did more than this; she appealed to the mother to wean herself from the grandmother: "Grandma has had her chance at motherhood. It's your opportunity now." When the therapist called attention to the father's basic sympathy with the patient's resentment of the grandmother, the father expressed the feeling that after all, "my daughter is fighting my own battle." He referred here, once again, to his original futile struggle to separate mother from grandmother.

After about a year of therapy, a further shift was observed. The patient reached out more actively toward her father. She mussed his hair and kissed his hand. The therapist called attention to the exaggerated and overintense way in which the patient expressed her urge to be close to her father. He asked her if she was devouring father, rather than kissing him. At the same time, he referred to father's fear of these aggressive approaches, his fear of any open dealing with sex, and his consequent shrinking away from contact. The father voiced his fright by telling his daughter to go find a boy of her own. The therapist dealt with this by interpreting that a daughter might also touch her father, that this was a different touch and need not be the same as the sexual touch of a wife. Inevitably, this led to an extended discussion of the fàther's lifelong fear of women, his relations with his own overpossessive mother, and his submissiveness to his wife and mother-in-law.

Returning to the incident with the "Formosan" waiter, it is noteworthy that the patient talked freely of this incident with the therapist but told her parents nothing. In her family, she felt that sex was not allowed, absolutely taboo. In her earlier years, when she directed any question about sex to her parents, she was given the "brush-off." The parents seemed embarrassed and evaded the issue. Instead, she was told to return to her studies or practice her piano. For example, she once asked her father how it felt to go on a date. Her father bypassed the question with a wisecrack; he quipped that a date, like a piece of fruit, gets squashed. The patient ceased to ask about sex.

Another aspect of this same problem was reflected in the patient's feeling about being an only child. Whenever she inquired about sisters and brothers, her parents evaded the question. Being an only child meant to her not only a lonely life, without companionship, but a proof that her parents disapproved of sexual activity. In fact, they rarely indulged. Whenever the therapist alluded to the patient's urgent curiosity regarding sex, she showed agitation and abruptly tried to cut off the conversation. On one occasion, she came to the session armed with a hammer. She towered over the therapist with the hammer, threatening to strike him if he persisted in talking of this taboo subject. The therapist countered her denial of sex with the remark that he was male, sexy. He could not help it. God made him that way. Gradually she relaxed and became less belligerent. She diluted her tension in this area by intellectualizing the whole subject. For example, one time, she delivered an oration on the role of genes in the human species.

Later, she came with a dream. In her dream, there was a considerable variety of nude pictures on the office wall, and a wild orgy was in progress. As the patient entered, the male therapist threw empty beer cans at her. While talking of this dream, the patient produced a deck of cards decorated with nude women. She pleaded with the therapist not to mention these cards to her parents; they would be horrified. Still later, she shared with the therapist a story she was writing in which a student nurse fell in love with a young intern. She spoke of planning a holiday, a real celebration. She would one day bring a bottle of champagne and she and the therapist would "have a ball."

Consistently, however, her admission of sexual interest was coupled with the threat of aggression. In one such instance, the patient took the therapist's hand and dug her fingers into his palm.

The therapist said to her that he wasn't sure whether her desire was to touch him or to scratch him. He pointed out that, while she wanted to come closer to him, she was frightened of impulses emanating from her and him. The patient admitted that while she was terrified, she also felt increasingly safer with him because he was in no way critical of her. The therapist indicated that they might talk freely of these urges but need not act upon them. Each time she enacted one of these scenes with the therapist, she referred back to her difficulties with her father. She expressed her conviction that her father was as frightened of sex as she was. She reacted vituperatively "against this man." The therapist countered the patient's denial of wanting to have anything to do with the father by calling her attention to their common interests and their resemblance to one another: she imitated his use of big words, his interest in biology, and his use of medical terms. Gradually, her denials weakened and she admitted her desire to reach out to her father.

In the family sessions, typical patterns of family interaction prevailed. They were re-enacted over and over and thus were entirely predictable. As the family members took their places in the interviewing room, the daughter sat at one end, the father at the opposite end. Between them sat the mother and grandmother. Later, when the grandmother no longer attended, it was the mother who kept daughter and father apart. As the sequence of interaction clearly revealed, the mother and grandmother not only intruded their physical beings between daughter and father but also their thoughts and words. Whenever it seemed that daughter and father might dissolve the wall between them through more direct interchange of feeling, the mother and/or grandmother intervened to block this. Each time they reinforced the barrier by reminding the daughter of her fear of men and the father of his rejection of his daughter. For example, when the father showed interest in joining his daughter in Queendom by way of a "special passport," the mother promptly reinforced the taboo against men. She instantly suggested that it might upset the daughter, that Queendom would no longer be as she preferred it: "No men allowed."

The therapist took an active role in counteracting the alliance of the two older women in barring every semblance of personal communication between the daughter and father. He undertook to put to the test of reality the daughter's and father's shared sense of catastrophic danger in any closeness between them. In this situation, the daughter displayed a characteristic ambivalence. She alternated between two extremes: a sudden spurt of reaching out to her father, followed by an anxious retreat, often reinforced by a gesture of walking out of the room. Father, in turn, showed a reciprocal quality of ambivalent conflict. He, too, revealed a flicker of interest, followed by anxious withdrawal. In his fright, he was all too willing for the therapist to take the lead for him in making contact with the daughter.

The therapist intervened in a special way. At an opportune moment, he suggested a rearrangement of places, so that daughter and father sat next to one another. He invited them to look squarely into one another's faces and express their feelings. He particularly challenged the father to come out of hiding, to show himself as a man and express directly his warmth for his daughter. The daughter and father stole furtive glances at one another, testing the dangers of contact. As they did this, the mother and grandmother persistently interfered. Finally, provoked by these repeated invasions, the therapist told them to shut up so that the daughter and father might get acquainted. Despite the shyness and fright of both daughter and father, some progress was made. By degrees, the mother and father joined in a mutual concern for the daughter, and father supported mother in emphasizing her difference from grandmother and her good intentions with daughter.

With this shift came an opportunity for the therapist to support the daughter in reality-testing her fantasy equation of sex and violence. He encouraged her to ask her parents more directly whether sex was allowed in this family. To this blunt question, both mother and father reacted evasively, "I hope so." Later, the father was more firm and answered, "Definitely, yes." At this point, the daughter projected a deep emotional appeal to the father to admit that he was human, real flesh and blood. She challenged his remoteness, his tendency to act like an impersonal robot with her. She craved from him a show of warm, personal interest.

The role of the therapist was active throughout. Into the emotional climate of the family he introduced those ingredients that were lacking: warmth and affection, an open and natural acceptance of sex, a linking of sex and affection, and more appropriate images of the family roles of man, woman, and child. The first step was to induce the parents to admit the malignancy of their daughter's illness. The next step was to offset the grandmother's persecutory intrusions and to neutralize her regressive, monopolistic possession of the mother. This required a melting away of the mother's fright and awe of the grandmother as an omnipotent and omniscient, dangerous person and the substitution of the therapist for the grandmother as a better parent figure. To bring this about, the therapist had to compete with the grandmother as being an omniscient, omnipotent, but also a wise, benign, and well-intended, grandparent.

By these means, the mother was gradually liberated from the

symbiotic, engulfing union with the grandmother. In a further step, the therapist moved in the direction of counteracting the mother's fear of the lethal powers of the aggressive "male monster" and supported her in a more adequate marital and parental joining with the father. The value of sexual gratification was supported. The father's male prerogatives were reaffirmed.

After a year and a half of continued treatment, the patient lost interest in her relations with Zena and Queendom. There was progressively less mention of hallucinatory communications with the inhabitants of this planet, and finally she ceased altogether to refer to these experiences. Gradually she seemed to resume her place in the real life space of her family on Earth. It became clear that she was progressively withdrawing her interest from her psychotic world and investing more and more of her feeling in her struggle to find a new place in her Earthian family.

At the same time, she began again to attend school. Her ability to concentrate on her studies was restored and there were no further failures in class. She worked better and, in fact, achieved an average of 85%. This was a striking change, remarked upon with amazement by her teachers. At the end of the year, she expects to graduate from high school.

At another level, she improved her relations with her peers. She began to talk with the young people in her class and developed a friendship with a girl friend. She was able to attend a school dance and have contact with boys as well as with girls. In the over-all picture, the patient showed marked improvement at home, in school, and in the larger community.

The following verbatim interview, which occurred in the twelfth month of conjoint family sessions and after sixteen months of combined individual and family treatment, was a follow-up interview conducted by the supervising and research psychiatrist.

Filmed Interview

VERBATIM RECORD	EVALUATIVE COMMENT
DR. A.: Well, Helen, how are you getting along with the old man these days?	Therapist continues to test danger of daughter's closeness with father.
HELEN: (much faltering of speech) I . . . uh . . . I . . . well, the less talk the better agreement.	
DR. A.: You mean that if you and Daddy were to talk freely, you'd get into trouble.	

(cont'd)

Filmed Interview (cont'd)

VERBATIM RECORD	EVALUATIVE COMMENT
HELEN: (hesitates to answer; starts and stops)	
DR. A.: More disagreement? More conflicts? More fighting?	
HELEN: Well, yeah.	
DR. A.: Is that right?	
HELEN: (to father) You know that's right.	
FATHER: Well, we still don't see eye to eye—let's put it that way. We still don't see eye to eye.	Father uses the existence of differences to fortify the emotional barrier.
HELEN: Well, he came back from Chicago. Everything was goody-goody for a while, but after he got through telling us about Chicago, then it was back to the same old routine again.	
DR. A.: What's the routine?	
HELEN: The same old grind.	
DR. A.: The same old gripe, did you say?	The therapist's use of the term "gripe" is not a slip on his part. His reinforcement of daughter's complaint against father is purposeful.
HELEN: Same old routine, same old grind.	
DR. A.: Grind, what is that?	
HELEN: Well, you know what a grind is. You get up in the morning, you go to work, you come home, you eat, you watch television, you go to sleep—you know what I mean.	
DR. A.: You mean he's like a machine?	
HELEN: Aren't we all in this modern, chaotic . . . it's all documentary.	Patient gets lost in diffusing the dehumanized quality of her father to all of society.
DR. A.: You mean in this modern, chaotic world we live in, people are no longer human beings? We all turn into machines?	
HELEN: In a way we are.	
DR. A.: Well, you have machines up in Queendom, but down on earth, well, I'm no machine. Am I a machine?	
HELEN: No.	
DR. A.: You've got a little allergy to somebody in the family	Therapist applies the emotional force of the term "allergy" to sharpen everyone's awareness of daugh-
HELEN: Yeah, something doesn't agree with me. I don't know.	

VERBATIM RECORD	EVALUATIVE COMMENT
DR. A.: Are you talking English (word not clear)?	ter's inability to tolerate the loss of human quality in her parents.
HELEN: I guess I'm coughing the whole thing up.	Helen's coughing tic is triggered by tension and
DR. A.: Well, as soon as I got you off the high level of generalization, as soon as I take you out of the atmosphere away from Queendom, when I bring you right down to earth in this family, you start coughing up.	signifies her unconscious effort to expel an object (male) that threatens dangerous invasion.
HELEN: I can't think of anything to say.	
DR. A.: I'm asking you a simple question: are you three together now? Is it all three for one and one for all, or are you apart?	Therapist shifts from an exclusive emphasis on joining with father to joining with the whole family.
HELEN: Well, I would say we're still pretty much . . . well, I guess there's more unity than there was the last time you saw us, but we're still not quite (unclear from here on).	
DR. A.: You mean the pieces in the jigsaw puzzle don't quite fit together in the right way to make the design.	The family members don't fit in a way that meets the patient's needs.
HELEN: Yeah, but there's a little more harmonization than there was the last time I saw you.	
DR. A.: Well, that's something.	
HELEN: (interrupting) But it's not a hundred per cent, not a hundred per cent.	
DR. A.: I'm not a perfectionist. I'll settle for a little improvement. Will you accept something better?	
HELEN: Yes.	
DR. A.: So there's a little more unity, a little more harmony, since we put Grandma out to pasture.	Therapist identifies the family member (grandmother) who epitomizes the obstruction to emotional integration of the next generation of the family.
HELEN: Yes.	
DR. A.: You said a little while ago that you wanted to marry her off. Want to get rid of her?	
HELEN: Well, no . . . well, I don't know. Well, I guess the little we see of her now is enough, because after all, she does need	Patient hints at emotions of ambivalence and guilt concerning exclusion of grandmother.

(cont'd)

Filmed Interview (cont'd)

VERBATIM RECORD	EVALUATIVE COMMENT
a family now that she's widowed and she's alone . . . you know, well, you know, she'll call Phyllis (mother) up. Well, she's making more friends now and that's more than I can say for myself.	
DR. A.: Well, you've gotten Grandma out of the family and into a separate apartment, but she's still in the family.	
HELEN: Yeah, she goes into the department stores where she lives, she's a little happier. She goes into the stores where she lives, it's a little livelier.	
DR. A.: It seems to me that you won't feel really safe until you get Grandma married off.	Patient wants grandmother far away.
HELEN: To someone who lives in California maybe.	
DR. A.: Well, you remember we talked about that. Grandma said you were getting her a boyfriend. You were acting the part of a "shadchen" (marriage maker). (Father laughs at this point.) You were going to fix her up with a guy. Still working on that little enterprise?	Father joins daughter in the half-jocular, hostile satisfaction of exiling grandmother.
MOTHER: Well, to tell you the truth, I still don't see where Grandma plays such a big part in this thing. I honestly mean that. We get off on Grandma, but this relationship (father and daughter) is still the same, whether she (grandmother) is in the house or out of the house. Their reaction to each other is the same, completely. When we were in Albany, it was the same and there was no Grandma there. When we were in many places where Grandma was far away, it was the same situation. I won't say that Grandma isn't a meddler, or anything like that.	This is mother's first entry into conversation. She overtly defends grandmother (covertly defends self) against the accusation of meddling in the relationship of daughter and father. Mother admits her ambivalence to grandmother.

VERBATIM RECORD	EVALUATIVE COMMENT
DR. A.: Well, yes.	
MOTHER: But not to the point . . .	
DR. A.: I exaggerate.	Therapist invites release of mother's hostility.
MOTHER: Yes.	
DR. A.: I exaggerate on purpose. You've got a little bit of your mother in you?	Therapist makes explicit and overt mother's intrusive role.
MOTHER: (beginning of her remarks unclear) I know my habits are very different from my mother's.	Mother again defends self, this time by asserting her difference from grandmother.
HELEN: They are.	
MOTHER: There are things that I resent about my mother and I certainly hope that I don't have the same . . .	
FATHER: The same qualities.	
MOTHER: . . . qualities.	
DR. A.: What are those qualities?	
MOTHER: Well, as Dr. F. knows, she's a very domineering person.	
HELEN: She's very intrepid, very intrepid.	
DR. A.: Intrepid?	
HELEN: Yeah, intrepid, audacious, a virago. It's one of my fancy words.	
DR. A.: Is that a Spanish word?	
HELEN: No. It's an English word. A virago means a woman who's more or less of a battle-ax, you know.	
DR. A.: Well, if you say battle-ax, I know what you're talking about.	
HELEN: Yeah. They call it a virago.	
DR. A.: (to mother) Well, you hope you're not aggressive, the same virago, the same old battle-ax as your mother (grandmother).	
MOTHER: I hope so, because those are the very things that I resent so much.	
DR. A.: Um-hmm.	
MOTHER: . . . her domination.	
DR. A.: (beginning not clear) But you do meddle a little bit. Just a little bit.	Therapist challenges mother's denial of being intrusive, like grandmother.
MOTHER: Oh . . . no, no. You mean the joke?	
DR. A.: Yes. You cut in between daughter and father (when daughter	

(cont'd)

Filmed Interview (cont'd)

VERBATIM RECORD	EVALUATIVE COMMENT
was retelling father's dirty joke).	
MOTHER: In what way?	
DR. A.: You didn't let her tell the story.	
MOTHER: (laughs) Well, it wasn't between the two of them.	
HELEN: It was a very humorous story.	
MOTHER: It was a joke among us. It wasn't between the two of them. Nothing gives me greater pleasure than when I can see there is some repartee there, really. That I can sincerely mean. (Between father and daughter)	Again mother makes a typical display of righteous denial.
DR. A.: Well, I was quite impressed when you came in. There was more coziness and more contact, feeling contact, now between Helen and her father than a year ago. Still, you did cut in on it a little bit.	
FATHER: Let me ask this question, Dr. A. Do you think she (mother) is cutting in to meddle, or is she cutting in to shield one of us from the other or each from the other?	Father comes to mother's support; he needs her to protect him from danger of violence.
DR. A.: I don't know. I can't find out.	
FATHER: For fear of our coming to blows. In other words, I don't think her motivation is one of wanting to meddle per se, as much as it is wanting to shield one from the other. You know, the buffer.	
DR. A.: Why? Are you going to hurt Helen?	Therapist challenges father as to his submerged violence.
FATHER: She knows I won't hurt her physically.	
MOTHER: He'd never do that.	Mother leaps to protect father from therapist.
HELEN: Physically, well, what do you mean—mentally, morally?	
FATHER: The point I'm trying to make now is that I think what you would feel is mother's meddling, and my mother-in-law's, I think it's based on different motivation. In my mother-in-law's case, it would probably be the	

VERBATIM RECORD	EVALUATIVE COMMENT
desire to dominate the situation. I think in her (mother's) case, it's as I said, to act as a buffer.	
DR. A.: She's protecting Helen from your violence?	
FATHER: Or vice versa. I don't know which it is.	
MOTHER: (breaking in) I really, I don't, don't think that you understood.	
DR. A.: Well . . .	
MOTHER: That I mean it when I say it really meant nothing to me when she told the joke in front of him. Will you believe that? I hope you do, because you've mentioned it several times, because I felt, you know, it was a little off-color. (Some over-talking here between Helen and her mother, and it isn't clear.) Well, I didn't know, all these people . . . there's a time and place.	Mother still defending self against therapist.
DR. A.: These people have heard dirtier stories.	
MOTHER: I know, but they don't come here to listen to that particular story. It's putting a little too much stress on it. But I know what it is you're trying to get at.	
DR. A.: Phyllis (mother), let me make a confession. I misunderstand all the time. (General laughter.)	
MOTHER: Don't give me that! Don't be sarcastic now!	
DR. A.: Feel free to correct me.	
MOTHER: You're being sarcastic!	
DR. A.: I don't know too much about your actual feeling . . .	
MOTHER: (breaking in) You know a great deal! I'm pretty sure of that!	
DR. A.: I don't know about how you act with Helen and Daddy.	
MOTHER: You're just wondering if someone doesn't come in between these two that causes them to act that way. It's as simple as all that.	

(cont'd)

Filmed Interview (cont'd)

VERBATIM RECORD	EVALUATIVE COMMENT
DR. A.: It was simple. He was the male monster and Helen had a terrible fear of men and boys. Men were all monsters.	
HELEN: You mean they were all another species.	
DR. A.: That's right.	
MOTHER: I know that Grandma wasn't in Albany for eight years. She came to visit us perhaps twice in all that time, but she couldn't have played too much of a part in it.	
DR. A.: Well, I don't know about that. How did you feel when you and Grandma were separated? You and your mother, how did you feel about that?	
MOTHER: Very happy. (She laughs.)	Mother turns about. With a release of sarcastic laughter, she admits her own need to be free of grandmother's domination.
DR. A.: When you were here and Grandma lived someplace else?	
MOTHER: (hesitatingly) Well, I was . . . of course, and when I . . . well, let's put it this way, I didn't miss her too much. I have my own interests. Believe me, I have enough interests. And I'm kept quite busy. If you think I'm hanging onto her . . ?	
DR. A.: When you said, "let's put it this way," there's more than meets the eye in that phrase.	Mother reveals her ambivalent dependence.
MOTHER: (breaking in) Do you think I'm holding onto her apron strings?	
DR. A.: I don't know. I don't know enough about you and your mother. How do you feel about it? You don't miss her at all? She calls you up.	
MOTHER: Yes, she does, now that we're living close by, she does call me up. She wants to be noticed. She wants attention.	
DR. A.: She doesn't want to be forgotten.	
MOTHER: She wants attention. She doesn't want to be forgotten. She hasn't any interest, very few interests,	

VERBATIM RECORD	EVALUATIVE COMMENT
she hasn't many friends in her new apartment, so she'll call me up whenever she gets an opportunity, whenever she feels she wants to talk to somebody.	Mother again shifts to her identification with grandmother.
DR. A.: Did she feel that she was sort of pushed out of the family?	
MOTHER: No, I think she wanted to, she wanted to go out.	
DR. A.: Well, she wanted to shove Helen out, off to boarding school, didn't she? (Mother laughs.) Isn't that true, she (grandmother) wanted to shove her (Helen) out?	
HELEN: I'm glad that I don't have a mother like that. She could dominate a person's life actually. Now she's going to pay for me to go to art school. I don't know.	
MOTHER: That's why she thinks she wants to get rid of her.	
HELEN: I don't know what's taking place in that crooked mind of hers.	Patient is suspicious of grandmother's motivation.
DR. A.: Your feeling about Grandma is that she brainwashed you.	Therapist picks up cue, underscores patient's fear of grandmother's manipulation.
HELEN: I don't know. She just goes off on little binges here and there.	
MOTHER: Well, it isn't that. As far as the art class is concerned, she just feels it would be an interest and she (Helen) is good in drawing.	
DR. A.: But, Mother. . . .	
MOTHER: (cutting in) She (grandmother) doesn't have too much to say.	
HELEN: But, mother, she's had her chance at motherhood. It's your opportunity now. She's been a mother already. I mean, doesn't she feel that she can loosen her apron strings a little bit, at least enough to breathe with?	Patient makes pathetic appeal for the right to breathe.
DR. A.: Did you catch Helen's message?	
MOTHER: Well, no, she still holds on tightly to her children. I know these things. Helen wants me to be completely free. Grandma	Mother again comes to grandmother's defense.

(cont'd)

Filmed Interview (cont'd)

VERBATIM RECORD	EVALUATIVE COMMENT
should get completely lost. Why? Because when Grandma talks to me, Grandma's taking some of my attention away, and she (Helen) doesn't like that. She doesn't want anyone to take any of my attention away. Not only Grandma. (Helen is talking in the background, but it isn't clear.)	Mother accuses daughter of jealousy of grandmother.
DR. A.: Helen sent you a message on the Zenascope. This is your chance, perhaps for the first time, to be a fulltime momma for Helen. A fulltime momma!	Again, patient appeals to mother—this is mother's chance to care for her own child.
MOTHER: Shall I tell my mother completely to get lost? So what should I do when she calls me up? Hang the receiver up? (Helen is constantly talking in the background, but it can't be understood.)	Mother evades daughter's appeal. She's too busy with self-justification.
HELEN: I told you when you passed an hour (on telephone with grandmother).	
MOTHER: Well, that's true.	
DR. A.: What kind of a momma is Phyllis to you now?	
HELEN: Well, she's getting a bit more patient. I like her. At times she exaggerates, she gets so high-strung at times, and we have our little differences, but I think we get along fairly well now.	
DR. A.: Are you closer to Momma now since Grandma's been out of the home?	
HELEN: Yes, I am. (Turning to mother) You know I am.	
DR. A.: Do you feel, looking back on it now, that somehow Momma was divided between you and Grandma, sort of torn between you and Grandma? (Helen's response is not clear.) You coughed again. That always means you're getting tense.	
HELEN: Getting tense?	

VERBATIM RECORD	EVALUATIVE COMMENT
DR. A.: Everytime I say something you don't like, you cough. Tenser, I should say. You're always tense. What's the matter?	Patient's cough seems now to be related to anxiety concerning closeness to mother.
HELEN: (faltering) . . . Uh . . . nothing.	
DR. A.: You had a thought. What was your thought?	
HELEN: Well, I think we're a little closer now that Grandma is a bit of a distance away, a little distance away, even if she's only five blocks away, we're a little closer.	
DR. A.: I saw you reach out to Momma. Did you want to hold her arm? (Mother laughs nervously.) Do you want to pat her? Do you want to do something?	Therapist challenges daughter and mother both to admit need for closeness and affection.
HELEN: I meant in reply to her, you know.	
DR. A.: (to mother) She sent you a little love message.	
MOTHER: I know. We have our moments of affection.	
DR. A.: (to Helen) Momma just reached out her hand to you. You didn't take it.	Mother and daughter join hands, but are extremely tense and uneasy.
MOTHER: (laughingly) Let's make him happy.	Mother is sarcastic, flip; she shows affection only to appease therapist.
DR. A.: For my sake? (Mother's laughter continues.)	
MOTHER: Every word is analyzed.	
HELEN: There comes a time when I have to be a little more independent. You know . . . a little more "iconoclastic." I like you, and all that, but I don't want to happen what happened with you (mother) and your mother (grandmother) previously. We can be close together. I still have to have some other diversion, you know.	Now daughter shows a rising anxiety as to the danger of closeness with mother, the same danger as exists in the symbiotic imprisoning bond of mother and grandmother.
MOTHER: And you know, the greatest thing for me is for Helen to be independent and not have to depend on me. I'm completely different from my mother. My mother would have liked me to	This is mother's disguised rejection of daughter. She moved to the extreme of detachment from daughter as a rebound from excessive, choking dependence *(cont'd)*

Filmed Interview (cont'd)

VERBATIM RECORD	EVALUATIVE COMMENT
be dependent. I want Helen to stand on her own. That's why I see no meeting of the minds at all between the two of us.	on grandmother.
DR. A.: Well, Helen, Mommy says that she feels different towards you.	
HELEN: Well, I feel (turning to mother) . . . Do you have enough confidence in me to feel that I could make the right decision at the right time, apropos?	Daughter again makes soft appeal to mother for acceptance.
MOTHER: Well, Dr. A. would like to know, have I ever kept you from making your own decisions, if you felt they were right, if they would help you? Am I one of the icons?	Mother feels on the spot with the therapist. She is too busy defending self against the male threat to receive her daughter's appeal. Instead, she wants to
HELEN: Are you one of the icons? Well . . . (falteringly) . . I don't get your opinion very often.	know if she, as one of the icons, should be destroyed.
DR. A.: Will you drop that, Helen. (Helen was handling the microphone and the sound wasn't clear.)	
HELEN: Well, I would say, you do have a certain amount of trust in me? Confidence? (to mother)	Daughter renews her appeal to mother.
MOTHER: You know I have. If she weren't locked up like she is, I would have a great deal . . . I mean, I see her potentialities.	Mother talks defensively to the therapist, away from patient. She does not listen to her child.
DR. A.: Yes.	
MOTHER: But there is that locked little room there, you know. And if she could free herself. But I do see potentialities. Very much so. It isn't something I say now because there are people listening. I say that constantly to you. Am I wrong?	Mother shows more of her ambivalent feelings. Continues defensively to plead for therapist's approval. Shows strong doubt of self.
HELEN: No.	
DR. A.: So, somehow you and mother are a little better joined.	Despite mother's ambivalence, therapist supports better joining of daughter and mother.
HELEN: Uh-huh. I'm happy she (mother) has her interests now. She's going to art school. She sketches now. That made me a little more interested in drawing.	Daughter gives mother half-hearted praise, but is choked with fear of the danger of closeness.

VERBATIM RECORD	EVALUATIVE COMMENT
DR. A.: Is there a better feeling that you share, the two of you now?	
HELEN: Yeah.	
DR. A.: Well, it's easier now, isn't it, since Grandma doesn't live with you?	
MOTHER: It's easier.	
HELEN: She (grandmother) had to have her say in everything, you know, like the U.N. General Assembly vote. She had to be the Speaker of the House, so to speak.	
DR. A.: It's very difficult to compete with Grandma's mouth.	Therapist supports defense against grandmother and, inferentially, against mother, too.
HELEN: She always had to put her two cents in.	
DR. A.: Uh-huh. So . . . what's doing with the male monster now?	With support for a better union of daughter and mother, therapist turns back to fear of father.
HELEN: Well . . . I don't know, I guess the male monster has his own problems. I don't know, I . . . (silence). What should I say about the male monster . . . he gets up, goes to work, comes home, sits down, and watches television . . . so I really don't know what's going on with him.	To patient, father is still a stranger.
FATHER: I think that what she wants to say is that there's still no togetherness there.	Father distances himself from relationship with daughter—"no togetherness there."
MOTHER: They still have nothing to say to each other.	
HELEN: As a matter of fact, once I made a little retort. I asked him sarcastically how many caps, how many gold inlays he put in today. He got very angry.	Daughter is caustic in a sad way about her father's remoteness.
DR. A.: Why aren't you telling that to the male monster? Why are you telling that to mother?	Therapist invites daughter to point her feeling directly to father.
HELEN: I don't know.	
FATHER: I guess she wants corroboration. (Both parents laugh.)	
HELEN: I really don't know what to ask him. Shall I ask him how many . . . I don't know what to ask him when he comes home . . . how many incisors he capped or how many inlays he put in	In a forlorn way, patient gropes with the question, how to reach her father.

(cont'd)

Filmed Interview (cont'd)

	VERBATIM RECORD	EVALUATIVE COMMENT
	(mother laughs very hard) . . . or how many bridges he worked on . . . I don't know what to say.	
DR. A.:	Well, Helen, I recall when you and I were talking about a certain type of man long ago, you felt maybe one day you could get a man for yourself, get married, have children.	Therapist stirs patient's hope of a man of her own.
HELEN:	Well, I don't know.	
DR. A.:	And I asked you about Daddy . . . whether he knew anything about sex, and you said he must, because he's always putting his finger into people's mouths, getting hold of people's teeth, therefore, he must know something about sex.	Therapist brings patient's fear of sex into the open.
HELEN:	I don't know.	
DR. A.:	What you are really saying . . . when he comes home from the office and you want to know what should you ask him . . . you're really saying what kind of a man is he? Don't you?	Therapist makes explicit patient's urge to know her father as a man.
HELEN:	Yes. I can't ask him how he gets along with his assistants, how he gets along with his nurses, how he gets along with teeth.	
DR. A.:	Well, take a look at him. What do you really want to know about Daddy?	
HELEN:	(hesitantly) Well . . . I want to know what kind of a person he really is, outside of his dentistry, outside of any business matters.	
DR. A.:	You want to know if he's really a person, really a human being.	
HELEN:	Yeah.	
DR. A.:	. . . not just a work machine.	
HELEN:	Not just a drilling machine or a cavity filler.	
DR. A.:	Not just a mechanic.	
FATHER:	A mechanical monster. (Mother laughs. Father joins in.)	Parents' laughter is a release of tension.
HELEN:	Whether you're flesh and blood.	

VERBATIM RECORD	EVALUATIVE COMMENT
DR. A.: So ask him. Are you alive, father?	
FATHER: Well, I don't know.	
HELEN: I have to remind you (father) that you're flesh and blood, that you breathe, that you eat, that you do other things, but you're flesh and blood, that you're not a robot, and that neither are we robots.	
DR. A.: Your daughter has to remind you that you have a throb in your veins, that you're not just a mechanical man.	
HELEN: A robot.	
FATHER: Especially now that spring is here.	
HELEN: What has spring got to do with it? You're the same way whether it's September or December, or whether it's May. (Mother breaks in laughing.)	
DR. A.: Well, what he's saying is that he's capable of a heart flutter in springtime.	
FATHER: That's right.	
DR. A.: Are you in love this spring?	
FATHER: (exaggeratedly) Oh, sure. (He and mother laugh.)	
HELEN: Are you in love?	
FATHER: Of course; all the sap starts flowing. (Mother continues to laugh. Father joins in.)	
DR. A.: Well, that's one thing robots can't do, have a heart throb.	Sap doesn't flow from robots.
FATHER: (Something, unclear, about spring not affecting robots.)	
HELEN: Well, that's something robots can't do. They have no heart throb, they are just made of metal.	
DR. A.: Well, as you look at this male monster, do you think he's capable of a heart throb?	
HELEN: I think he's capable of . . . well, other things, too.	Patient makes vague allusion to father's capacity for sexual love and making babies.
DR. A.: Like what?	
HELEN: I know he's flesh and blood; at times he may seem to be inanimate, inert.	Patient backs off from area of danger, to father's usual

(cont'd)

Filmed Interview (cont'd)

VERBATIM RECORD	EVALUATIVE COMMENT
DR. A.: Inanimate and inert?	deadness and, once again, a
HELEN: Yeah.	moment later, he's alive,
DR. A.: Like those mechanical beings up in Queendom you described to me.	"scintillating."
HELEN: Oh, not even like that. Like that lamp over there or that telephone or even that table. But I know that deep down he's a nice person; he's ingenuous, he's scintillating, he has a heart of gold, he's an all-round good fellow.	
MOTHER: She's looking for his personal attention. More attention.	
DR. A.: (to father) She wants to see your spark.	Therapist challenges father to show his "spark."
MOTHER: When he tells a story, she doesn't want him to tell the story to me. She wants him to tell the story to her.	Mother shows rivalry.
DR. A.: Father, she accuses you of hiding your manly talents.	
FATHER: Well, you see, basically, and, of course, Dr. F. encourages this very definitely, she feels apart from the family. She doesn't feel included in the family circle.	Father talks to therapist, away from daughter, exactly as mother did earlier.
DR. A.: Father, you're starting to make a speech again. (Helen broke in here, but what she said wasn't clear.)	Therapist counteracts father's tendency to intellectualize.
MOTHER: Dr. A. knows that, but he wants to know why you feel that way.	
FATHER: Well, I'm sure you are aware of that phase of it.	
DR. A.: Helen looked at you and said that if she were to judge by surface impressions, you would seem to be an utterly inanimate, unfeeling, mechanical man, a robot. You say no. Comes springtime, you fall in love all over again.	
HELEN: And then every winter, he goes back. You know.	
DR. A.: Helen looks at you and says you hide from her. Your man-	

VERBATIM RECORD	EVALUATIVE COMMENT
liness . . . (Helen breaks in. It isn't clear.) (to Helen) Do you want to talk? (to father) She wants to see you.	
HELEN: I know. I know. He's a man. I know all these things. It's when he comes home.	
DR. A.: But you don't really know.	Similarly, he counteracts the patient's intellectualizing.
HELEN: But when he comes home, he is so tired he wants just to read his paper and eat. You know . . . he's too tired to talk. You know . . . I mean, he's pooped. You know.	
DR. A.: He's just nursing his body.	
HELEN: Yeah.	
DR. A.: Where's his spirit?	
HELEN: I don't know . . . but . . . (Long pause.)	
DR. A.: She wants to see your spark, Father.	
HELEN: It's like a vegetable. (Turns to therapist) When do you . . . I see you alone? (Mother laughs.)	Patient is discouraged, also fearful. She seeks escape in asking again to see therapist alone.
DR. A.: Well, at the moment you make me uneasy. At the very moment we talk about the question of what Poppa's hiding from you, his manly spark in springtime, he declares for all the world he is a man, he can be romantic, he can get excited about a girl, in the springtime especially, is that right?	
FATHER: Yes.	
DR. A.: At that moment, you (Helen) want to break it up. You want to talk to me privately. Do you want to send him (father) walking?	
HELEN: That was rather rude of me.	
DR. A.: I'll talk with you alone, but let's explore this a little bit, talk a bit further, can we?	Therapist neutralizes patient's fear and resistance.
HELEN: Well, I don't know. I think you're getting down a little too deep. Once you pass the clothesline . . . well . . . I don't know . . . I think you're getting a little too deep . . . you	Patient refers directly to her fear of exposure, of self and of father.

(cont'd)

Filmed Interview (cont'd)

VERBATIM RECORD	EVALUATIVE COMMENT
know, like an oil well that's going down.	
DR. A.: You mean you're getting scared. You mean it sounds almost like I'm about to undress him before you?	
HELEN: Well, I don't know. (Pause.) Well, perhaps it happens elsewhere, but it never happens in this group.	
DR. A.: You mean there's no sex in this group?	Therapist continues to challenge resistance.
HELEN: I mean, let's be a little more conservative. (General laughter.)	
FATHER: May I impose upon you?	
DR. A.: Sure, what do you mean "impose" upon me? (Father requests a cigarette from doctor. Dr. A. also offers one to Helen.) Does Helen smoke?	
HELEN: I don't smoke. I don't drink, don't have sex. I'm just . . .	
DR. A.: You don't smoke, don't drink, you don't have sex. Well, you can do without drinking and smoking, but I don't know about the other.	
HELEN: Well, I'm naughty in other ways. I tell lies.	Therapist continues effort to bring sexual problem into the open.
DR. A.: Is it naughty to have sex?	
HELEN: (Grunts and falters for an answer) I don't know.	
DR. A.: Well, you see, we're back at the point where we were earlier. It's a very important problem, because in this imaginary world you've created for yourself up in Queendom, no sex allowed, no males allowed . . .	
HELEN: Everyone is self-sufficient.	
DR. A.: They're all mechanical beings up there, created in a factory? They reproduce only by binary fission?	
HELEN: (to father) By the way, how is Chicago this time of year?	Patient is mildly evasive, while making a joke of it.
FATHER: Beautiful.	
HELEN: Anything to change the subject. (Mother laughs.)	

VERBATIM RECORD	EVALUATIVE COMMENT
FATHER: We're getting a little deep. We're probing and beginning to reach the nerve. This is the only way we'll reach. . . .	
DR. A.: I think we have to reach a decision as to whether sex is allowed in this family down on earth or not? Yes or no?	Therapist wants a commitment: is sex allowed, yes or no?
HELEN: Well, I don't understand. I thought . . . What do you mean by sex? I just can't understand . . . I thought we were all meant to be together no matter what sex we are.	Patient evades.
DR. A.: Oh, I can't agree with you that it doesn't matter what sex one is. It matters to me very much that I wear pants, it matters to mother that I wear pants. (Father and mother laugh. Mother makes a comment that is inaudible over the laughter.) It matters very much. You and Helen agree. No undressing.	
MOTHER: Well, it all depends. If I were in art class, I would be very happy.	
HELEN: Or nature . . . a nature club.	
DR. A.: Let's pretend that this is a nature club for a moment. Why don't you ask your parents if they allow sex in this family?	Therapist induces patient to face parents directly with the sex question.
HELEN: (to parents) Well, do you?	
MOTHER: Well, *I hope* we're normal in that way.	"I hope we're normal"—a typical ambiguity.
DR. A.: Well, yes or no? (Mother and Helen both start to talk. Helen apologizes for interrupting.)	
HELEN: I know your brother and sister-in-law sure enjoy sex.	Patient puts parents on the hot seat. Others enjoy sex, why don't they?
MOTHER: Helen's afraid we don't because there's only one child in our family.	
HELEN: They have five, you know.	
DR. A.: They keep pretty busy. (Mother laughs.)	
MOTHER: You see, she's always resented so much the fact that she's an only child.	Mother intellectualizes.
HELEN: Oh, well.	

(*cont'd*)

Filmed Interview (cont'd)

VERBATIM RECORD	EVALUATIVE COMMENT
DR. A.: Helen asked you a direct question. Is sex allowed or isn't it allowed in this family? Yes or no?	
FATHER: Yes, of course.	
HELEN: That's like saying is eating allowed in this family, is digestion allowed in this family or isn't it. Or is breathing allowed in this family.	Patient affirms that sex is natural, like eating and breathing.
DR. A.: That's right. Do you want to know from your Pop? You can ask him.	
HELEN: (to father) Is sex allowed?	
FATHER: Definitely.	
HELEN: Definitely?	Helen, turned to parents' unsureness and vacillation, disbelieves father's assurances. She is right; he is simply complying with therapist's wish that he be definite about sex. Almost immediately, the unsureness returns, in the standard, stereotyped form. Mother is again defensive, self-justifying in an obsessional, literal way.
FATHER: Of course.	
HELEN: You mean no red tape?	
FATHER: Your mother and I are normal married people, *I hope.*	
DR. A.: Do you mean you have sex together?	
HELEN: Oh dear, I didn't think it would be anything like this.	
MOTHER: I just wonder about this, because it's never been taboo in our family, that we wouldn't tell an off-color joke. I mean, the way I answered at first wasn't because I was afraid for them. I know there are families like that, where it's completely taboo, where they never mention it, where they never tell a dirty joke.	
HELEN: Your mother (grandmother) was pretty conservative, wasn't she.	
MOTHER: Yes, but she loved them (dirty jokes).	
DR. A.: Grandma likes jokes?	
MOTHER: Of course she does. And she likes all kinds of stories.	
HELEN: You mean "Little Miss Conservative"?	
DR. A.: Is that what you call Grandma?	
HELEN: Conservative Rose.	
DR. A.: You mean as far as sex is concerned, you think she was a	

reactionary? You mean she was agin it? (Helen hesitates to answer.) She was pretty bossy. Did she permit sex between your mother and father?

HELEN: Well, she says things . . . that . . . well, I wouldn't have the audacity to say. She comes out with remarks here and there that I wouldn't have the audacity to say.

DR. A.: Well, give me an example.

HELEN: Well, do you remember the time where she said when you and father were first married?

MOTHER: Oh, yes, I know what you're trying to say. Go ahead.

HELEN: Father was busy with his practice and you were busy helping him? And she was the instigator in the case, that, I mean . . . that . . . well . . .

A vague allusion that grandmother claimed credit for urging parents to have a child.

MOTHER: I know what you're trying to say.

DR. A.: Don't say it for her.

MOTHER: All right, I know what she wants to say. Go ahead.

DR. A.: Don't put words into her mouth.

Mother interrupts repeatedly; due to her anxiety, she shut off daughter's flow. She has the urge to think and talk for her.

HELEN: . . . that you didn't care for a family . . . I mean . . . that you didn't care to have children . . . and she was the one . . . she was the inspirer, the instigator . . . I don't know.

MOTHER: She made a senseless statement.

HELEN: Well, that was a senseless statement. I'm surprised that she even had the audacity to say it.

MOTHER: I gave . . .

HELEN: You gave her hell for it.

Mother again defensive. Do mother and daughter have an unconsicous confusion as to whose daughter Helen is (mother's or grandmother's)?

MOTHER: You know, she is so anxious to get Helen to care for her, that she makes these completely irrational statements. They're as far off . . . (mother breaks off).

DR. A.: So, there is some actual basis in fact.

HELEN: She said that you and father didn't want children, for the time being.

(cont'd)

Filmed Interview (cont'd)

VERBATIM RECORD	EVALUATIVE COMMENT
MOTHER: She (grandmother) said it was because of her we had Helen, because of her . . . her influence.	
HELEN: I don't know . . . her something or other.	
MOTHER: . . . influence. She said that to Helen once and I gave her holy hell. You're a witness. What did I say to Grandma?	
HELEN: I don't know. You gave her a piece of your mind.	
MOTHER: It was really so stupid! My husband and I never consulted my mother whether we should have a child or not, and my husband and I both wanted Helen very much. I don't know where she came in the picture at all.	Mother shows usual righteousness.
DR. A.: Well, today, this morning, Helen, do you think you could get a straight answer about sex from your two parents?	Therapist returns to the question: is sex allowed in this family?
HELEN: Could I get a straight answer from them on sex?	
DR. A.: Yes.	
HELEN: You mean if I asked them to explain the facts of life, would they do so without a blush of embarrassment? Would they tell it to me freely? Would they . . .	
DR. A.: Would they give it to you straight?	
HELEN: Would they uncover any mysticism I might have had or would they . . . or would they keep it all a hush-hush, top military secret?	
MOTHER: It's not a question of misinformation. Helen knows more about it. She knows everything.	Again, mother shows her obsessional literalness. She has a "school-marm" attitude to sex.
HELEN: I read this in books, you know.	
FATHER: I'd like to explore this a little further (to Dr.).	
DR. A.: I know it isn't just a question of sheer facts, Momma. (Mother laughs.)	
MOTHER: Interfering again?	
DR. A.: Yes.	

VERBATIM RECORD	EVALUATIVE COMMENT
FATHER: I'd like to explore this with you. Please continue (to therapist).	Father urges therapist on. He depends on therapist to take initiative for him.
DR. A.: I think it's very important that Helen has the feeling that she can talk with you honestly and undefensively, in a simple, direct way, about sex. That she can ask you questions. That your attitude would be that you would want to answer. It isn't just a question of the information. It's a question of the quality of the relationship, the feeling that counts, whether you make it a deep, dark, mysterious and dirty secret, or whether you discuss it openly.	
MOTHER: Well, we've discussed it hundreds of times . . . where babies come from, and so forth. It's not a taboo question. How many times have we talked about it?	
HELEN: I know. I know there are many people who are very conservative, prudish like.	
DR. A.: Are you calling Momma a prude?	
HELEN: (to mother) Do you approve of S—E—X?	
MOTHER: (laughingly) Oh, very much so.	
HELEN: I mean . . . if you could change nature . . . you know . . . would you do so? Would you make it possible to reproduce like an amoeba, you know, without sex . . . an amoeba, you know, splits in two.	
DR. A.: Are you for it or agin it?	
MOTHER: I just hope I've never shown her that I've been agin it in any way.	Again a righteous protest.
DR. A.: If you want to get a straight answer, ask them a straight question.	
HELEN: Well, why about sex? I could . . .	
DR. A.: Well, do you want to know the way in which they feel about you as their daughter? Will they give you a straight answer, or	

(cont'd)

Filmed Interview (cont'd)

will it be hush-hush? Or will
Momma get embarrassed and
act like a prude? Or will Daddy
act shy, like he's afraid of losing his pants or something?

HELEN: I don't know about him. I certainly would! (Mother laughs.)

DR. A.: So, you'd be shy?

FATHER: So, you're the one that's conservative?

HELEN: Maybe I'm the one that's conservative . . . I don't know.
(General laughter.)

DR. A.: Daddy's right, you're the prude.

HELEN: I don't know. I get the impression that he can talk about the
stocks and bonds, he can talk
about retirement, old age pen-
sions . . . but, but, sex? . . .
you know . . . I mean . . .
men and women? . . . you
know what I mean.

DR. A.: Well, ask him a question!

FATHER: When you ask me any questions, do I ever dodge them?

HELEN: Do you ever dodge them?

FATHER: Well, did I ever give you any
misinformation?

DR. A.: You did.

FATHER: Did I?

DR. A.: I'll remind you, Helen. You
told me a little story once, you
came to Daddy, you asked him
what is it like to have a date.

HELEN: Did I ever ask that question?

DR. A.: Yes. You told me that Daddy
made a joke of it. He said a
date is like fruit, you squash
the date.

HELEN: He beat around the bush maybe? And ignored it maybe?

DR. A.: Yes. Would you like to ask him
the same question again?

HELEN: I, well . . . I don't know, because . . . it's . . . it doesn't . . .
oh, gee!

DR. A.: Well, would you go into the
library, please? (to the parents)

| | EVALUATIVE |
| VERBATIM RECORD | COMMENT |

MOTHER: I was just going to mention that he (father) gets embarrassed if she (daughter) touches him and I think that gives her a feeling of inadequacy and doubt as to how to act to other boys, because every time she touches him, in any way, he draws away, you know.

DR. A.: Do you, Father? Do you shrink everytime Helen touches you?

MOTHER: I think that's very important.

HELEN: You know, he moves to another couch.

MOTHER: Well, she probably thinks if he's going to be like that, what is it going to be like with another boy?

DR. A.: How does he act when you (mother) touch him?

MOTHER: Well, not like that at all. He feels at ease with me, but he feels that she should be at ease with boy friends, not with her own father.

DR. A.: Well, when you touch father, he doesn't fade away.

MOTHER: No, because he feels that's the proper relationship.

DR. A.: That's proper, but when your daughter touches you, that's improper. Is that the way you feel, Father? Well, it's a different touch when Helen touches you.

Discussion

We have described an acute psychotic reaction in a 16-year-old girl, studied and treated within the matrix of her family group for a period of eighteen months. In this case, some of the primary features of psychotic experience were shown to be reversible. During the period of therapy, the patient moved in and out of her psychotic world. The dominant shift was a movement away from the psychotic world in space, back to her real life space in her Earthian family. In this connection, a number of significant questions must be considered.

The psychotic reaction of this young patient germinated in a set of disturbed family relationships. By what criteria do we define the disturbance of this family? What components of this disturbance are specifically pathogenic for the patient and bear a direct relation to the precipitation of an overt psychosis? What other pathogenic components in this family are relatively nonspecific for psychosis but have other consequences for the emotional health of the family as family and for the members as individuals?

Let us try first to discern those components of the pathogenic make-up of this family group that may bear a specific relation to psychotic development in the daughter. The emotional make-up of this family unit revealed a family pair, mother and grandmother, regressively joined as one and asserting an exaggerated, righteous goodness and sacrifice. The quality of this union was such as to require the expulsion of a dangerous and bad element. To begin with, this bad element was epitomized as the "male monster," the father, who was seen as alien and dangerous, invading the bond of the two older women with sex and aggression. Sex itself was equated with violence. Sex and body contact in general were sharply reduced. The all-powerful governing grandmother established a taboo on a true sexual union of father and mother. Sex was symbolized as a dirty and destructive contaminating force and dissociated from warmth and affection. To save his own life, father joined with the older women against the only child. He did not provide for this child the needed antidote to the destructive invasive force of the two older women.

The daughter came to symbolize the alien and dangerous element in this family. She became the "bad seed" and was expelled. She had only two choices: retreat into a psychotic world or commit suicide. In either instance the end-result would be self-destruction; she would comply with the overwhelming expulsive force in the family and wipe herself out.

In the interactional processes observed in the family interview, it was noteworthy that when mother and grandmother came to life, i.e., asserted their aggressive dominance of the situation, the patient tended to die off emotionally, to withdraw. When, by contrast, the therapist supported the patient against the invasive force of the older women, the patient came to life. In turn, whenever Helen expressed herself with animation, the older women seemed to die off. In this setting, the father seemed paralyzed and lost. Passively, he followed the therapist's lead in an ingratiating, submissive way, or made a feeble, short-lived attempt to join with his daughter which he could not sustain except with the active support of the therapist. In effect, then, when one part of the family raised its voice aggressively, the other part lay down and died, and vice versa. In this connection, it is interesting to speculate as to a possible essential difference in the quality of emotional interaction in the family that breeds a psychotic member and, by contrast, the family that mainly breeds neurotic members: the neurotic family implicitly lays down the taboo, *the child must not be different;* whereas in the family that breeds a psychotic, the taboo is: *the child must not be.* This family has a covert fear of new life, a prejudice against birth, growth, movement, any newness in life. This child lost the right to breathe; she was choked off.

Of great interest in this case is the possible diagnostic significance of the human relations scheme which the patient designed for her psychotic universe in Queendom. The social pattern which the patient created for her psychotic community in outer space seems to cast a long shadow on the pathogenic distortions of her real family on Earth. It is fascinating to speculate on the meaning of the contrast between the way of life in Queendom and the way of life in her Earthian family. What may this contrast signify for the illness process itself? What may we usefully infer from the value clash which is dramatized in the contrast of the two worlds? What is the same and what is different in the two universes? In Queendom, the patient designed a way of life which merged elements of her Earthian family with other elements of change which she seemed to require as a defense against the disintegrative anxiety of her illness. In her psychotic world, she remade life in a special way, altering the whole value system of the community in Queendom. To recapitulate briefly, she removed whatever was dangerous and ugly in her Earthian family life and introduced magical forms of self-protection. Queendom represented an effort at magic repair, a compensatory design. It erased the Earthian threats, but, beyond that, did not point the way toward growth and health. It was, however, more bearable than the pattern of her Earthian family. Such considerations as these may be relevant to the correlation between the interactional distortions of the family group and the development of psychosis in an only child.

Another question emerges: what components of pathogenic disorder exist in this family group that are relatively nonspecific for psychotic development in an offspring and yet have extensive consequences for the remaining nonpsychotic personalities in the family? In this parental partnership, there is a conscious joining in an allegiance to the goals of security, harmony, loyalty,and intellectual pursuits. There is, however, a profound contradiction between the conscious value striving of this parental pair and their actual way of life. The conscious pretext of peace and harmony is thin. It is virtually a fiction. In actuality, the parental couple slides into a pattern that is routinized, mechanized, static, half dead. Their relationship is extraordinarily lacking in vitality and growth. In the joined obsessional effort to control the dangers of uncurbed aggression, sex and spontaneity of expression are reduced to a minimum. It is apparent that a basic shared anxiety concerning destruction pervades the whole family and rigidly constricts its range of development. The goals of sexual fulfillment and forward growth of the family, in terms of a child, are almost totally sacrificed to the interest of sheer survival. In this setting, all members suffer in their emotional health. Grandmother becomes fixed in the role of the martyred persecutor. Mother becomes anchored in an obsessionally vapid existence. Father, severely castrated, moves off into a detached, mechanized, static preoccupation with intellectual matters. The child is given no right to eat, breathe, or grow.

In a family of this type, there is a progressive patterning of pathogenic roles, the grandmother in the role of persecutor, the mother in the role of the chronically immature child-wife projecting toward her own child only a ritual concern, the father in the potential role of protector and rescuer of the child but too impotent and frightened to be effective. Therefore, in this family group, there is no effective integration of any member into a role as healer of family conflict and no effective integration of anyone in a creative or growing role. There is only progressive reinforcement of a sick pattern of prejudice, scapegoating, victimization of daughter and father, and a mounting force toward regression.

With these pathogenic trends in mind, the therapy moved toward the following objectives:

1) To break the regressive symbiotic alliance of mother and grandmother.

2) To counteract grandmother's role as omnipotent destroyer, to puncture her hypocritical pretense of always being "right" and of loving the granddaughter better than the parents did.

3) To wean mother from grandmother, eliminating the need for complicity with her, and to encourage mother to accept the "male monster," and, for the first time, to join him in marriage; to counteract the image of sex as violence.

4) To join with and fortify father in undertaking a role as "family healer" in order to provide the needed antidote to the destructive invasion of mother and grandmother.

5) To save daughter and father from their roles as scapegoats.

6) To induce mother and father to accept their daughter.

7) To overcome the fear of touch contact between mother and father.

8) To permit daughter to touch father in a different way, thus neutralizing the fear of incest and violence.

9) To induce the parents to admit the value of growth, open, free, emotional growth; to neutralize their perception of the child as the "bad seed"; to support the daughter in finding a healthy role as child in this family; to protect her right to be born, to grow, to assimilate a natural, rather than an omnipotently destructive, image of sexual union and childbirth.

References

ACKERMAN, N. W. (1960). Family-focused therapy of schizophrenia. In S. C. Scher and H. R. Davis (Eds.) *The out-patient treatment of schizophrenia.* New York: Grune & Stratton, pp. 156–173.

ACKERMAN, N. W. (1961). Schizophrenic patient and his family group. In M. Greenblatt, D. J. Levenson, and G. L. Klerman (Eds.) *Mental patients in transition.* Springfield, Ill.: Thomas, pp. 273–282.

7

LYMAN C. WYNNE

Some Indications and Contraindications for Exploratory Family Therapy

All psychoanalysts and psychodynamically inclined therapists have a deep interest, I assume, in the understanding of family relationships. Ever since Freud described the family constellation in terms of the oedipal situation, the psychoanalytic process has included as one of its central tasks the untangling of the web of current and past family relationships. In individual psychoanalytic and psychotherapeutic treatment, the primary concern is, however, with the internalized, intrapsychic representations of the patient's family relationships, rather than with the *direct* observation and study of actual, ongoing family transactions. In this chapter, I shall consider some of the circumstances under which direct psychotherapeutic work with family units seen conjointly may be indicated or, on the other hand, contraindicated.[1] The problem I raise is not whether

---

[1] Most of the ideas and observations presented here have emerged during discussion of family therapy problems with my colleagues, staff, and consultants at the National Institute of Mental Health, especially Drs. Juliana Day Franz, Irving M. Ryckoff, Leslie Schaffer, F. Gentry Harris, Alexander Halperin, Harold Searles, Roger Shapiro, Mr. Stanley Hirsch and Miss Carol Hoover. I am

family relationships are interesting or important—I assume agreement on this point—but rather from what vantage point and for what purposes psychotherapeutic contact with family units may be useful.

I approach this problem with an investigative spirit, not with the intent of making doctrinaire pronouncements or promulgating an ideologic, family-therapy party line. Let me state at the outset that I do not regard family therapy as a psychiatric panacea, but as a valuable addition to our psychiatric repertory. On the one hand, I consider family therapy as the treatment of choice under certain conditions, which I shall attempt to specify. On the other hand, certain limitations, some of which are intrinsic to family therapy and others of which are imposed by external, practical considerations, restrict the range of problems for which this treatment approach is appropriate. Comparable considerations apply to every form of psychiatric treatment; through exploration of the especially advantageous and disadvantageous conditions for using each approach, we may eventually be able to become both more specific and more comprehensive in making treatment recommendations than is presently possible.

Characteristics of Exploratory Family Therapy

In this chapter I am especially concerned with indications and contraindications for one form of family therapy: long-term, exploratory, conjoint family therapy used as a main mode of therapy. This form of treatment brings into sharp relief special characteristics and potentialities of conjoint family interviewing which remain latent or masked in less intensive and less prolonged work with families. As the term implies, exploratory family therapy relies heavily upon the exploration and clarification of the nature and sources of family difficulties as a means of resolving these difficulties. The immediate, on-going transactions of family members with one another and with the therapists are regarded as the most significant starting-point data to be explored and understood.

Exploratory family therapy, especially if prolonged and intensive, is greatly facilitated by the provision of a stably structured treatment set-up. This includes a schedule of regular appointments with regularly attending participants. It also includes a "therapeutic culture," induced by the therapists, in which the conjoint sessions gradually

indebted to them for their invaluable contribution to my thinking, but it should not be assumed that they agree with all details of the formulations presented here.

become a safe place and time to express directly and verbally feelings which have otherwise been blocked or displaced or have erupted into action.

The intent in exploratory family therapy is to establish a treatment setting within the limits of which interaction takes place as freely as possible. Under these conditions, familial styles of communication may become apparent, including patterns of controlling and organizing interaction, as well as modes, of becoming disorganized and experiencing disconnectedness. Many or most recurrent interaction patterns are unnoticed by the participants, who are caught up in their perpetuation. This applies especially to nonverbal exchanges and to the sequences in which interaction takes place. No one in a family is apt to be aware of a recurrent pattern in which, for example, the mother becomes confusingly disorganized and takes over the center of attention immediately after father and daughter have been exchanging reciprocally solicitous glances. Here the therapist or therapists add a new ingredient by being able from time to time to step back from, and to comment upon, the interaction patterns.

Especially in the early phases of exploratory family therapy, much of the therapist's activity necessarily consists of helping the family to notice their immediate, ongoing behavior, to become aware of the sequences and patterns into which this behavior falls. As a therapeutic technique, this activity of the therapist is not interpretation in the psychoanalytic sense but clarification. As in psychoanalysis, the therapist's comments may bring into consciousness that which has been out of awareness, but in family therapy the focus is more on the *unnoticed but observable* rather than on the *unnoticed but inferable*.

Inferences about unconscious motives and about links between present and past events may usefully be expressed by the family therapist on certain occasions, especially in late stages of therapy. However, the special opportunity of exploratory family therapy is to make maximal use of directly observable interactional data and the immediate impact of the interaction. Here I include the impact upon the therapist's own subjective experience as he comes into contact with the varied facets of the family. With most families, discussion of the past is an intellectualized exercise unless considerable work has first been done in noticing and understanding current experience and interaction within the sessions themselves.

By way of summary contrast, exploratory family therapy differs in emphasis from other forms of conjoint family interviewing: *Family diagnosis* is a necessary, evaluative precursor to exploratory family therapy. The diagnostic study may include home visits, psychological testing, history-taking, and interviews with individual family members and various family subgroups. However, the intent of conjoint family interviews as a part of family diagnosis is not to provide definitive treatment but to help formulate a well-considered treatment strategy, which may or may not include extended exploratory family therapy. In any event, a diagnostic process of this kind involves having a relatively brief look at various family patterns without attempting to stabilize a treatment structure for their detailed exploration and resolution.

Marriage and family counseling is conducted in a variety of ways, ranging from psychoanalytically oriented psychotherapy, to nondirective listening, to advice-giving and the manipulation of living arrangements. Ordinarily, even when conjoint family meetings are included in the counseling process, the primary treatment strategy is not, as it is in exploratory family therapy, to observe directly intrafamilial interaction and to understand the patterning and dynamics of this interaction.

Conjoint family interviews adjunctive to individual therapy may be valuable in selected situations but differ in orientation from exploratory family therapy in which a deliberate effort is made to look at the over-all balance of the family. For the purposes of exploratory family therapy, the difficulties of a particular individual family member are not lastingly the focus of attention (although the feelings or behavior of an individual may be a *temporary focus*, in order to illustrate and understand an aspect of a pattern in which other family members share).[2]

Exploratory Family Therapy at NIMH

Most of the observations and suggestions of this chapter are derived from work in the Family Studies program at the National Institute of Mental Health and may be better understood after a brief description of the clinical side of this program. Ordinarily, the families in treatment consist of two parents and their adolescent or young adult offspring. Ordinarily, one of the offspring has been identified by the referring physician or by the family as the "patient" because of schizophrenic or neurotic symptoms for which he may be hospitalized for periods of weeks to years. Other persons are included if they fall within the family's "psychological boundaries," a concept which will be discussed later in this chapter.

---

[2] Further observations about the special characteristics of exploratory family therapy have been described previously by Wynne (1961), and Schaffer, Wynne, Day, Ryckoff, and Halperin (1962).

Usually in the NIMH program two therapists work together with each family unit. However, as variants, we have tried family therapy with a solo therapist and with three therapists. The therapists are all psychodynamically oriented: psychoanalytic psychiatrists, other psychiatrists in the late stages of their training, clinical psychologists, and psychiatric social workers. Most commonly, a psychiatrist who also sees the presenting patient in individual therapy works with another psychiatrist or a psychiatric social worker who has no individual contacts with the presenting patient.

In order to gather ideas about the usefulness of various combinations of individual and family therapy, we have tried, at the one extreme, seeing family members *only* in conjoint family therapy with no individual therapy for anyone, and, at the other extreme, seeing each family member in individual therapy in addition to the conjoint family therapy.

Most families are seen in hour-long sessions twice weekly, but others may be seen one or three times weekly. Although nearly all of the families are seen at least once in their home during the initial evaluation of treatment plans, the regular family therapy sessions are held in our hospital interview rooms. Each family entering the NIMH program is informed that meetings are routinely tape-recorded and may be observed through a one-way mirror by professional colleagues who are always known to the therapists.

As the therapist or supervisor in this NIMH setting, I have observed some sixty families in conjoint family therapy, apart from consultations and evaluation sessions. Additionally, I have also seen a number of other families and couples conjointly as part of more conventional practice outside of the research setting. The maximum length of time I have seen one family in conjoint family therapy, mostly on a schedule of three times a week, has been for five years.

Although this experience with family therapy has been quite diverse, it should not be regarded as providing a systematic research evaluation of family therapy as a technique. In the NIMH Family Studies, our systematic research has focused upon family dynamics in relation to psychopathology, especially schizophrenia, and not upon technique or results of therapy. Our more exploratory clinical studies have used treatment approaches, including exploratory family therapy, which we have expected both to be therapeutically useful and to deepen our understanding of family dynamics. Thus, the ideas presented here constitute a distillate of clinical impressions, deserving further evaluation and subject to revision and expansion but sufficiently extensive to warrant comparison with the experience of others.

General Indications for Exploratory Family Therapy

As a broad, preliminary generalization, exploratory family therapy may be indicated for the clarification and resolution of any structured intrafamilial relationship difficulty. In using the term "relationship difficulty," I refer to problems in the transactional patterns, in the reciprocal interaction, among family members to which *each* person is contributing, either collusively or openly.

Only transiently are human relationships not "structured" or patterned, so that this specification eliminates only those family difficulties which involve new or nonrecurrent catastrophes or illnesses. From the practical standpoint, a nonexploratory approach may be indicated to cope with the immediate events of such crises. However, most intrafamilial psychiatric crises appear to be part of a recurrent or continuing pattern, a patterning which may usefully be explored in conjoint family therapy. In addition, the manner in which a family reacts to any sort of crisis may be chronically maladaptive even though the immediate content of the crisis may be new.

Intrafamilial relationship difficulties always have current intrapsychic aspects as well as intrapsychic and relationship roots in the past. It is reasonable, in my opinion, to treat the intrapsychic aspects with traditional individual psychotherapeutic and psychoanalytic approaches, sometimes after a period of conjoint family diagnosis or therapy. It is equally reasonable, though less traditional, to treat the intrafamilial relationship aspects with conjoint family therapy, sometimes after a period of individual diagnostic study or therapy.

As the transference ordinarily becomes established in individual psychoanalytic treatment, various manifestations of the patient's early family relationships become reactivated, focused, and available for analytic scrutiny. However, there clearly are psychiatric conditions in which a useful transference relationship is established not at all or only with difficulty. For some of these conditions, which I shall specify, exploratory family therapy provides a preferable or an alternative approach.

In general terms, exploratory family therapy should be considered, as I see it, for the treatment of relationship problems in which all of the participant family members have a vital and continuing stake, on either a conscious or unconscious level. Ideally, a central part of each family member's life should be absorbed in wrestling with, fending off, or coping with the shared problem.

Such involvement is best evaluated in a series of conjoint sessions conducted on a diagnostic or trial basis before a plan to go ahead with extended exploratory family therapy is decided upon. In our program at the National Institute of Mental Health, we routinely spend the first two to three months evaluating treatment alternatives with a family. Sometimes even during the referral process there are explicit statements about the existence of a "relationship" problem. In other instances such a problem can be inferred from the way in which some members of a family are acting "on behalf of" another. Any of these indications may be a basis for setting up initial sessions on a conjoint, evaluative basis. These initial sessions provide an opportunity to consider the kind of reciprocal expectations the family members have toward one another and whether the family as a whole is enmeshed in a problem for which more extended conjoint therapy may be indicated.

Conjoint evaluation sessions are ordinarily a good deal easier to set up earlier rather than later in the course of therapy. We usually ask the whole family to meet together in the first session; then we can have evaluation interviews with individuals, pairs, or family subgroups, and still easily return to therapy with the family as a unit. If an intense therapeutic relationship is first established with an individual family member, and if there has been no early, evaluative contact with the family as a unit, both therapist and family are likely to have difficulty later in shifting to an orientation to the over-all family patterns and to shared family problems.

In general, it seems unfruitful to try to embark upon exploratory family therapy if the evaluative conjoint sessions indicate that the presenting problem does not have *current* emotional and behavioral meaning and consequences for the family members. For example, there is not sufficient basis for active exploratory family therapy if some of the family members merely have politely narrated historical facts to report about the problem. Difficulties in current family relationships or interaction, as revealed in the conjoint sessions themselves, serve as a springboard for exploratory family therapy.

Sometimes, even in the conjoint sessions, one or more family members may at first appear indifferent or unaffected. Others may come to the initial conjoint sessions voicing reluctant grumbles or giving only compliant lip service. The literal content of these initial forms of interaction may be misleading. If the therapist goes ahead with an exploratory family approach on a trial basis, he may find that the appearance of indifference or grumbling belies a deep involvement.

One way for the therapist to begin to explore such initial behavior is to wonder if this person may be expressing the unspoken feelings or wishes of other family members as well as himself. In effect, the therapist raises the question whether the grumbling, compliance, silence, or whatever, serves a purpose or function for the family as a whole. For example, it may represent a style of warding off or of encompassing the "outsider" therapist. This inquiry may lead into consideration of feelings and difficulties family members have about making relationships which go across family psychological boundaries. Then, too, the therapist may observe that the interaction between himself and a family member is also manifest between family members, as an aspect of *intrafamilial* relationship difficulties.

If the family members actually become involved in working in conjoint treatment on their problems together, this appears to be a better criterion of "shared involvement" than their verbal avowals or disavowals. Certain family members may continue to assert for months or even years, whenever they are anxious, that "the problem," as they see it, resides *only* in the individuality of some other family member and that they are *only* coming out of a wish to help this person. Yet, behaviorally, these same family members may be vigorous participants and speak, when more relaxed, of the value and meaningfulness of the family therapy both for themselves as individuals and for their family.

Thus, exploratory family therapy by no means is indicated only when all the family members acknowledge verbally their personal motivation for the treatment. The expectation of such acknowledgment by a family therapist is certain to arouse defensiveness and is contrary to the view that, *during the conjoint family sessions,* "the patient" is the family, not *any* individual.

In summary then, difficulties in current family interaction, as revealed in the conjoint sessions themselves, serve as the clearest indication and the most lively springboard for exploratory, reconstructive family therapy.

EXAMPLES OF INDICATIONS

Without attempting to make a comprehensive inventory, I shall describe here a number of problems for which exploratory family therapy seems especially suited. These problems are not mutually exclusive but tend to be found in combinations with varying emphases in different families.

1) *Adolescent Separation Problems.* In the Adult Psychiatry Branch program at NIMH, special attention has been given to the problems of late adolescence, both in the Family Studies Section and in the studies headed by Dr. Roger Shapiro on adjustment difficulties of college freshmen.

As Erikson has stressed (1956), a central issue of late adolescent development is the consolidation of a stabilized sense of personal identity, linked to, and differentiated within, the psychosocial environment. Difficulties at this stage in psychological differentiation and identity formation commonly present themselves as "separation" problems:

a) identity crises, including acute schizophrenic episodes, often precipitated by the first major separation from the intrafamilial environment, such as going away to college;

b) rebellious, sometimes delinquent, moves by the adolescent to establish himself apart from his family and its value system;

c) failure to emerge from a symbiotic dependency relationship with a parent (with the complaint about this situation usually coming from the other parent or other offspring).

Traditionally, these various problems are regarded as indications for individual psychotherapy with the adolescent. In ordinary psychiatric practice, initial and supplemental sessions with the parents are usually conducted apart from those with the adolescent. When the adolescent is primarily involved in working through the unresolved difficulties of his childhood and his parents are not currently deeply enmeshed with him, a traditional individual treatment arrangement does seem to me reasonable and appropriate. However, preliminary evaluation in *conjoint* family sessions is, in my view, nearly always useful in order to consider directly to what extent the parents share in the adolescent's ambivalence and confusion about his separating from them and going ahead with new extrafamilial roles. More often than not, in my experience, the parents are suffering as deeply, or more so, than the adolescent from their conflicted feelings about these changes. In terms of selecting treatment alternatives, the conjoint sessions may assist in distinguishing those problems which have an active, continuing residue chiefly in one family member from those problems in which the difficulties continue to be reciprocally shared. It is in the latter situation that extended exploratory family therapy appears to me to be especially indicated.

The subgroup of problems which are commonly called symbiotic, with mutually intrusive parent-child relationships, are most suitable of all for this form of treatment. Bringing the symbiotically enmeshed family members together is, in effect, an acknowledgment of the fact that the relationship is worthy of understanding because it serves significant functions. The conjoint treatment approach attempts to identify and analyze these functions rather than legislate them away through hospital or treatment arrangements, which too often merely create an external appearance of separation.

2) *The Trading of Dissociations.* There is a large and important group of family problems for which conjoint family therapy is indicated in which the intrafamilial problems are complementary and

interlocking. This significant kind of problem is so complex that the discussion of it here must take place by way of illustration. The general form of these problems is the following: Each person sees himself as having a specific limited difficulty which he feels derives from another family member and which he announces can only be alleviated by the other family member. While the claims appear to have some basis in fact, the person about whom they are made does not recognize the possibility that he himself makes any contribution to the problem. However, this other family member may be highly perceptive about corresponding difficulties which are similarly unacknowledged (dissociated) by the first, or another, family member. Thus, there is an intricate network of perceptions about others and dissociations about oneself in which each person "locates" the totality of a particular quality or feeling in another family member. Each person perceives one or more of the others in a starkly negative, pre-ambivalent light and experiences himself in a similar but reciprocal fashion, with the same abhorred quality in himself held dissociated out of his awareness. What is distinctive about this pattern, and therapeutically difficult, is the trading of dissociations: the fixed view that each person has of the other is unconsciously exchanged for a fixed view of himself held by the other. The interlocking result is similar to the system of reciprocal role-expectations which sociologists have described in intrafamilial relationships. However, here I refer to a system or organization of deeply unconscious processes, an organization which provides a means for *each* individual to cope with otherwise intolerable ideas and feelings.

The psychodynamic mechanisms operative here have been described under a variety of headings: projective identification (Bion, 1957; Klein, 1946), externalization (Brodey, 1959), etc. In the present connection, I wish to emphasize especially the ways in which the involvement may be shared by the whole family, is organized in a "social subsystem" (Parsons and Bales, 1955), and is, to a degree, enduringly established.

It should be stressed that the reciprocal and shared trading of dissociations both serves to *keep out* of each individual's awareness of himself the dreaded qualities and ideas and also serves to *retain* these qualities within his purview, at a fixed distance from his ego. The individual's fear that the dissociated experience might become unmanageable is thus reduced, but at the same time the problem is perpetuated, especially insofar as the interactional process helps make this a real and abiding part of the other person's behavior.

The trading of dissociations means that each person deals most focally with that in the other which the other cannot acknowledge.

Thus, there can be no "meeting," no confirmation, no mutality, no shared validation of feelings or experience. Here we have, of course an aspect of schizoid and schizophrenic experience, or, more accurately, failure of experience.

As a clinical example, in one family, here described highly schematically, the father, mother, and son each had dissociated into unawareness his or her own intensely destructive feelings for the others, but were keenly perceptive of the evidence for such feelings in the others. The father saw himself as having frustration but no real animosity toward his son, who was a caricature of the occupational failure which the father struggled to avoid feeling himself to be. However, the son and mother were acutely aware of the angry contempt contained in the criticism which the father heaped upon the son, which the father regarded as "helpful concern and advice."

The son, in turn, was blandly casual, at the time treatment began, about his academic and occupational failures with which his father was so preoccupied. However, the son sharply noted numerous indications that the father felt, but could not acknowledge, despair and failure about his own career. The mother, in turn, saw the father and son as dependent, helpless, squabbling boys needing her to manage the most minute responsibilities for them. When she brought up in family therapy one plan after another for them, they accepted her decisions quietly, but nevertheless spoke of her activities as meaningless "busy work." They failed to see their very real dependency on her, but belittled her feelings of loneliness and emptiness, feelings which she dissociated until family therapy made it possible for her to recognize them.

Further clinical details could document the processes underlying and sustaining the pattern of relationships within this family, but perhaps this brief outline, for purposes of this chapter, will suggest something of this common variety of problem for which family therapy seems especially indicated. It should be noted that the full complexity of a pattern of this kind usually becomes apparent only after a number of months of therapy.

In such a situation the intrapsychic dissociations of each family member are stabilized and reinforced by locating the dissociated aspects of each individual in the overt behavior of another family member. There he can regard the dissociated qualities as real and worthy of concern and efforts at change. In this kind of family problem no family member experiences himself as having an intrapsychic problem for which he might seek individual psychotherapy or psychoanalysis. Indeed, when such individuals do consult a psychiatrist, they are commonly regarded as not suitably motivated and treatment is not recommended. The person then goes on his way dissatisfied with the other members of his family and with what psychiatry has to offer them, but remains quite content with himself.

From the standpoint of individual diagnosis, many of these problems fall into the large group of ego-syntonic character disorders. Although sometimes these disorders can be converted through individual therapy into ego-alien problems about which the patient gradually becomes motivated in the course of the therapy, it is my impression that they drift in vast numbers into the recesses of psychiatric attention. Yet their pathologic impact upon others may be very considerable indeed. It is my suggestion that family therapy provides a means for bringing into treatment individuals who have very serious characterologic disorders indeed, but who would not come near a psychiatrist who insists on labeling them as individual patients.

3) *Collective Cognitive Chaos and Erratic Distancing.* Exploratory family therapy also seems indicated with the families of those schizophrenics who manifest bizarre, disruptive intrusions of so-called "primary process" thinking. These families commonly manifest what can be called "collective cognitive chaos," or as Dr. Margaret Thaler Singer and I have described it in another connection, "transactional thought disorder" (Wynne and Singer, 1963a). From still another vantage point, Schaffer et al. (1962) have described the subculture of these families as having an "institutionalization of fragmentation" of deep psychodynamic significance for each of the family members and for the family as a social subsystem.

In these families each person's individual statements, apart from the transactional context, may appear sufficiently normal so that one would not ordinarily question the rationality of specific, isolated statements. However, the over-all transactional sequence may be utterly bizarre, disjointed, fragmented. Even if the parents are psychotic to some degree, the over-all transactional disorder in these families often exceeds the severity of the individual parental disorder. This discrepancy between individual parental disorder and transactional family disorder can be grasped only with the greatest difficulty from individual diagnostic or therapeutic contacts with the family members. A number of clinical illustrations of this phenomenon have been described in previous publications (Wynne, 1961; Schaffer et al., 1962; Wynne and Singer, 1963a).

All the family members seem caught up in this chaotic communication, which is the "symptom" of their familial "pathology." They chronically have been unable to step back from this chaos, comment on it, or interrupt it in any useful fashion. Here the family therapist has a useful function to perform. As he gradually begins to grasp the nature and impact of these kinds of problems, his capacity to intervene actively is a matter of the greatest importance and complexity. Exploratory family therapy is the only means available, so far as I can see, for observing and treating the shared aspects of familial cognitive chaos.

In family problems, as well as otherwise, cognitive and communicative difficulties go hand in hand with difficulties in emotional "distancing" (Wynne and Singer, 1963a; Singer and Wynne, 1965). Families with chaotic thinking and communication characteristically have highly erratic, unstable styles of relating and of establishing "proper distance" with one another. At one moment they are remote and emotionally detached, and the next, intrusive or engulfing. The cognitive "focal distance" appropriate for a given task or communication thus shifts bewilderingly; blurred and fragmented thinking is inevitably associated with erratic distancing.

In principle, the family therapist's role can be, from time to time, to intervene, forcibly if necessary, and to assist the family in focusing upon specific issues, upon what was said and meant in a particular exchange. Thus, he may gradually help create a new model or pattern for thinking, communicating, and establishing appropriate distance or closeness.

In practice, we do not fully know what the potentialities of exploratory family therapy are with this kind of family. It is clear that inexperienced and passive therapists are swamped by these families. It is also clear that substantial therapeutic headway is possible, with more experienced and active therapists, in working with quite chaotic families after neither family nor individual appear to have benefited from previous individual therapy. However, it remains to be evaluated whether exploratory family therapy (or any presently available mode of treatment) is indicated for the *most* extremely disorganized families in which some family member or other perpetually disrupts valiant efforts of skillful therapists to bring order out of chaos. Perhaps a "total push" in-patient treatment of the entire family is necessary in such instances.

In any event, the family therapist is able to become acquainted with a treatment dilemma of which the individual therapist ordinarily remains blissfully unaware. As Schaffer et al. (1962) stressed, *any* therapeutic interest in pattern and meaning is basically antithetical to the subculture of these families in which meaning is either feared or not conceived as possible. An underlying subjective experience of patternlessness and meaninglessness pervades these families. A therapist's efforts to discover or create and to point out underlying meanings (*for him*) run head on against the family's underlying assumptions. It appears to me that the family therapist's perception of this chaotic kind of experience in the family, and at least part of the time, in himself, is a necessary beginning for genuinely therapeutic work with the family. However, the prospects of successful treatment outcome, and thus the assessment of treatment indications, are matters deserving prolonged scrutiny.

4) *Fixed Distancing, with Eruptive Threats and Episodes.* In other families for whom exploratory family therapy is indicated, the presenting problem is not erratic distancing but a relentless, deadening fixity of distance in relationships and a perseveratively rigid manner of organizing thoughts and perceptions. Whimsical, poignant, anxious, angry, or simply narrative accounts are all likely to be viewed in these families from the same fixed vantage point.

For example, in one family, a son was manifesting increasingly explosive restlessness and anger during a family session and expressed these feelings, while looking at the wall clock, by making a ten-second countdown ending in a loud, "Blast-off!" His mother, with characteristic literal-mindedness and detachment from direct encounters with her son, turned to the therapist and said: "I don't understand why Tommy has always been interested in clocks."

The members of these families regularly suffer from a shared sense of being unable to reach one another on any sort of human, feeling level. Each family member is painfully aware of his own need and wishes for relatedness, but each feels that the others block and do not allow intimacy or affection. They are, on the one hand, inextricably caught up with one another, yet, on the other, are unable either to separate or to develop mutuality (Wynne, Ryckoff, Day, and Hirsch, 1958). They appear to be held apart at a more or less fixed psychological distance.

The dynamics underlying this presenting problem vary. Often, however, the fixed distancing is the result of enduring, shared efforts to exclude from family life certain major kinds of feelings which are experienced as unmanageably threatening. Some of the shared mechanisms for maintaining these exclusions have been described in previous publications under the headings of "pseudomutuality" and "pseudohostility" (Wynne, 1961; Wynne *et al.*, 1958). When these mechanisms are massive and pervasive, and when, in addition, family psychological boundaries have few openings into emotionally significant extrafamilial experience, the child who grows up under these conditions is going to have great difficulty in recognizing and integrating a major variety of feelings and experience. For example, in some families anger and hostile feelings are quite massively excluded, in other families lustful feelings, and in still other families, feelings of tenderness and gentleness. When such feelings intrude themselves into the child's awareness as he moves into later adolescence or adulthood, as he undergoes biologic and psychological maturation, and as he becomes more exposed to these feelings in extrafamilial settings, he is apt to have an abrupt, shattering breakdown, sometimes schizophrenic in quality. On the family level, the breakdown is both dreaded and collusively supported as a direct and vicarious relief from the tense and vigilant, but immobilized, earlier family experience.

While an individual and a family are in the midst of coping with an acute schizophrenic episode, conjoint family therapy is sometimes exceedingly valuable in helping the family get in touch with previously excluded or denied experience which has erupted during the episode. On the other hand, the sealing-off and re-excluding family mechanisms often move so rapidly that only very intensive family therapy during this period can keep pace. Often, by the time the family is referred for treatment and can be seen conjointly, a new level of pseudomutuality or pseudohostility has been established, usually at an altered psychological distance. However, there may be a sufficiently bizarre quality to these shared restitutive changes or sufficient anxiety may be created by the return or threatened return of the psychotic process that there may be a high level of shared motivation to engage actively in the family therapy.

If the sealing-off process has gone farther, so that a new gap or scotoma has been established, with the disturbing ideas or feelings being prominent by their omission from recognition, the family therapy will proceed a good deal more slowly. However, because it is so striking when *all* the members of the family leave out certain kinds of feelings, discussion and clarification of the nature of this gap may be more easily and effectively brought up by the therapist working with the family than when he works with the individual. Usually, at least one family member is partially able to notice these feelings or ideas and can, with help, gradually pave the way for freer perception and communication by the rest of the family.

The possibility that these family members have tender or affectionate feelings for one another is especially regarded by them as utterly incredible. Suggestions by a therapist that occasions for such feelings might come up are at first regarded as a preposterous matter for perplexity or scorn. Families weighed down with a sense of pointlessness about relating appear to live together, move about together, and yet from an emotional standpoint experience themselves as disconnected, with the very possibility of emotional contact regarded as unreal. When the family therapist can start to uncover and help make tolerable the long-stifled, masked, or transformed capacities of these family members for tenderness and affection toward one another, very considerable therapeutic gains sometimes ensue. I am especially indebted to Dr. Harold Searles for helping me become alert to this aspect of family experience (Searles, 1958).

5) *Amorphous Communication.* A kind of family problem for which exploratory family therapy is possibly indicated is a pervasively amorphous, vague, undirected form of communication (Wynne and Singer, 1963b), particularly prominent in the families of so-called undifferentiated simple and "process" schizophrenics, but not exclusively limited to schizophrenics. Families of certain neurotic characters also have this tendency, although with lesser degrees of severity. In the family therapy and apparently also in the rest of their lives together they are not so much afflicted by frankly contradictory, double-binding expectations but rather by vaguely defined expectations. Statements are not stated and then disqualified but are instead never clearly enough stated so that one would know when a disqualification has taken place. The offspring in these families are usually not frankly delusional or bizarrely disturbed, but rather show a very marked and generalized impairment of basic ego skills, including the use of language.

Psychotherapists, both with individuals and families, have generally found these kinds of patients and their families thoroughly dull and uninteresting, if they see them at all, even in consultations. More prolonged contact is apt to plunge the therapist into the depths of therapeutic despair (Farber, 1958). Therapists naturally veer away from the profound feelings of pointlessness, the drifting unclarity of expression, the absence of those illuminating flashes which temporarily redeem work with more lively psychotics and their families.

Precisely because these patients have been so neglected, because they are so numerous, though quiet, in the back wards of large mental institutions, and because of the theoretical significance of this form of disorder (Wynne and Singer, 1963b), family therapy, as well as other modes of treatment, deserves further trial. It is my impression that these patients as individuals become more intelligible (and more interesting) when seen as part of their family matrix. However, the potentialities of *extended* family therapy with families of these patients has not yet been adequately pursued, at NIMH, or elsewhere, so far as I am aware.

Without regarding this brief survey as at all comprehensive, I hope, nevertheless, to have conveyed something of what I mean by problems which are unconsciously shared in a family unit and for which conjoint, exploratory family therapy is especially indicated.

OTHER FACTORS AFFECTING THE INDICATIONS

In general medicine and surgery, a number of conditions or factors other than the nature of the presenting illness determine whether a particular form of treatment is indicated at a given time. The patient may be allergic to an otherwise desirable drug; his cardiac status may be incompatible with an exhausting surgical procedure; the only available surgeon may be inadequately trained to perform a difficult operation with a reasonable chance that the patient might survive.

For exploratory family therapy there is an analogous array of considerations which should be evaluated in order to decide whether this form of treatment is indicated on a practicable basis in a specific situation. Three varieties of such considerations will be discussed here: (1) the physical and psychological availability for treatment of the appropriate family constellation; (2) the phase of the over-all psychotherapeutic process in which the conjoint family therapy is undertaken; and (3) the characteristics of the therapists who are available for the conjoint family therapy.

1) *Family Constellation Available for Therapy.* A very special and significant problem in exploratory family therapy is to ascertain who the "patient" is, that is, who constitutes the relevant family group that should be brought into treatment. Should married off-spring and their spouses be included? Grandparents? Pre-adolescent offspring? If a key family member can, or will, attend only irregularly or not at all, should a conjoint family approach be undertaken without this family member?

As I have already implied, the most important consideration in selecting and maintaining an appropriate constellation of family members for exploratory family therapy is that they have a network of continuing, emotionally significant relationships with one another. This network or system of relationships, however, malfunctioning and troublesome, is holding these people together in a pattern of reciprocal obligations and expectations. The family therapist thus endeavors to establish a relationship, not with an individual nor with an aggregate of individuals, but with an interpersonal *organiza-tion* having both a history together and potentialities of a future to-gether. In Parsonian sociologic terms (Parsons and Bales, 1955), the treatment relationship is with the social subsystem.

The special characteristics of a family constellation in treatment can be illuminated by a comparison with conventional group ther-apy. The differences are striking. Too often, in my opinion, family therapy is regarded as a variant form of group therapy, as reflected, for example, in the unfortunate term, "family group therapy," presumably because of the superficial similarity of numbers of individuals meeting together. Family therapy, when carried out on an exploratory level, has distinctive features which are obscured if it is regarded as a form of group therapy.

First of all, the motivation which brings family members into conjoint therapy is quite different. Family members are not necessarily aware of individual motivation for personal change, but rather agree to and want to meet with their family members because they are entangled in a web of troublesome relationships with them. Group therapy participants, in contrast, usually have never even seen the other group members before and agree to meet together because of a wish for personal change. Later, the situation may be reversed as a *result* of treatment: Family members may discover personal dissatisfactions and the wish to change aspects of themselves, not just others; group therapy participants may develop an emotional investment and entanglement in the group structure. However, the criteria for selecting participants are very different. Personalized motivation for change is a bonus in selecting family therapy participants, while it ordinarily is a precondition for getting individuals to begin to come to group therapy.

This distinction perhaps makes more clear the importance of the previously mentioned stricture that family therapy participants be emotionally invested and entangled with one another, not just interested in this family constellation from a detached or intellectual standpoint. This shared entanglement is the functional equivalent in family therapy of the individual inner distress which gives impetus to individual psychotherapy and conventional group therapy.

A second, closely related distinction between the kind of constellation treated in family therapy and in conventional group therapy lies in the historical continuity of the family social organization and the discontinuity of the group therapy constellation. In those families which are appropriately treated with exploratory conjoint therapy, there is a deeply unconscious basis for a shared family ideology and set of values which may have become more or less idiosyncratic for the particular family as a subculture. In this respect, individual psychotherapy and family therapy are rather close to each other. Both the individual psychotherapist and the family therapist are presented with an *historically established*, on-going unit or system—personality, in the case of individual therapy, and the family social organization, in the case of family therapy.

In conventional group therapy, in contrast, the therapist can only endeavor to *create* such a system. The group therapy "system" which is created in the course of therapeutic interaction cannot have, and perhaps should not have, the historical continuity and depth of reciprocal expectations which have naturally arisen as the family nurtures and infuses its characteristics into the cognitive and emotional bones, the ego structure, of at least some of its members, i.e., the offspring.

It may be helpful to describe here an example of a family in which historical continuity and current emotional entanglement did *not* exist and for whom, therefore, exploratory family therapy was *contra*indicated. In this family the husband's illness with a brain tumor apparently had precipitated an acute schizophrenic episode in the wife. She had been married for a number of years and had a couple of children; she was mainly involved emotionally with her family of marriage rather than with her family of origin. A staff member who wanted to work with an acute schizophrenic in family therapy set up "family therapy" sessions with this woman and her parents. However, she no longer had a really meaningful system of relationships with her parents, even though the three of them complied with the request that they meet together. This arrangement was not useful therapeutically; in fact, it was a disturbing distraction to getting around to more useful, more specifically indicated individual therapy.

In selecting the appropriate family constellation for exploratory family therapy, it is important not be be bound down by literal and legalistic definitions of the "family." Although those persons who live in the same household together are most commonly the appropriate constellation to see together, the possibility of exceptions should be considered in the preliminary evaluative phase of the work with every family. Sometimes grandparents, spouses of offspring, and other members of the extended family are active participants in the current family dilemma, whereas in other instances, members of the nuclear family, such as very young offspring or married offspring who live elsewhere, may not be centrally involved in the family impasse which is the focus of treatment.

Thus, my suggestion is that the constellation of persons seen in family therapy be those who are *functionally* linked together, within discernible *psychological* boundaries. These persons are not necessarily limited to the nuclear family (parents and their immediate offspring). This point is undoubtedly much more important in those cultural groups in which the extended family is more significant than it is in urban, native-American families.

An example of the inappropriate use of family therapy occurred early in our experience through a failure to assess properly the location of the psychological boundaries around the family system. This family, Asian in background, was referred to us by a man who told us he was the interpreter for the family. We found that the family could speak English well enough for us to understand, and we regarded the interpreter as something of a busybody interloper. However, it turned out, as we now would predict, that the whole venture was sabotaged by this nonbiological family member, the interpreter, who from a standpoint of the psychological setup was very much a family member and had been for over twenty-five years. This was one of the first families we saw conjointly and we excluded him from the family sessions which we had set up. After a number of sessions with this particular family, two sisters of the schizophrenic son stopped participating because, we discovered, of the intervention of the "interpreter." The sisters were sufficiently involved in the parent-son relations so that it was not fruitful to proceed without them. This example illustrates the importance of taking time to evaluate where the psychological boundaries of the family are and not taking at face value conventional definitions of the "family."

A family in which the constellation brought into treatment was more adequately assessed is the following: In this family the presenting patient was a 20-year-old daughter, a schizophrenic inhabitant of a large mental hospital which had referred the problem to us because of acting-out between the girl and her father. The father had worked his way into the ward past all varieties of visiting regulations, and was getting involved in behavior which the nursing staff regarded as pretty frankly incestuous. The mother also complained about this father-daughter relation. At first we did not hear about a fourth member of this family, a sister, aged 22, who was unmarried and living at home. When we raised the question of having this sister take part in an initial family diagnostic session, the father demurred and indicated she was not concerned with the problem. However, we asked that she come and later found she was indeed a key figure in the family organization.

It became apparent that this was indeed a system of relationships in which the "well" sister was very intensely involved in a rivalrous relation with the patient. There was a balance of power in the family between the father and the schizophrenic daughter, on the one hand, and the mother and the well sister, on the other hand. If we had seen this family without the well sister present, the family therapy would have been, I am quite certain, a fiasco. Only by having an opportunity to assess and work with this balance of power was it possible to look at the family dynamics in deeper detail and to understand contextually various segments of the family relationships.

It should be obvious by now that not all disturbed families, legally designated as such, constitute social subsystems for which family therapy is indicated. The term "subsystem," as Parsons has explained (Parsons and Bales, 1955), implies that the family has a degree of internal organization and a certain level of self-regulatory functioning, but is not really self-sufficient and enduringly independent of the larger social system and society in which it is embedded. However, the degree to which families for long periods of their existence are organized in *relatively* self-regulating, self-sustaining systems varies widely, both within Western cultures and probably elsewhere.

It is my clinical impression that disturbed families are differently integrated into the larger social system than are better adapted, "normal" families. Psychologically and sociologically disturbed families tend to have either (a) absent or defective subsystem boundaries, or (b) psychological boundaries with an abnormal impermeability, maintained partly through shifting the boundary location without really opening up genuine transactions with the broader community. This phenomenon has previously been described under the heading of the "rubber fence" in relation to certain families of schizophrenics (Wynne *et al.*, 1958). The members of these latter families may have transient relationships with extrafamilial persons and use them as intermediaries from time to time. Sometimes individual family members may have relationships outside the family which are unacknowledged by the other family members. However, as members of these families, they do not have stabilized, *acknowledged* relationships with the wider community. They do not receive intrafamilial recognition and support for these extrafamilial relationships. Thus, the family boundaries surround the intermediaries or massively exclude them, but in either event, there is no pattern for negotiating stable relationships beyond the psychological family boundaries.

Cross-cultural psychiatric investigations now being undertaken in our program may reveal, I suspect, that the difficulties related to family boundaries are particularly prevalent where the isolated, nuclear family is the predominant form of family organization. Where extended family organization is more highly valued and structured, it seems to provide culturally recognizable means for individuals to move from within the immediate nuclear family into the broader community. Thus the notion of family boundaries takes on a different meaning in such situations.

Those situations in which family boundaries *are* tightly organized, or are shifting in location and are really psychologically impermeable, are precisely those for which conjoint family therapy appears to be especially indicated. The therapist in a sense represents some contact with an extrafamilial figure whom the family may try to incorporate and digest. If the therapist can survive as a distinct individual, he may provide a new experience for the family as a meaningful emotional contact with an extrafamilial figure. In situations in which it is difficult or impossible to define family boundaries, diagnostic and evaluative family sessions may be useful, but extended exploratory family therapy may not be possible. The available family constellation will in such circumstances be too indeterminate.

The principle of working with a stably defined family social subsystem as the "patient" unit is closely linked to the psychoanalytic principle that stability of the treatment set-up facilitates the analytic treatment process and, indeed, makes possible exploration in some detail and depth. Comparable to the psychoanalytic situation, I feel that the family constellation with whom the therapeutic work is being carried out should be specified and maintained with as much rigor as possible, *if* the particular dynamics of this constellation are to be as fully explored as possible. I have already indicated the desirability, for certain diagnostic and research purposes, of seeing the family in various combinations. This, however, should not be confused with the goal of working with a *particular* family constellation in depth.

As in the psychoanalytic treatment situation, expectable stability in the treatment relationship helps build up a shared sense of trust. This is based upon the gradually growing experience of the participants that the family therapy unit will continue to meet together even when disturbing and disruptive feelings or thoughts have been communicated. If the therapist randomly changes the treatment constellation, the development of this trust and freedom in communication may be impaired. In addition, allowing family members to miss sessions whenever they find them slightly inconvenient or somewhat disturbing, or haphazard shifting of the treatment arrangements for any reason, tends to be collusive with acting-out tendencies within the family. If changes in the treatment arrangements are planned or permitted, the implications and consequences for the unfolding of the treatment process should be clearly recognized. If only a portion of those persons who are psychologically involved in a family network or constellation can regularly attend the conjoint sessions, family therapy as an exploratory venture in depth over time is limited in scope. In some cases these limits are so marked that individual psychotherapy or other treatment approaches may be indicated in preference to family therapy even when the kind of problem presented by the family seems suitable for family therapy.

2) *Phase of the Psychotherapeutic Process.* Another condition

affecting whether exploratory family therapy is indicated in a specific instance is the phase of the psychotherapeutic process. I find useful a view of the psychotherapeutic process as passing through a series of phases in which first one problem area and then another comes into focus. For example, one focus for therapy may be intrapsychic conflict, such as an individual's struggle to deal with the inhibiting effects of anachronistic anxiety upon his sexuality. Another focus may be a cognitively confused power struggle permeating all of a family's relationships. As various foci of these kinds come into view, long-range changes in the nature of the "presenting" problem and the nature of the emotional organization of the individual family members and the family as a whole may make appropriate a shift of main focus from family therapy to individual therapy or the reverse. These shifts, if carefully considered, need not involve the random, haphazard changes in treatment arrangements which I have discussed above as limiting the effectiveness of any form of psychotherapy.

An example of long-range shifts depending on the phase of treatment occurred in the work with a family in which Drs. Juliana Day, Leslie Schaffer, Irving Ryckoff and I participated. In this family the parents and two sons, aged 21 and 23, were seen together. The parents were in constant conflict and had come to the kind of impasse I have called pseudo-hostility (Wynne *et al.*, 1958). This constitutes a shared defense against recognizing or experiencing potential tenderness, affection, or sexual attraction. For twenty-five years this couple had been talking about getting a divorce but had never gotten around to it. The elder son, who was the presenting patient, was constantly involved in negotiating between the parents and in rescuing the marriage. This left him in constant turmoil, with a melange of obsessional, schizophrenic, and depressive symptoms. He had started individual psychotherapy three times without being able to make effective use of it.

In conjoint therapy with this family, we noticed and were able to comment upon the way that every time the parents began to quarrel, or later, to express positive feelings, they turned away from each other to the elder son. Reciprocally, he actively interceded with pithy attacks on one or the other until their quarrel or incipient love-making was temporarily disrupted. Despite the regularity with which this interaction pattern was manifest, none of the family members had been aware of it and could not have described it verbally in individual therapy.

In passing, it is of interest that the elder son was literally conceived in order to fill this mediating role between the parents. Within a year after the parents were married, the mother felt that the marriage was going to break up. The husband had been previously married and divorced without having children. In a deliberate effort to hold the marriage together, the wife omitted the use of a contraceptive and became pregnant. The elder son was in effect a child savior. Only after extended therapy was he able to relinquish this gratifying but anguished role and were the parents able to attenuate their need for him.

The younger son in this family had not been so caught up in this conflict. His role differed. Although he was a quite emotionally isolated young man, his problems were not predominantly intrafamilial relationship problems. Soon after the family therapy began he went away to college, was married, and dropped out of the family picture.

Over a period of about two and one-half years of conjoint therapy the family interaction gradually changed. The elder son began to stand apart from the parental struggle, and, at the same time, the parents were occasionally talking to each other rather than only *about* each other. However, these changes did not stabilize until several other "levels of interaction," long-standing in the family life, made their appearance in the conjoint therapy. If the son failed to intervene actively, the tempo and intensity of the parental quarrel characteristically heightened, at which point the son diverted their attention in another fashion. He would stretch out horizontally with a profoundly aggrieved facial expression, a combination of rage, paralyzed withdrawal, and ostentatious boredom. The parents, who had long familiarity with his behavior, would become preoccupied with divergent interpretations of its cause. At any rate, their quarrel again shifted focus from each other to the son.

Although the son was inclined to describe himself, as the hapless victim of the parental struggle, his behavior, as the therapists noted, has a distinct element of actively sharing in, and contributing to, the struggle. He acknowledged considerable perplexity about his involvement, and when the therapists proposed that he explore his personal distress more fully in individual therapy (with another therapist), he readily agreed.

He entered psychoanalytic therapy on a four times a week basis. As he gradually focused more and more on his personal, intrapsychic problems, the family sessions increasingly were concerned with the marital problems of the parents. First, however, another family interaction pattern made its appearance, once again a pattern of long-standing. When the son quietly but clearly was becoming more involved in extrafamilial interests, his mother became alternately furious and depressed. She attacked him for being disinterested in her, not caring about her any more, and so on. At first he retreated from his outside interests and again spent more time at home.

Eventually, however, it was apparent that the son was no longer really a part of this family's emotional organization in the same sense that he had been originally. He was dating a girl regularly in spite of his mother's objections. He was succeeding in his college work, which he had not been able to do previously despite high intellectual capacity.

As he went ahead with his individual therapy and his own life and as the parents became more intensely and directly involved with each other, the therapy changed its focus. After these changes in the kind of problem and the kind of family psychological constellation were fully apparent, the conjoint sessions were discontinued. Marital therapy with the two parents took its place, and the son went ahead with his individual therapy which was completed with a very satisfactory result.

In the course of time, the mother, who was rather more reflective than the father, began to notice that some of her sources of difficulty with her husband stemmed from her early life experience with her father and from her identification with her mother who had been in a rather similar marriage. The intensity of involvement in the marital struggle attenuated. She said she would like to have some individual therapy because she would like to work more intensively on problems which did not directly involve her husband. Although some of these things had been dealt with in the family and marital sessions, it now did seem as if the focus of emotional tension had shifted. We arranged for individual therapy for the wife, and eventually all the conjoint sessions were discontinued, with individual therapy taking their place as the problems became progressively more intrapsychic.

Here, then, was a situation in which family therapy seemed to be highly indicated during a particular phase of the over-all treatment process in which the family members were very caught up with one another. Individual therapy, attempted previously but unsuccessfully with the son, appeared to be facilitated by the conjoint therapy. The mother would never have considered the possibility of individual therapy for herself without the experience of family therapy first.

However, this example should not be taken to mean that the facilitation of individual therapy is a primary criterion of successful family therapy. This outcome may be appropriate for certain families, but for others, increased understanding and reduction of tension in family relationships may usefully occur without individual therapy for anyone.

In some situations individual therapy may prepare the way for family therapy, rather than the reverse. Two kinds of problems in which this phasing seems advisable are the following:

a) Some depressed and masochistic individuals take over, indeed soak up, blame for any and all family difficulties, absolving the others of any responsibility (and denying that they have any power). In my experience, such a person has always been the mother-wife. These individuals, who have a high propensity for introjection, commonly have families who support and fit in with the individual by directing at her a barrage of projective accusations and contempt. Sometimes the shared insistence on this view is so intense at the beginning of therapy that the family seems motivated only to perpetuate it. If diagnostic conjoint sessions indicate that the family members are not at all prepared to think about or look at their shared contribution to the problem, then a period of individual therapy can help the presenting patient become aware of wishes to be something other than a scapegoat. However, conjoint family therapy may, at a later phase, speed understanding and facilitate change in the ways that she unconsciously invites abuse and the other family members fulfill her expectations in actuality, not only in fantasy. The distinction between fantasy and actuality has often become incredibly garbled in these families. After a family has become concerned with this issue, conjoint therapy may be very useful. However, a phase of individual therapy, before or concomitant with the family therapy, may facilitate recognition of the shared nature of the problem.

b) As I have suggested earlier, conjoint family therapy may sometimes be valuable in helping cope with the intrafamilial aspects of an acute schizophrenic episode in an offspring. On the other hand, those acute schizophrenics who are still in panic and who have not yet established a relationship with a therapist may not be able to tolerate the complexity of family interviews. This is less of a problem than usually anticipated by those who are inexperienced in family therapy; a vigorous therapist who clearly takes charge of the conjoint interviews can do a great deal to bring anxiety down to a therapeutically useful level. Nevertheless, there do appear to be situations in which regular conjoint therapy is best delayed for a month or two until after the panicked schizophrenic offspring has begun to develop some degree of trust in an individual therapist. Then if this therapist participates in the family therapy with a co-therapist, the psychotherapeutic process may unfold quite smoothly. However, it should be made clear to presenting patient and family, at the time of the *initial* conjoint evaluation, that the family may be asked to meet regularly in conjoint therapy later on.

3) *Kind of Available Therapists.* Finally, I shall discuss the very important issue of the kind of therapists available for exploratory family therapy. In general, as one might expect, the more skillful the psychotherapist or psychoanalyst, the better family therapist he will be. However, there are certain additional characteristics and qualifications which are desirable in the family therapist. The absence of these characteristics and skills in the therapist imposes certain limitations and sometimes contraindications on the use of exploratory family therapy.[3] Even though a family problem exists for which family therapy would be indicated under *ideal* circumstances, this approach may not be indicated under *actual* conditions. including the unavailability of a suitable family therapist, as well as the unavailability of the appropriate family constellation during a suitable psychotherapeutic phase.

a) COUNTERTRANSFERENCE PROBLEMS. Whenever work with a particular family continues over a prolonged period, an especially high level of awareness of countertransference pitfalls is desirable. Through unconscious or deliberate selection of particular kinds of individual patients and avoidance of others, a psychotherapist can systematically avoid persons in roles which give him especial countertransference difficulties. For example, a therapist who has not fully resolved his problems with authority figures may omit older males from his practice. However, in his relationship to the constellation of persons seen in family therapy, the therapist cannot so easily bypass partially unresolved countertransference problems. He must retain the capacity to be empathic with each of the family members and still be able to step back and reflect about the nature of the over-all transactions.

Either overidentification with a particular family member or a failure to appreciate, understand, and empathize with individuals in a particular family role may create difficulties. The therapist new to family therapy often feels in an impossible double-bind with conflicting demands from the various family members and from his expectations of himself. Some therapists seem to deal with this experience by becoming more tightly constricted in the expression of their feelings and in the reflective utilization of their fantasies;

---

[3] The term "contraindication" is used in medicine to refer to any condition of the patient which makes the indicated medication or treatment inadvisable. In family psychotherapy the "patient" is, or becomes, the family unit or, more precisely, the family-therapist unit, for it is the relationships between all of these persons and the behavior and subjective experience of all of them, including the therapist, which constitute the data that is under scrutiny. Therefore, any "condition" of the family-therapist unit (including characteristics of the therapist) which makes family therapy inadvisable, though it would be otherwise appropriate, constitutes in a broad sense a "contraindication" to family therapy.

other therapists, however, do manage to regain confidence in their own resiliency and that of the family, even in the face of these emotional dilemmas.

Gradually, during the last several years, there seems to be a diminution in an earlier tendency in family studies and family therapy to perceive offspring as primarily victimized by their parents. Clearly, as an abiding, constricted perception, this view involved an overidentification with the offspring and a failure to grasp the nature of the reciprocal processes in family relations.

A special problem created by overidentification with one of the family members in family therapy is that this quickly leads to disruptive alignments and splits in the family therapy group. In individual therapy overidentification may simply, for a while at least, lead to a lack of therapeutic progress. In family therapy other family members experience the patient and the overidentified therapist as aligned together and split off from the rest of the family therapy group. Illustrations of this phenomenon have been described elsewhere (Wynne, 1961). If this continues unrecognized and uninterpreted, some of the participants will soon be unwilling to continue. In both individual and family therapy, of course, maximal self-awareness by the therapist will greatly facilitate favorable therapeutic movement.

A particularly difficult countertransference stumbling-block in family therapy comes up in problems of competition with the father of the family. Often the parents are already defensive and threatened by feelings of failure over the fact of psychiatric disturbance in the family, but, in addition, the father's culturally assigned role as a decision-maker and responsible leader of the family may in effect be taken over by the therapist. Particularly, the male therapist needs to be aware of the implicit humiliation which a father may experience simply by observing a therapist who deals decisively and effectively with the other members of the family. If the therapist is regarded warmly or affectionately by one family member, this may be experienced by other family members as evidence of their own unlovability. Open recognition and discussion of such issues can be greatly clarifying and reassuring, whereas unacknowledged competition with a family member by the therapist can make that family member's position untenable and lead him to withdraw or disrupt the therapy.

It is at least conceivable that some of the special countertransference problems in family therapy may be partly the consequence of the traditional emphasis upon dyadic relationships in psychoanalytic and psychotherapeutic practice. Although the oedipal situation is after all multipersonal, it is possible that the dyadic treatment relationship in traditional practice tends to underestimate the impact and full complexity of triadic and multipersonal problems. If it is true that in the usual personal analysis psychiatrists and psychoanalysts have not very adequately worked on and resolved their own anxieties and difficulties about being with groups, this may add to the countertransference difficulties of family therapists, as well as conventional group therapists. In this regard, training and experience in conventional group therapy may be of considerable help to the family therapist, and vice versa, with experience in either form of therapy broadening the perspectives and range of self-awareness of the individual psychotherapist and psychoanalyst.

I have suggested already that the problems of working with families on a diagnostic and short-term basis are quite different from more intensive long-term therapy. One difference is the relative ease with which countertransference difficulties can be overlooked or brushed aside in shorter or less intensive contacts with families. The focus is apt to be on such matters as the diagnostic evaluation itself, the planning of further therapeutic or other activity, the immediate resolution of a crisis, etc., so that skewed reactions by the therapist may not have obvious consequences.

Similarly, if the therapist changes the therapeutic set-up frequently, either the interview schedule of the constellation of people meeting together, neither countertransference nor transference issues are allowed to unfold and become clarified. The therapist can even deceive himself into believing that these issues do not arise in family therapy. Even though both the structure and content of transferences in family therapy differs from that in individual psychotherapy or psychoanalysis, these same phenomena do occur, because it is part of human psychology that this should be so, and they can become clear and structured if the therapist allows them to come into view. Only fragments of transference phenomena will be apparent unless there is a stabilized set-up for the family therapy. I feel that the tendency to disregard transference-countertransference phenomena in family therapy is the result of not establishing treatment conditions on a sufficiently stabilized basis so that the patterning of the transference-countertransference can come into focus. To be sure, it is much more complex than in individual therapy, especially as a result of original transference figures being present.

This issue deserves much more extensive and intensive exploration than has as yet been accomplished. My colleague, Dr. Leslie Schaffer, has suggested that we need to find out how fully a "regressive family transference neurosis" can be established; optimal conditions would include a rigidly maintained constellation of participants, a high frequency of sessions, say, four times a week, and freedom from the distraction and diffusion of other forms of therapeutic intervention carried on concomitantly. Those experiences which I have had which most nearly approximate these conditions, did, in fact, lead to a better defined transference-countertransference picture than in other family therapy situations.

A common pitfall in family therapy occurs when the therapist decides he should see individually a family member toward whom he has unresolved positive or negative feelings. Rationalizing this change on the grounds of "flexibility," he disrupts the unfolding, and mutes the impact, of feelings which could most appropriately be explored within the conjoint treatment set-up, not fearfully evaded. It seems to me highly desirable to scrutinize very carefully *every* move to change the family treatment set-up, whether long-range, as described in the previous section, or very transient, in order to consider whether the change may be mainly stimulated by countertransference difficulties of the therapists or emerging transference phenomena in family members.

b) SUSTAINED INTEREST OF THE THERAPIST. A practical problem of some importance in prolonged family therapy is that the tasks of maintaining alertness to countertransference problems (self-observation) and of observing the very complex transactions in the therapy are emotionally wearing and exhausting. As with therapists working intensively with individual schizophrenics, there tends to be a fairly high attrition rate among therapists willing to continue with this kind of professional activity. At least part of the problem is a matter of the amount of energy that a therapist is willing to expend over long periods. Special interest in work of this kind, especially with regard to research objectives, may be necessary to sustain the activity with highly disturbed families over long periods.

In addition, it is not easy to develop a *workable* orientation to families as units (social subsystems). Many therapists conduct family therapy in a manner which suggests that they continue to be primarily concerned with the individual presenting patient or, sometimes, some other individual family member. In effect, they do individual therapy in a family setting. Although at certain times it is desirable to direct most of the verbal attention to a particular family member, the therapist who is doing family therapy of the sort I have been describing will retain an underlying alertness to the nonverbal reactions of the other family members and will be considering in the back of his mind how the individual material fits into the overall family patterns. An orientation to families as units is, I believe, not so much a matter of the skill of the therapist as of his "set," his way of thinking about therapy and human relationships. It should be acknowledged that some therapists are primarily oriented to intrapsychic issues and to the dyadic patient-therapist relation.

Conjoint family therapy conducted by therapists who cannot, or do not wish to, shift from this traditional "set" will not capitalize upon the full potential of the conjoint treatment situation.

c) ACTIVE, LIMIT-SETTING CAPACITIES OF THE THERAPIST. A third characteristic of therapists which is more important in family therapy than in individual therapy is that the therapist needs to be comfortable with the aggressive, active, limit-setting aspects of his role. Edward Hoedemaker (1960) has written a very valuable paper on this subject in which he has contended that an intrinsic aspect of even the classical psychoanalytic situation is the limit-setting functions of the analyst. Ordinarily, with well-acculturated neurotics who know what to expect of the analytic setup, very little overt limit-setting needs to be done. With acting-out, borderline, psychotic patients, more activity is required of the therapist. In family therapy, the necessity of activity by the therapist is regularly a problem. The therapist who is apprehensive about setting limits and defining conditions for the therapy is going to have even more difficulty in working with families than with individuals.

In some instances the family social system is so tightly organized and integrated that the therapist finds himself treated as an outsider and he may have difficulty making entry into this system. This situation is somewhat analogous to treatment of ego-syntonic character disorders; comparably, some families present what might be called *family-syntonic disorders*. Especially with such families, activity of the family therapist is a necessary stimulus to change. Family therapy, like the psychoanalysis of individual character disorder, requires special orientation to the opening up of closed-off issues.

Because many families will continue talking with one another even though the therapist does nothing, it is easy for the family therapist to be passive and even to rationalize a belief that his inactivity is desirable. Repetitious talking or squabbling can be a means of avoiding reflective therapeutic work. The mere fact that a family is willing to keep coming and keep talking does not necessarily mean that this is therapeutically useful. With families which are all too highly patterned in their use of homeostatic mechanisms, the therapist who "lets the family work out their own problems" will be confronted by a staggering monotony and failure to change.

d) CAPACITY OF THE THERAPIST FOR RESTRAINT. Activity by the therapist, of course, should not be confused with acting-out. The temptations and pressures to be indiscriminately active are often even greater than in other forms of therapy. Sometimes this takes the form of giving poorly considered advice; sometimes, laying down reckless ultimatums; sometimes, badgering one or other family member endlessly.

A more subtle and more common form of this difficulty is the use of premature interpretations or clarifications. A great deal of observable dynamic material is often very impressive to the family therapist. It is easy for him to assume that the family members are noticing at least some of what is going on. The family therapist needs to use all of his empathic capacities to understand the form in which the various family members are experiencing what is going on so that he does not leap ahead in ways which either are simply confusing to them or which provoke heightened defensive operations. A problem in family therapy is that the material, both verbal and nonverbal, which is available for clarification and interpretation, rapidly out-distances what the family members are ready to allow into their awareness. In individual therapy the data known to the therapist accumulates at a pace more nearly that which the patient can assimilate.

A Few Suggestions for the Training and Orientation of Potential Family Therapists

With all the strictures that I have been describing, the reader may have incorrectly assumed that I believe that exploratory family therapy is so difficult that no one is qualified to do it. On the contrary, although I regard the issues and problems raised as worthy of attention, they are by no means insurmountable. Many of the difficulties can be reduced to a manageable level by quite workable means, such as establishing as definitely as possible the conditions for treatment with each family, clarifying the therapist's expectations about such matters as who is expected for the sessions, and maintaining an orientation to those problems which are shared concerns of the *entire* family rather than to intriguing but distracting side issues.

I have already indicated the importance which I attach to reducing, if not eliminating, the countertransference pitfalls in family therapy through the psychoanalytic experience of the therapists. I have also suggested that experience in conventional group therapy may help curb the individualistic bias of most therapists.

In addition, while therapists are developing experience with a conjoint family approach, the liberal use of colleagues, supervisors, observers, and co-therapists to discuss the issues which come up can be of great assistance in avoiding some of the pitfalls I have discussed.

The problem of co-therapists is a whole subject area which I cannot discuss in detail here. In our program at the National Institute of Mental Health we have used two therapists with most families, as a training and research device. Therapeutically, we have also found that in families with many members, and in families which are especially fragmented and disorganized, the use of co-therapists does help the therapist to survive. He can be freer in his reflective capacities, not have to be defensively managerial, and can call upon the resources of the additional pair of eyes and ears in keeping up with the events of the therapy.

Even though the same events may be observed, the emotional reactions of different therapists may vary and, additively, help build up a more adequate picture of the various facets of the family situation. Because emotional reactions are not likely to be simultaneous in more than one therapist, the problems of disruptive alignments and splits involving the therapist can sometimes be reduced with the use of co-therapists. Nevertheless, after the therapy is a going concern and the therapist has some sense of the nature of the family with which he is working, the use of a solo therapist is quite practicable, if necessary, except in the most disturbed families.

Finally, I would like to state that it appears easy to exaggerate the possible hazards in family therapy. The likelihood of bringing about drastic or precipitous changes unintentionally is actually extremely low. Examples which I have heard cited of major changes occurring as a consequence of family interaction turn out to be actually a repetition of a long-standing family pattern, new only to the therapist, or to involve gross errors in the treatment approach, especially excessive passivity on the part of the therapist and a prior failure to establish a treatment plan. In family therapy, as in individual psychotheray and psychoanalysis, the appearance of symptoms in the treatment situation is necessary and appropriate. The important consideration is whether a treatment structure has been set up for containing and working with the symptoms. This has obviously not been done when therapists and family become alarmed and drop the conjoint family approach as soon as significant psychopathology emerges, either in the form of symptoms or resistance.

I have been far more impressed with the difficulty of bringing about genuine and lasting change in family patterns than in the dangers of unintentionally disorganizing them. Inept comments may make various family members angry or upset, and the therapist and the family members may become quite uncomfortable, but this is not the same as bringing about lasting change. The homeostatic, self-regulatory capacities of families as social subsystems, especially if one is actually meeting with the whole family rather than a piece of it, are very considerable. Indeed, *families have a staggering capacity to remain the same*. Hence, the caution which persists in some centers about trying out family therapy approaches may reflect in part an underestimation of the strength of patterning in human relationships

Individual psychotherapy and psychoanalysis, conventional group psychotherapy, and conjoint family therapy each have distinctive kinds of patient-therapist relationships, leading to distinctive problems, goals, and indications. I have attempted here to summarize my current views, subject to revision, of some of the issues pertinent to an appraisal of the place of family therapy in the psychiatric repertory.

References

BION, W. (1957). Differentiation of the psychotic from the non-psychotic personalities. *Int. J. Psycho-Anal. 38*, 266–275.

BRODEY, W. M. (1959). Some family operations and schizophrenia. *A.M.A. Arch. gen. Psychiat. 1*, 379–402.

ERIKSON, E. H. (1956). The problem of ego identity. *J. Amer. Psychoanal. Ass. 4*, 56–121.

FARBER, L. H. (1958). The therapeutic despair. *Psychiatry 21*, 7–20.

HOEDEMAKER, E. D. (1960). Psycho-analytic technique and ego modification. *Int. J. Psycho-Anal. 41*, 34–46.

KLEIN, M. (1946). Notes on some schizoid mechanisms. *Int. J. Psycho-Anal. 27*, 99–110.

PARSONS, T., AND BALES, R. (1955). *Family, socialization and interaction process.* Glencoe, Ill.: Free Press.

SCHAFFER, L., WYNNE, L. C., DAY, J., RYCKOFF, I. M., AND HALPERIN, A. (1962). On the nature and sources of the psychiatrists' experience with the family of the schizophrenic. *Psychiatry 25*, 32–45.

SEARLES, H. F. (1958). Positive feelings in the relationship between the schizophrenic and his mother. *Int. J. Psycho-Anal. 39*, 569–586.

SINGER, M. T., AND WYNNE, L. C. (1965). Thought disorder and family relations of schizophrenics. III. Methodology using projective techniques. *Arch gen. Psychiat. 12*, 187–200.

WYNNE, L. C. (1961). The study of intrafamilial alignments and splits in exploratory family therapy. In N. W. Ackerman, F. L. Beatman, and S. N. Sherman (Eds.) *Exploring the base for family therapy.* New York: Fam. Serv. Ass. of Amer., pp. 95–115.

WYNNE, L. C., RYCKOFF, I. M., DAY, J., AND HIRSCH, S. I. (1958). Pseudomutuality in the family relations of schizophrenics. *Psychiatry 21*, 205–220.

WYNNE, L. C., AND SINGER, M. T. (1963a). Thought disorder and family relations of schizophrenics. I. A research strategy. *A.M.A. Arch. gen. Psychiat. 9*, 191–198.

WYNNE, L. C., AND SINGER, M. T. (1963b). Thought disorder and family relations of schizophrenics. II. A classification of forms of thinking. *A.M.A. Arch. gen. Psychiat. 9*, 199–206.

8

CARL A. WHITAKER

RICHARD E. FELDER,

JOHN WARKENTIN

Countertransference in the Family Treatment of Schizophrenia

There has been a conspicuous increase of late in the discussion of countertransference problems encountered in the general field of psychotherapy. Recent studies have included specific research based on tape recordings, detailed observation of interaction, films, and linguistic analyses of communication. These studies consistently indicate that the therapist is much more involved in the therapeutic process than we have previously dared to realize. The increasing tendency to treat patients in the setting of their family has also activated new insights into the therapist's involvement. The use of two therapists with one patient expanded into the use of two therapists with a married couple and has gradually given us such courage that we are now treating the family group. As a result, this experience has led to the treatment of the schizophrenic in his family setting. This chapter proposes to discuss the therapeutic problems involved in this effort, specifically those that emerge in the therapist himself. No effort will be made to evaluate the patients' problems or the process of psychotherapy as such.

In letting himself get involved in the family of the schizophrenic patient the therapist inescapably must be able to resonate to the group and also to identify with first one and then another of the members. He then challenges them to disconnect some of the octopoid vectors that they have been living with and reconnect in such a manner that each can find a new separateness and be free to interact with the therapist. In breaking into the family, the therapist is clearly activating his own open valences. The therapist must bring to bear in this new setting those securely interdigitated defensive patterns which were associated with his own original family setting, not just those related to his parents as individuals. Presumably these latter transferences were worked through in his own analysis. There is a hidden danger, for he is relating to a family and yet he has never experienced therapy in the setting of his original family.

As the therapist faces a schizophrenic and family in treatment, countertransference problems of even the experienced therapist become more obvious than in other forms of psychotherapy (Whitaker, Felder, Malone, and Warkentin, 1962). When he accepts the family as his patient the therapist begins to expose the immature residuals of his own person. No matter how the therapist tries to participate with mature warmth, he will reveal some infantile or pathologic responses in spite of himself. During the interview itself he may not sense what has happened, but he can discover the slips from a study of taped records or with the help of a colleague.

Setting and Treatment Approach

The work reported here was done in a private clinic where the nine therapists maintain a close working relationship. They are in daily multiple therapy and consultative work with each other and in the process have developed a shared ideology of psychotherapy.

The theoretical framework of the authors is designated *experiential* psychotherapy (Malone, Whitaker, Warkentin, and Felder, 1961). By this term we denote a pattern of sequential overlapping between the transference relationship and the existential relationship, the existential relating dominating the later stages of psychotherapy. Every effort is made to increase the expressive and emotive aspects of the therapist-patient relationship within the limits of clinical judgment (Auerbach, 1963). This approach to the schizophrenic and his family necessitates increased specific involvement in the countertransference aspects of treatment. By countertransference we denote the distorted feelings of the therapist. We include in these not only the counterfeelings which develop in the therapist to the transference feelings from the family which is his patient, but also those from the subgroups within the family. We also include in the term countertransference those affects which develop in the therapist and have to do with his direct transference. The group or subgroups or individuals may symbolically represent to him someone in his own past, i.e., his brother, his father and mother, or his family group. We also include under the term countertransference the identification process which takes place in the therapist so that, for example, he becomes so involved that the schizophrenic patient is something of an alter ego to him and he sees the schizophrenic patient as though that person were the therapist himself. Finally, we do not differentiate between overt and covert feelings in the therapist, since in either case the therapist is anxious. Yet, if his feelings are expressed to the family they may be more useful to the family than if they stay hidden (Whitaker, 1958).

Parenthetically we must warn that countertransference is non-therapeutic but that the depth of involvement which it evidences is necessary in the successful treatment of any psychotic patient. A mature therapist can attain such depth if he is willing and able to resolve the countertransference pathology so that his relating will be free and in the patient's interest. The overt expression of the therapist's "pathology" to the family must be controlled by his clinical judgment of its danger. However, unwillingness to share it is frequently based on his pride and embarrassment, and in this event only produces a secondary type of confusion in the relating.

In this paper we are discussing the treatment of a family group seen as a unit even though the overt symptoms are expressed through a clinically sick child. In our development as a clinic group we have spent many years working with groups, working with couples, and using multiple therapy in all the areas of psychotherapy. We utilize multiple therapy as a method of resolving the countertransference tendencies of the therapist and making him increasingly competent to deal with those defense patterns which weaken his therapy. Our study of countertransference has been made largely on the basis of taped interviews and observations which emerge from the multiple therapy setting where each therapist is able to be an observer of the dynamic patterns emerging in the other member of the therapeutic team. In contrast, his own countertransference is usually not apparent to the therapist during the interview.

In our clinic the father or mother ordinarily calls for the initial appointment, at which time we ask that the entire family come in together. We do not see the schizophrenic patient by himself at any time, nor do we see the parents without the patient. We decide in the first interview whether to include siblings. We treat the family as a unit and insist that unless the entire unit is present we have no "patient." We sometimes dramatize this structure by calling our patient the interlocked group or, graphically, a "people salad." Each member is confined in a network of interlocking relationships which is like a jello salad with each person embedded in it. For instance, on one occasion the father in a family interview, when asked if he planned to buy a new car, said, "*We* didn't have that on *my* mind."

The description of family treatment is a difficult job, since one is really facing a whole new definition of the primal scene which now becomes not a sexual scene but a total two-generation interactional unit. We assume that the schizophrenic child is the sacrificial lamb who, in order to meet the family need, is being repeatedly put through the crucifixion gesture. In family psychotherapy it becomes our job to help the child complete the therapy of the family so that each member can be free. If the therapy is successful, then the result must bring about freedom in the parents from their involvement in the "people salad" that includes the child and the two parents.

In contrast with individual psychotherapy, we are here presented with the actual home relationships which in ordinary psychotherapy are transferred to the therapist. The child is relating to his actual mother and his actual father, and the three of them are involved in a group to which the therapist is related in a separate manner. In other words, individual therapy is based on a symbolic relationship; group therapy is based on a social matrix; and family psychotherapy is based on that biosocial unit which is the basis for our entire society. No wonder the therapist has for years past not dared to walk into the middle of this situation and try to alter it. The dynamics of the family unit arise from the neurotic interlocking between the parents, a love which is both real and symbolic and reinforced by the affect developed in this union by the birth and growth of children and the experiences of many years of living together. In contrast to family psychotherapy, group psychotherapy involves a transference relationship between the members and toward the therapist; these relationships develop in a gradual, symbolic cathecting. In family therapy, the relationship within the group has been operating for many years; it is deeply invested with affect and is not only systematized but well defended in many different directions. The family comes to the therapeutic situation with greater power than the therapist has; and the therapist himself is an outsider. The process of family psychotherapy is one by which this powerful group is for the first time beginning to make deliberate efforts to break up interlocking defenses and patterns that hinder growth.

Dynamics of Process

The process of change in psychotherapy is a major subject and is not to be covered in this chapter. However, we must note that the process of change as described for the individual patient and the process taking place in the psychotherapy of a family are quite different. Family psychotherapy is also different from psychotherapy of a married couple. *A family as defined here consists of at least two and usually three or more persons who compose a two-generation unit.* The very fact of this two-generation spread changes the dynamics of the therapeutic process. In addition, the presence of a cultural breakdown of the family as an institution, as evidenced by the psychotic patient, adds a new vector to the complexities of family dynamics. The natural homeostasis of the family unit is, however, reinforced during psychotherapy by the group allegiance which Bion describes as developing in "the face of a battle" (Bion and Richman, 1943).

We all know that stability prevents change, but the fluidity of groupings and regroupings within a family also prevents change. This fluidity is as protective as the compliance of the man who never disagrees with anybody. Any anxiety in a member is compensated for by reassurance of the member or attack on the therapist by another member of the family or by a subgroup of the family. The therapist as an added force may even freeze the interaction at any one point and cause group panic and the sudden fixing of allegiances, just as he may expose new counterbalancing antagonisms and symbolic identifications. With the therapist as obstetrician a few of these hidden alignments exposed during the panic are delivered into consciousness. When the homeostasis is thus disturbed, a secondary flurry of recompensation may develop and still other interpersonal alliances are exposed and hopefully integrated into the dynamics of the whole.

Family therapy, then, includes a break-up in family loyalty, with the development not only of new subgroups but also of emerging tension systems which have been covered for many years. In family psychotherapy, the therapist must unite with and help with this disruptive effort and the subsequent new alignments. *If the therapist is to be at all useful to the family, the stress of such deep involvement must eventuate in a primitive countertransference-like attachment* (Rosen, 1953).

Countertransference Patterns

We have said that countertransference is unconscious during the time that it is operative; however, it may be forced to the therapist's attention during the experience, or he may become aware of it soon afterwards. When the therapist approaches the psychotherapy of the family, he brings certain specific attitudes which are already part of his personal response to any therapeutic situation. Because he is accustomed to treating one patient, he approaches a family situation as though in search of a person to treat. This is a natural result of his past experience, but it sets the stage for countertransference problems. Actually, then, the therapist may approach the therapeutic situation with more anxiety and more affect than does the family. They are a self-contained group set to relate defensively; they have experienced many years of conflict with others who challenge their integrity as a group. They have resisted such attempts and have a deep unconscious conviction of their own power. So the therapist is off balance, and the patient, in this case an entire family, is very much in balance; it has stability and certain group and subgroup methods of handling stress.

Some data seem to indicate that the therapist uses his work with the family as a way of experiencing some of his own tensions about the social structure in which he grew up. He could not change the community in which he grew up; therefore, he will change this part of the social structure. In this fashion is his missionary zeal stirred. He may at least change this family.

Although we have elected to use the conventional term "countertransference," it may be that most of the distorted affect in the therapist should be labeled transference. He is reliving his early life experience in a sense not possible in his analysis or even in his present home. He can exercise infantile omnipotent control of this family, can become lost in this family group, or can run away from home like Huck Finn. He has the ideal "as if" family, and the temptation to "act-out" is all but irresistible.

One therapist, after working with a family for thirteen months in a multiple therapy setting, suddenly in the middle of the hour had a fantasy of cutting off the head of each of the parents. This countertransference problem had undoubtedly been present for many interviews, and it is our conviction that if it had *not* been shared, it would in effect have weakened the therapeutic relationship. Since it was shared, it was one step in teaching the family to alter their own patterns by sharing feelings which seem too horrible to reveal.

To us the only effective counter for this kind of countertransference seems to be a co-therapist who can help make the personal needs of the therapist a current problem of the treatment situation. One therapist would be eaten alive and lost in the "people salad."

1) ENGAGEMENT PHASE

In the initial phase of his relationship to the family the therapist is facing an excessive anxiety. He develops a plan for this new family, *his* new family. Maybe he is going to be the parent to this group and make them over in the image of his fantasy, his first family. Whatever his plan is, it is likely to be different from what he later discovers himself doing in his relating to the family. In his effort to commit himself to the family, he is very likely to become lost in it and absorbed as a member of the family. If so, he has already developed a transference. He may experience this transference as an impulse to assault the family homeostasis. He tries in effect to break the family in much the same way that John Rosen (1953) talks about "breaking the back of the psychosis" with the individual schizophrenic patient. He may fail miserably because of his involvement, as did the therapist in the following case fragment:

MOTHER: Well, Doctor Jones, what is your idea on sending Pat to a private school, and what type and where?

THERAPIST: I don't think the problem is with the school. I think you are right when you say his problem has existed for years and that the school only catches the problem already present.

MOTHER: Well, Doctor Jones, all right, the thing is, if there was any end in sight in taking him out of school, all right, but he can't stay out indefinitely, and he has been out two months this year.

THERAPIST: Do you see what you're doing as you talk?

MOTHER: No, I have no idea.

THERAPIST: Do you, Dad?

FATHER: No.

THERAPIST: Do you, Pat? (patient, 16-year-old) (No answer.)

THERAPIST: John? (younger brother)

JOHN: No.

THERAPIST: I was pointing out that the problem is right here in the office.

JOHN: (interrupts) Right here?

THERAPIST: Yes. And then Mother immediately switched our talk back to "what shall we do about school?," as though the problem were at school.

MOTHER: The problem is getting an education for him.

THERAPIST: I don't think so. That's what I'm saying. I don't think that's the problem. The problem is that he has to put his dirty shoe on my $80 chair, and his father doesn't do a damn thing about it. That's the problem. (Therapist is angry about dirt and with father.)

FATHER: What can you do? (Meaning what can *you* [the therapist] do.)

MOTHER: How can you take anything that big and put clean clothes on it? You lay them out and tell him to put them on and he doesn't put 'em on and he pays no attention to you whatsoever.

THERAPIST: I think that's beginning to narrow down the problem all right.

The therapist's effort to get away from the subject of school to the present situation failed. In trying to point out an immediate problem between patient and father, the therapist not only failed but became a part of the family's depersonalization of the patient ("anything that big" and "put clean clothes on it"). Mother would not have talked this way if the therapist had not, in the face of his own anxiety, participated in the family's hostility to the "patient." Listening to the rest of the interview, one is aware that the therapist remains impotent, inundated by the fixed family dynamics, and unable to extricate himself. Had two therapists been present, the other therapist would probably have been able to insure that the first therapist could have been stable in his own setting and in being himself. Thereby he would not have needed to "belong to" the family just because he was deeply concerned for its movement. *The therapist decompensated into "wishing" and "trying" prematurely.* A half-step would have been: "How much of your family problem seems to be here in this room, right now?," or "Did any of you pray for me in this interview?" or, "Does my office seem like a place for you, Dad, to fight your family to a finish?"

2) INVOLVEMENT PHASE

As the therapist becomes increasingly involved, he may find himself identifying with the child of the family and attacking the mother as though he were going to protect the child from her malicious impulses. In a secondary way, he may also be endeavoring to replace her in the child's inner life and to become himself the mother in the family structure. On the other hand he may identify with the mother and endeavor to double-bind the schizophrenic child in the same way she has done, either because of his effort to capture a patient or because of his competitive feelings with the mother. For example:

MOTHER: Well, I guess there are things that come up that you don't want to do. But there has been a time when you wouldn't do anything you were asked to do.

SON: I don't feel that's . . .

MOTHER: If I feel the need of asking you to do anything now, I would ask you just like I would any of the rest of them that was around. I tried to give advice and tried to teach you all while you were young—in other words, and after you get grown I feel if you don't know it from me—so I might as well not give too much advice. I have to give you a little about some things because of—well, I reckon you don't think it through.

SON: I think it is very important that you give an opinion about this business. We don't have any idea of knowing what you think. In other words, if you don't say anything, we are at the place we've always been because we don't have anyone to say to us authoritatively if we are right or wrong, exactly where we were.

THERAPIST: (Clearing his throat) Well . . .

SON: I know it is an improbable thing, but I am sure we would both like to know what you think about it. If I am wrong in my feelings—I mean, I know I am not wrong in my feelings. I know how I feel—but if I am wrong in my thinking, I have to find that out too.

THERAPIST: That's right. That is the reason why I don't comment. Because I am here to try to help you understand each other and have an experience with each other in which I can participate and possibly make this experience different from others you have had with each other. I don't have an opinion as such that occurs to me. If I have anything that is useful in participating with you, I won't hesitate to say it.

SON: I can't feel like she thinks the way she does about things, and I still don't feel the way I do.

THERAPIST: I'm sure that's true. I expect *that* to continue for a long time. I don't expect either of you to change overnight.

SON: I admit to you that we were both upset going back home last time and probably will be this time.

THERAPIST: I would like to say that much about it and I can give you that kind of opinion. This is the kind of opinion I think I am useful for. (Clears throat.) I think whenever you get upset by being in here that it is going to help you. Anytime you are upset by what happens in here, you can congratulate yourselves on the way home by having accomplished something, because just as long as this is just a peaceful talk, it isn't going to make you more able to go to work.

MOTHER: Well, maybe I'm wrong about this. He says I'm never positive so I can't be positive about this but I can say what I think and what the actions has made me think. If I were to tell Howard he was wrong about something he wouldn't pay any attention to me, he wouldn't think it was, he would think he knew. If you were to tell him something was wrong, give an opinion about something, he has a right to respect what you say more because you taught in this and you know about it, I don't. On the other hand, I feel like that as long as I have been here, if I hadn't learned a little of the true experience I must have been awfully dumb to start with. And with all the things I've seen and experienced myself, and I don't want to give any of them the wrong advice at any time because they might take it. I don't think they will. I don't think Howard is going to take much of my advice if I give any but I just wondered if it's not that way.

SON: I keep wondering, although there is a wide gap in our ages, how two people can have the same situation and get such different results from it. I feel that one of us is not looking at it right.

MOTHER: Well, I do too and I don't feel like it is all me. Maybe I'm too complacent and maybe not complacent enough. I will go a long way to keep from having an argument with a neighbor.

SON: I say you would.

MOTHER: I don't know of anything my neighbors have done to me. That is what I have been trying to tell you. You say I will take anything and I don't think I have.

SON: Would you say that you have never had an argument with anybody about anything?

MOTHER: Oh, I have had plenty of arguments.

SON: I've never heard you make a statement that can be construed . . . (both talking)

MOTHER: I have never had occasion to have an argument where you were present that I know of. The fact of the business, I stay home all the time and don't see very many people . . .

SON: Which is something else.

MOTHER: Which is just a little while at a time. It is just another habit, because I've stayed home so long now I don't want to go and I think I am entitled to that. The fact is I have never cared to get out in public much and I had to go to work and that was enough.

SON: Would you make a comment, would you generalize it and say what a relationship between a mother her age and a son my age, what should they do? I don't mean specifically, but generally. I want to know.

MOTHER: Tend to their own business I guess. I don't believe you asked me though. In other words, that is putting it pretty flat.

SON: What are my private affairs and what are her private affairs—what things should we, two people, mother and son, not as a personal element . . .

THERAPIST: I think the personal element is very important.

SON: Well, you refuse to say.

THERAPIST: Howard, I am not interested in setting up a theoretical mother and son, but a real one. I will be glad to say what I think you are talking about this morning; the fact that you feel dependent on her and resent that, which is the normal relationship between mother and a little child of four. Where the child is dependent on the mother, she supplies his food, she is the most of his world. But he resents this because he wants to be a big man and be out in the world, and that part I can see in this relationship so far.

Mother and son have taken over and are going around in a closed circuit. Son tries to involve the therapist, mother starts to interfere, then changes her mind. Son doesn't like therapist's comment ("I think the personal element is very important") and provokes him ("Well, you refuse to say") as he provokes mother. Therapist becomes mother and answers sweetly, but double-binds (and thus confuses) the patient ("I am not interested in setting up a theoretical mother and son," etc.), but before the end of the paragraph he is speaking to the patient, of the patient, in the third person. The transition from "you" to "he" is very subtle.

As a third bind, the therapist may, of course, become impotent and soft and endeavor thus to carry the balance of power as the father does; the therapist then stimulates the child to become sacrificial at one moment or stimulates the mother to be overtly dominant and symbiotically double-bound at the next moment (Winnicott, 1958).

As this involvement phase continues, the therapist is often bound in such a way that he begins to isolate himself from the group artificially to prevent further absorption into this "people salad." He may think of this isolation as becoming objective or interpretative. We conceive of it as a split in the family so that the therapist is simultaneously related to the child and related to the parental couple. Family therapy is a unique kind of experience for the psychotherapist and something which he may be unable to perceive because he is dealing not in a symbolic, historical situation but in a current dynamic system. We have been so impressed by this experience in the therapist's countertransference that we have been tempted to generalize and say that every therapist is dynamically the product of the distortions of another family, his own family of origin. If this supposition is true, the therapist faces the possibility of reinfection. His own sense of reality may be weakened, his ego defenses reinforced for protection, and his loss of integration may become a fact instead of a danger.

A significant part of the distortion in his relationship to the family is involved with his positive identification with the patient. We psychiatrists have for many years idealized the schizophrenic patient, idealized his insightfulness as being magical and omniscient, as though we believed his delusion of grandeur. We have idealized his mysteries, whether neologisms or symbolic formulations which we could not interpret. We even equate the schizophrenic's insightfulness with therapeutic capacity as though his insightfulness meant that he would be the ideal therapist in our fantasy of what would make *us* mature. We absurdly assume that the schizophrenic patient understands life better than his parents do, and because of this assumption we wallow in an induced hostility to the parents.

In addition, because of our training, we have a deep appreciation for, and preoccupation with, the symbolic experience; but we distort the communication within the family and accuse the family of creating a "sick" person. Because we idealize this sick person as noted above, we may thus formulate a rather nice double-bind for the family, and, of course, this is returned in kind: the family then can double-bind the therapist, usually on a nonverbal level.

It is not unusual for us to picture the schizophrenic patient living in the framework of his sacrificial effort toward a family and to bypass entirely his narcissism. We say in effect, "You are wonderful." The patient says, "You are wonderful, too." And with this kind of feedback system we overidentify with the patient and become lost in a standard transference-countertransference jam. Another time we say to the patient, "Get better but keep the craziness you have. It is your creativity, and we admire you for it." In fact, it may well be that sometimes we become so preoccupied with the artistic enjoyment of symbolism that we use it for its own sake and form a little artistic entente with the patient. At another time we may idealize the schizophrenic child by saying, "He is the only honest person in the family." This compliment is obviously false since the family pattern is certainly unified.

Another countertransference pattern is an extension of the above in which we asexualize the schizophrenic child. Our picturing him as transcending sex is in itself a way of rejection and avoids any sexual countertransference affect. One of the other countertransference problems is associated with the therapist's tendency to become destructive of his own person. It is as though he accepts the patient's code of being sacrificial and becomes himself sacrificial as the patient is to the family. He says, "Here am I, Lord, take me." Our idealization of the schizophrenic may at times spill over to an idealization of the family itself. We tend to close off our third ear so that it is unable to hear the psychopathic maneuvering which takes place in this kind of therapeutic situation. It is obvious that schizophrenics are very adroit at maneuvering people; they maneuver deliberately and they maneuver with real affect. If the therapist loses sight of these two patterns, he becomes enmeshed in the situation.

The therapist sometimes develops a pattern of countertransference which has to do with his own identification with the mother. She says to the child, "How can you do this when I work my fingers to the bone?," and he says almost in direct echo, "How can you all be unappreciative of me when I have sacrificed myself for you?" He is saying to them, "You must appreciate me, else you are not worthy of my love."

This situation reconstructs the child's original dynamic setting and entangles him in a very primitive manner. Thus involved, the therapist faces a very serious countertransference problem. He may resonate to and enjoy the relationship to the family as a unit as he did with his own family group. He is not a working therapist but the child of the family.

In contrast, at times the countertransference problem builds up negative tension patterns within the therapist. These may simply disrupt his function, or they may develop to such a point that he resolves them by means of an affect explosion into the family setting.

"This family just will not go along with my plan for them." At another level, he may become lost in the subgroup power struggle within the family either by attaching himself to the parental group or to some other subgroup (mother-son or father-son) or by attaching himself to one of the individual members of the family group. In any of these eventualities he is involved in such a way that he becomes therapeutically impotent. If he avoids the Scylla of overinvolvement, he is immediately faced with the Charybdis of isolation. Finally, the therapist may become countertransferred in such a manner that he deftly switches from one side to another in a type of alternating transference which not only keeps him from becoming aware of his involvement but also keeps him from being an adequate therapist.

Thus we see the therapist in a loaded situation. The family is intact and he is enacting only a functional role. His normal warmth in relating to an individual suddenly becomes a countertransference vector. His affect must be attached to the family unit, yet he may not belong to it. He must help the family to break up their group loyalty, to develop new subgroups, and gradually to sense their right to "belong" yet not lose their identity in the group. (Is it possible that *any* subgroup is healthier than the whole family?) Through all this process he must be "in," yet not "of," the family and its subgroups. He must be available to each person of the family, yet belong to none; he must belong to himself (Whitaker, Warkentin, and Malone, 1959).

3) DISENTANGLEMENT PHASE

It seems very difficult to understand the final phase of treatment of the family. Experience is limited, the situation is complex, and even the multiple therapist tends to become unavailable as an observer because of the significance of the experience to him as a person (Whitaker, Warkentin, and Johnson, 1950). If family psychotherapy has progressed to the stage of disentanglement, failure is a relative term. Many families do not stay in treatment until they have gotten all that is possible out of psychotherapy, in our view, but does that mean the case is a failure? The "break" out of treatment which stops the interviews may originate in the marriage of the patient, father getting a new job and moving to another city, or the gradual withdrawal of the family unit from treatment. We try to participate in any such movement. We express our reservations and our satisfaction, our sense of loss and our relief; yet through it we maintain their right to decision. This is the right we have trained them to take. Only time will tell whether the pattern will recur.

If the therapy of the schizophrenic and his family has been successful and the "people salad" has been altered, there develops in the middle phase of treatment a situation in which there are three separate people who have a rather tenuous relationship to each other. Each of them is becoming an entity, and they may be "out of phase" with each other, i.e., no longer reinforcing each other's pathology. If the disentanglement phase is effective, there must develop a stable parental subgroup which forms a base to which the child can relate in a voluntary manner. He is free to attach himself to his primary parental group and detach himself at will. The twosome is available to him but is not enmeshing him. The parents in turn can enjoy his attachment, and when he is separate they can enjoy each other to a greater degree. They feel free to fight for the marriage as the central concern to them. The patient is secondary. Finally, the parents can each be separate, yet a part of the marriage.

We see then that to maintain his separateness throughout the therapeutic process, the therapist must avoid not only the countertransference problem of overinvolvement but also the countertransference problem of isolation. As a prototype he must be a part of the group. He must be involved and not merely carrying a role with the family, yet he must avoid being absorbed into their quicksand kind of meshing.

Resolving Countertransference Problems

The resolution of countertransference problems has at least two foci. There are certain specific countertransference problems that are resolvable in specific ways; yet in the over-all sense, countertransference problems, inasmuch as they are implicit, are best resolved by a general reorganization of the relating of the therapist and the "patient." Thereby, the dynamics which keep the countertransference operative are gradually dissipated. The most obvious way of resolving countertransference is prevention. The prevention of countertransference is aided in an over-all way by several specific moves. The most obvious is an adequate therapeutic experience for the therapist so that he comes to the treatment process with a maturity and freedom to become involved in the relationship without losing his own integrity or without becoming pathologically transferred to the treatment situation. He needs an adequate background also in the sense of a training experience in which he has grown as a person. He should have an opportunity to experience his patient needs in more than one setting, for example, as a patient in group therapy, in an opportunity to do therapy with small children, or in an opportunity to face his own tendencies toward countertransference in a multiple therapy setting. Adequate supervision of this varied therapeutic work also helps prevent countertransference problems. The simple therapeutic settings also help him learn how to work through countertransference affects and help him grow by this struggle. This background of growthful experience as a person should, of course, be complemented by a fairly lengthy experience as a psychotherapist. He thereby may have become a "professional" therapist rather than someone who still does psychotherapy for the love of it—what we call an amateur. It is important that the psychotherapist let himself become involved in his work to the extent that it becomes stressful. Through stressful experiences he adapts himself and increases his strength to function in his professional role.

Since the therapist must live and work with one foot outside the social structure, it is very important that he be secure in his membership in a professional group. A research institute or a hospital staff may supply this security. If not, his isolation from the community may be a serious burden. If he has a group of colleagues, his freedom to walk in the valley of the shadow of psychosis will be increased. It may be that family treatment of schizophrenia is impossible without this kind of support.

One of the most significant assets in the prevention and the resolution of countertransference affects is the strength the therapist has in his own family life outside the office. A psychotherapist who is deeply related on a constructive and satisfying level to his own wife and children is much more likely to function as a competent person in the treatment of a sick family than one who is living in deep stress at home.

If the therapist is adequate in the above areas, countertransference factors are likely to be resolved if the therapist can muster the courage to bring to the therapeutic interview a type of extreme honesty and affect-sharing. His honesty and sharing is the model around which the family can pivot; they can compare their own method of relating and be tempted to be more nearly honest themselves and more sharing of their feelings than before. In effect, the therapist's self-image serves as a prototype for the family and its individual members. The therapist should obtain supervision of his relationship to the family, either by way of tape recording or through actual participant-observation by a colleague. In fact, even a technical ploy on the part of the therapist to bring his own affect concerns to the family may alter his affective involvement.

As prevention, we have found it ideal to utilize multiple therapy in the treatment of these families. It may be that as we become more and more adequate, multiple therapy will not be necessary. "When I get over my head I want a co-therapist to push me on through or debunk my distorted effort" (Whitaker, 1958).

TECHNIQUES FOR RESOLVING COUNTERTRANSFERENCE

On a technical level, there are several things which we think of as helpful in the resolution of countertransference patterns. It is valuable if the therapist can maintain an over-view of the family as a whole. His affective relationship to the family group is one effective way of keeping himself from becoming countertransferred to subgroups or individuals in the family. At the same time he must ride the other horn of this dilemma and be involved with the individuals and the subgroups. Thus the resolution necessitates a type of fluidity and strength in his moving in and out of the family situation. To be strong and fluid the therapist must "be," and in his "being" stand and move in his own personal uniqueness and his own spontaneity. Continuity in relating is less valuable than authenticity. In essence, the therapist finds himself involved in a series of oedipal triangles, and he must be competent and free to disrupt these triangles from time to time in a very deliberate fashion and to recreate them or allow himself to be pulled into them in the same free rhythm with which he may elect to back out and destroy them. When he does this, of course, he becomes a professional therapist carrying on a professional role, which by itself is not enough to constitute a therapeutic relationship but is a necessity in the resolution of the various countertransference slivers which inevitably develop.

Technically, the therapist can also help in the resolution of countertransference by deliberately leaving the initiative for the conduct of the interview to the family members themselves. This kind of withdrawal sometimes is very clearly a process of rejection of the entire situation and as such may precipitate tension patterns which will then have to be worked through, but it is a process that can be invaluable at times. A fairly standard example is that of an interview when the entire family is depressed. The therapist is tempted to step in and reassure them, to participate in the depression and its resolution, and to be himself their saviour. However, frequently when he steps in he is expressing his own countertransference. Technically, it seems more valuable to activate the depression, to push the family depression to a new depth, and to come through it rather than to back out of it. It is as though the therapist denies his loyalties to each member of the family and asserts his relationship to the group as a whole.

An awareness that the parents' marriage is a figment may prevent one unreality tendency. To see them as premarital adds a freedom to help them become a healthy subgroup.

If the treatment involves multiple therapy, it is possible at times for the therapist to resolve his countertransference problems by retreating to his relationship to the other therapist, and the therapeutic process then becomes a process of two groups relating to each other. The therapist is thus free to have his major loyalty to his own group and break up his overidentification with the sick family. It may even be that this relationship between the two therapists with its "incestuous" understructure resolves some countertransference problems by making the incestuous relationship between the members of the family less guilt-producing and more satisfying.

In the usual family pattern the mother, with father as her collaborator, accomplishes her purpose by using one sacrificial goat—the patient; with the single therapist she may be able again to structure a sick "family"; with two therapists she is helpless. They form their own group. Since the therapists have their greatest affect with each other, the family is left with their own misery and may thereby rededicate themselves to the therapeutic effort.

If the treatment of the family is not by multiple therapy, then the technical maneuver of bringing a consultant into the interview may serve the same result. If the therapist has no consultant he may well become lost in the group dependency of the family. In breaking the congealed "people salad" by the addition of another person, the therapist may become free to move in and out of his involvement with the family rather than be frozen into it. In contrast, we suspect that attempts at resolving this kind of countertransference by supervisory discussion are ineffective since the experience is unavailable to the therapist for overt discussion. However, the use of taped interviews may produce enough reactivation of the original setting so that the therapist is able to resolve some of his countertransference problems by listening to the tape with a colleague. This suggestion may seem overcautious unless we all agree that the therapist's involvement is not neurotic or technical. He is investing his own deep psychotic-like feelings, those of the primary process itself. This investment is one of the differentials between family psychotherapy and group psychotherapy. Family psychotherapy involves primary process dynamics, whereas group psychotherapy uses to a large degree secondary process dynamics. The therapist's feeling participation must follow the appropriate pattern.

Concluding Remarks

While the therapist of this generation has had no personal experience of being the patient in his family setting, the next generation of psychotherapists may well include some individuals who got part of their psythotherapy in their family group and who, in so doing, resolved not only their transference problems but also the transference problems of their relationship to their entire family group as a unit. In the meantime, the preparation of a therapist for working with the extremely powerful families who have as their presenting symptom a schizophrenic child necessitates an extensive personal therapeutic analysis and much experience in being a professional psychotherapist. Furthermore, the therapist must be significantly related to his own family and with enough security there so that he is not emotionally liable to major countertransference jams. We assume he also needs the security of a group of colleagues to whom he is deeply related and with whom he can work in multiple therapy.

An extensive experience in supervised family psychotherapy, whether the supervision is individual or group, might make it possible for the therapist to avoid many countertransference problems in family psychotherapy. His training should also develop the capacity to diagnose family dynamics. This latter experience is probably not attainable in the individual consultation room or the ordinary hospital training, but must be obtained either in a Mental Hygiene Clinic or in work with families in a social agency. Only in this kind of training will he develop a security in the strength of the family group so that he will approach this family with respect rather than with disgust, curiosity, or fear.

We trust it is clear from the above discussion that the psychotherapist who gets involved in this kind of work is in essence developing a kind of split within himself. He must be simultaneously involved with the family and separate from it; he must be an entity in himself and at the same time a member of the group, and a primary group at that. He must be able to identify with the child in the family without himself becoming a child. He must be with the parents, yet not a parent. This capacity emerges from experiences which make this kind of openness and this kind of involvement something he can move into and out of rather than avoid. His training should help him know that the family is more powerful than he is and at the same time make him able to participate in the family situation and its alteration without being overwhelmed by its strength or without trying to utilize the group for himself.

In this latter sense, the work with families is the ultimate challenge, the ultimate excitement, the most dangerous and at the same time the most deeply satisfying work that a psychotherapist can attain. It is a real life and death struggle, and "the life you save may be your own."

References

AUERBACH, A. H. (1963). Application of Strupp's method of content analysis to psychotherapy. *Psychiatry 26*, 137–148.

BION, W., AND RICHMAN, J. (1943). Intragroup tensions in therapy, their study as a task for the group. *Lancet 2*, 678–681.

MALONE, T. P., WHITAKER, C. A., WARKENTIN, J., AND FELDER, R. E. (1961). Rational and nonrational psychotherapy. *Amer. J. Psychother. 15*, 212–220.

ROSEN, J. (1953). *Direct Analysis*. New York: Grune & Stratton.

WHITAKER, C. A. (Ed.) (1958). *Psychotherapy of chronic schizophrenic patients*. Boston: Little, Brown.

WHITAKER, C. A., FELDER, R. E., MALONE, T. P., AND WARKENTIN, J. (1962). First stage techniques in the experiential psychotherapy of chronic schizophrenic patients. In J. H. Masserman (Ed.) *Current psychiatric therapies*, vol. 2. New York: Grune & Stratton, pp. 147, 157.

WHITAKER, C. A., MALONE, T. P., AND WARKENTIN, J. (1956). Multiple therapy and psychotherapy. In F. Fromm-Reichmann and J. L. Moreno (Eds.) *Progress in psychotherapy*, vol. I. New York: Grune & Stratton, pp. 210–216.

WHITAKER, C. A., WARKENTIN, J., AND JOHNSON, N. (1950). The psychotherapeutic impasse. *Amer. J. Orthopsychiat. 20*, 641–647.

WHITAKER, C. A., WARKENTIN, J., AND MALONE, T. P. (1959). The involvement of the professional therapist. In A. Burton (Ed.) *Case studies in counseling and psychotherapy*. Englewood Cliffs, N.J.: Prentice Hall, pp. 218–257.

WINNICOTT, D. W. (1958). Hate in the countertransference. In *Collected papers*. New York: Basic Books, pp. 194–203.

9

RONALD D. LAING

Mystification, Confusion, and Conflict

You can fool some of the people some of the time . . .

Marx used the concept of mystification to mean a plausible mis-representation of what is going on (process) or what is being done (praxis) in the service of the interests of one socioeconomic class (the exploiters) over or against another class (the exploited). By representing forms of exploitation as forms of benevolence, the exploiters bemuse the exploited into feeling at one with their exploiters, or into feeling gratitude for what (unrealized by them) in their exploitation, and, not least, into feeling bad or mad even to think of rebellion.

We can employ Marx's theoretical schema, not only to elucidate relations between classes of society, but in the field of the reciprocal interaction of person directly with person.

Every family has its differences (from mild disagreements to radically incompatible and contradictory interests or points of view), and every family has some means of handling them. Here one

---

Part of the clinical material contained in this chapter also appeared in Laing and Esterson (1964).

343

way of handling such contradictions is described under the rubric of *mystification*.

In this chapter I shall present in discursive form this and some related concepts currently being developed in research and therapy with families of schizophrenics, neurotics and normals at the Tavistock Clinic and Tavistock Institute of Human Relations, London.[1] I shall compare the concept of mystification to certain closely related concepts, and I shall give brief descriptions of certain aspects of some of the families investigated in order to demonstrate, it is hoped, the heuristic value of the theoretical discussion and its crucial import for therapy. This paper will not, however, discuss the practical aspects of therapy.

The Concept of Mystification

By mystification I mean both the *act* of mystifying and the *state* of being mystified. That is, I am using the term both in an active and in a passive sense.

To mystify, in the active sense, is to befuddle, cloud, obscure, mask whatever is going on, whether this be experience, action, or process, or whatever is "the issue." It induces confusion in the sense that there is failure to see what is "really" being experienced, or being done, or going on, and failure to distinguish or discriminate the actual issues. This entails the substitution of false for true constructions of what is being experienced, being done (praxis), or going on (process), and the substitution of false issues for the actual issues.

The *state* of mystification, mystification in a passive sense, is possibly, though not necessarily, a *feeling* of being muddled or confused. The act of mystification, by definition, tends to induce, if not neutralized by counteraction, a state of mystification or confusion, not necessarily felt as such. It may or may not induce secondary conflicts, and these may or may not be recognized as such by the persons involved. The feeling of confusion and the experience of conflict have to be distinguished from mystification, either as act or state. Although one of the functions of mystification is to avoid authentic conflict, it is quite common for open conflict to occur in mystifying and mystified families. The masking effect of

[1] Investigators: R. D. Laing (Chief Investigator), Dr. A. Esterson, Dr. A. Russell Lee (1959–1961), Dr. Peter Lomas, Miss Marion Bosanquet, P.S.W. Dr. Laing is a current Research Fellow of the Foundation's Fund for Research in Psychiatry. Dr. A. Russell Lee's participation was made possible by the National Institute of Mental Health, Bethesda, Md. (Grant No. MF-10, 579).

mystification may not avoid conflict, although it will cloud over what the conflict is about.

This effect may be enhanced if the seal is placed on mystification by mystifying the act of perceiving mystification for what it is, e.g., by turning the perception of mystification into the issue of this being a bad or a mad thing to do.

Thus, the mystified person (or persons) is by definition confused, but may or may not *feel* confused. If we detect mystification, we are alerted to the presence of a conflict of some kind that is being evaded. The mystified person, in so far as he has been mystified, is unable to see the authentic conflict, but may or may not experience intra- or interpersonal conflict of an inauthentic kind. He may experience false peace, false calm, or inauthentic conflict and confusion over false issues.

A certain amount of mystification occurs in everyday life. A common way to mystify one person about his or her experience is to confirm the content of an experience and to disconfirm its modality (regarding perception, imagination, fantasy, and dreaming as different modes of experience, a theory developed elsewhere [Laing, 1962]).

Thus, if there is a contradiction between two persons' perceptions, the one person tells the other, "It is just your imagination," that is, there is an attempt to forestall or resolve a contradiction, a clash, an incomparability by transposing one person's experiential modality from perception to imagination or from the memory of a perception to the memory of a dream ("You must have dreamt it").

Another form of mystification is when the one person disconfirms the content of the other's experience and replaces it by attributions of experience conjunctive with self's view of the other (cf. Brodey's [1959] concept of the "narcissistic relationship").

A child is playing noisily in the evening; his mother is tired and wants him to go to bed. A straight statement would be:

"I am tired, I want you to go to bed."

or

"Go to bed, because I say so."

or

"Go to bed, because it's your bedtime."

A mystifying way to induce the child to go to bed would be:

"I'm sure you feel tired, darling, and want to go to bed now, don't you?"

Mystification occurs here in different respects. What is ostensively an attribution about how the child feels (you are tired) is "really" a command (go to bed). The child is told how he feels (he may or may not feel or be tired), and what he is told he feels is what

mother feels herself (projective identification). If we suppose he does not *feel* tired, he may contradict his mother's statement. He may then become liable to a further mystifying ploy such as:
"Mother knows best."
or
"Don't be cheeky."

Mystification may be over issues to do with what *rights* and what *obligations* each person in the family has in respect of the others. For example, a boy of fourteen tells his parents he is unhappy, and they reply:

"But you can't be unhappy. Haven't we given you everything you want? How can you be so ungrateful as to say you are unhappy after all that has been done for you, after all the sacrifices that have been made for you?"

Mystification is particularly potent when it involves this rights-obligations system in such a way that one person appears to have the *right* to determine the experience of another, or, complementarily, when one person is under an *obligation* to the other(s) to experience, or not to experience, himself, them, his world or any aspect of it, in a particular way. For instance, has the boy a right to be unhappy, or must he be happy because if he is not he is being ungrateful?

Implicit in Marx's formulation is that before enlightened action can be taken, the issues have to be demystified.

By issue we mean, as in law, "the point over which one affirms and another denies" (*Oxford English Dictionary*). The issue, in our material, frequently is how to define the "real" or "true" axis of orientation: the point at issue is what is to be the issue. Quarrels are often about what the quarrel is about: what is going on is a conflict, or a struggle, to agree or determine the "main issue." In the families of schizophrenics, one of the most fixed aspects of the extremely rigid family system is often a particular axis of orientation, which is the lynch-pin, so it seems, that keeps the whole family pattern in place.

In some families, every action of different members of the family is evaluated in terms of its particular axis or axes of orientation. An action of a family member thus plotted may become the issue, or the issue may be, as stated above, what is the valid axis of orientation to hold.

Judith, aged 26, and her father frequently quarrel. He wishes to know where she goes when she leaves the house, who she is with, when she will be back. She says that he is interfering with her life. He says that he is simply doing his duty as a father. He says she is impudent because she does not obey him. She says he is being tyrannical. He says she is wrong to speak in that way to her father. She says she is entitled to express what views she likes. He says, provided that the views are correct and that they are not correct, etc.

Anyone, including the investigator, is free to make an issue out of any part of the interactivity of the family. The issue may be agreed upon among all the family members, but the investigators may not see the issue in the same terms as do the family members.

Our axis of orientation both as researchers and as therapists is to pick out what the axes of orientation and issues are for each member of the family in turn. These may be expressed explicitly or be implicit. Certain members of a family may conspicuously fail to recognize any axis of orientation or to pick up the existence of any issues other than their own.

In order to recognize persons and not simply objects, one must realize that the other human being is not only another object in space but another center of orientation to the objective world. It is just this recognition of each other as different centers of orientation, that is, as persons, which is in such short supply in the families of schizophrenics we have studied.

There are as many issues as people can invent, but we have come to regard the issue of person perception as central in all the families we have studied. Although this issue may be central as we perceive it, we have to recognize that it is not necessarily seen or accepted as such by the family members themselves.

If active mystification consists in disguising, masking, the praxes and/or processes of the family, in befogging the issues, and in attempting to deny that what is the issue for oneself may not be so for the other, we have to ask how we decide what to us is the central issue, if our perception of the central issue is disjunctive with the perceptions of the family members themselves.

The only safeguard here is to present the perspectives of everyone in turn (including our own) on "the shared situation," and then to compare the evidence for the validity of different points of view. For instance, one can pick out certain axes of orientation in terms of which the actions of the family are evaluated by particular others:

June's mother described the following changes in June's personality that came on (aged 15) six months before what to us were the first signs of psychosis. A change in her personality had occurred in the last six months after she had been to a holiday camp, and away from home, for the first time in her life.

According to her mother, June was:

BEFORE	AFTER
boisterous	quiet
told me everything	does not tell me what is going on inside her
went everywhere with me	wants to be by herself
was very happy and lively	often looks unhappy; is less lively
liked swimming and cycling	does not do this so much but reads more
was "sensible"	is "full of boys"
played dominoes, drafts, and cards at night with mother, father, and grandfather	is not interested in these games any more; prefers to sit in her room and read
obedient	disobedient and truculent
never thought of smoking	smokes one or two cigarettes a day without asking permission
used to believe in God	does not believe in God

In the six months between her first perception of such changes in June and the onset of what we recognized as a psychotic breakdown, June's mother had gone to two doctors complaining about these changes in June, which she regarded as expression of an "illness" and perhaps expressions of evil. "It's not June, you see. That's not my little girl." Neither doctor could see evidence of illness or evil in June. Her mother actively attributed these changes in June, that to us were normal maturational, culturally syntonic expressions of growing up and achieving greater autonomy, etc., to expressions of a more and more serious "illness" or of "evil." The girl was completely mystified, because although becoming more autonomous, she still trusted her mother. As her mother repeatedly told her that her developing autonomy and sexual maturation were expressions of either madness or badness, she began to *feel ill* and to *feel evil*. One can see this as *praxis* on her part to attempt to resolve the contradiction between the *processes* of her own maturation and her mother's barrage of negative attributions about them.

From our standpoint, June appears mystified. She feels she has a lovely mummy, she begs forgiveness for being such a bad daughter, she promises to get well. Although at this point she is complaining that "Hitler's soldiers are after her," not once in many interviews does her mother make any other complaints about June except to attack as bad or mad those processes of development that we regard as most normal about her.

That is, her mother's only axes of orientation, in terms of which she saw and evaluated the changes in June, were good-evil, sane-mad. As June began to recover from a psychotic breakdown, her mother became more and more alarmed that June was getting worse, seeing intensified evidence of evil in her concurrently with our evaluation that she was achieving greater ego strength and autonomy.

Mystification entails the action of one person *on the other*. It is *trans*personal. The *intra*personal defenses with which psychoanalysis has familiarized us, or the various forms of "bad faith" in Sartre's sense, are best distinguished at present from ways of acting on the other. It in the nature of the mystifying action of persons on each other, rather than of each on himself or herself, that we wish particularly to consider in this paper.

The one person (p) seeks to induce in *the other* some change necessary for his (p's) security. Mystification is one form of action on the other that serves the defenses, the security, of the own person. If the one person does not want to know something or to remember something, it is not enough to repress it (or otherwise "successfully" defend himself against it "in" himself); he must not be reminded of it by the other. The one person can deny something himself; he must next make the other deny it.

It is clear that not every action of the one person on another, in the service of the one person's security, peace of mind, self-interest, or whatever, is necessarily mystifying. There are many kinds of persuasion, coercion, deterrence, whereby the one person seeks to control, direct, exploit, manipulate the behavior of the other.

To say: "I can't stand you talking about that. Please be quiet," is an attempt to induce silence over this topic in the other, but no mystification is involved.

Similarly, no mystification is involved in such statements as:

"If you don't stop that I'll hit you."

or

"I think that is a horrible thing to say. I'm disgusted with you."

In the following instance, a threat of something very unpleasant induced the boy to deny his own memory. The tactic is not, however, one of mystification.

A boy of four stuck a berry up his nose and could not get it out. He told his parents, who looked and could not see it. They were disinclined to believe that he had got a berry up his nose, but he complained of pain and so they called the doctor. He looked and could not see it. He said, showing the boy a long shining instrument, "I don't see anything, but if you say it's still there tomorrow, we shall have to take this to you." The boy was so terrified that he "confessed" that he had made up the whole story. It was not until twenty years later that he summoned up the courage to admit even to himself that he had actually put a berry up his nose.

By contrast, the following is an example of mystification.

MOTHER: I don't blame you for talking that way. I know you don't really mean it.

DAUGHTER: But I do mean it.
MOTHER: Now, dear, I know you don't. You can't help yourself.
DAUGHTER: I can help myself.
MOTHER: No, dear, I know you can't because you're ill. If I thought for a moment you weren't ill, I would be furious with you.

Here the mother is using quite naively a mystification which is at the very heart of much social theory. This is to convert praxis (what a person does) into process (an impersonal series of events of which no one is the author). This distinction between praxis and process has recently been drawn in an extremely lucid way by Sartre (1960).[2]

We unfortunately tend to perpetuate this particular mystification, I believe, when we employ the concept of family or group "pathology." Individual *psycho*pathology is a sufficiently problematic concept, since without splitting and reifying experience and behavior to invent "a psyche," one can attribute to this invention no pathology or physiology. But to speak of family "pathology" is even more problematic. The processes that occur in a group are generated by the praxis of its individual members. Mystification is a form of praxis; it is not a pathologic process.

The theoretically ultimate extreme of mystification is when the person (p) seeks to induce in the other (o) confusion (not necessarily recognized by o) as to o's whole experience (memory, perceptions, dreams, fantasy, imagination), processes, and actions. The mystified person is one who is given to understand that he feels happy or sad regardless of how he feels he feels, that he is responsible for this or not responsible for that regardless of what responsibility he has or has not taken upon himself. Capacities, or their lack, are attributed to him without reference to any shared empirical criteria of what these may or may not be. His own motives and intentions are discounted or minimized and replaced by others. His experience and actions generally are construed without reference to his own point of view. There is a radical failure to recognize his own self-perception and self-identity.[3] And, of course, when this is the case, not only his self-perceptions and self-identity are confused but his perceptions of others, of how they experience him and act toward him and of how he thinks they think he thinks, etc., are

---

[2] For an exposition of this theory, see Laing and Cooper (1964).
[3] In most forms of psychotherapy the therapist attributes motives and intentions to the patient which are not in accord with those the patient attributes to his own actions. But the therapist (one hopes) does not mystify the patient, in that he says implicitly or explicitly: You see yourself as motivated by A and intending B. I see you, however, as motivated by X and intending Y, and here is my evidence, drawn from my personal encounter with you.

necessarily subjected to multiple mystifications at one and the same time.

The Function of Mystification and Some Related Concepts

The prime function of mystification appears to be to maintain the status quo. It is brought into play, or it is intensified, when one or more members of the family nexus (Laing, 1962) threaten, or are felt to threaten, the status quo of the nexus by the way they are experiencing, and acting in, the situation they share with the other members of the family.

Mystification functions to maintain sterotyped roles (Ryckoff, Day, and Wynne, 1959) and to fit other people into a preset mold, Procrustean fashion (Lidz, Cornelison, Terry and Fleck, 1958). The parents struggle to preserve their own integration by maintaining their rigid preconceptions about who they are and who they ought to be, who their children are and ought to be, and the nature of the situation that characterizes family life. They are impervious (Lidz et al., 1958) to those emotional needs in their children that threaten to disrupt their preconceived schemata, and they mask or conceal disturbing situations in the family, acting as if they do not exist (Lidz et al., 1958). Imperviousness and masking are very common concomitants of mystification in the present tense when, for instance, they are backed up by transpersonal action on the other person, when, for instance, attempts are made to induce the other to believe that his emotional needs are being satisfied when clearly they are not, or to represent such needs as unreasonable, greedy, or selfish because the parents are unable or unwilling to fulfil them, or to persuade the other that he just thinks he has needs but has not "really," and so on.

Needless to say, no mystifying-mystified relationship can be a reciprocally confirmatory one in a genuine sense. What may be confirmed by the one person is a false front put on by the other, a prefabricated schema on the one person's part that the other is induced more or less to embody. Elsewhere I have tried to describe the structure of certain forms of such unauthentic relationships (Laing, 1960, 1961).

Such concepts are close to the concept of nonmutual complementarity developed by Wynne and his co-workers. The intense pseudomutuality described by these workers, "the predominant absorption in fitting together at the expense of the differentiation of the identities" (Wynne, Ryckoff, Day, and Hirsch, 1958, p. 207) is very much in line with our findings.

Mystification appears to be one technique, highly developed in the families of schizophrenics, to maintain the rigid role structure in such pseudomutual nexuses. We are currently investigating the extent to which, and the manner in which, pseudomutuality and mystification occur in the families of nonschizophrenics. Lomas (1961), for instance, has described the family of a girl diagnosed as an hysteric in which unauthentic fitting together and rigidly maintained sterotyped roles of an engulfing nature were clearly in evidence.

Searles (1959) describes six modes of driving the other person crazy, or techniques that tend "to undermine the other person's confidence in his own emotional reactions and his own perception of reality." I have slightly recast Searle's six modes of schizogenesis into the following form.

1) p repeatedly calls attention to areas of the personality of which o is dimly aware, areas quite at variance with the kind of person o considers himself or herself to be.

2) p stimulates o sexually in a situation in which it would be disastrous for o to seek sexual gratification.

3) p simultaneously exposes o to stimulation and frustration or to rapidly alternating stimulation and frustration.

4) p relates to o at simultaneously unrelated levels (e.g., sexually and intellectually).

5) p switches from one emotional wave length to another while on the same topic (being "serious" and then being "funny" about the same thing).

6) p switches from one topic to the next while maintaining the same emotional wave length (e.g., a matter of life and death is discussed in the same manner as the most trivial happening [Laing, 1961, p. 131–132]).

Each of these modes of schizogenesis is liable to induce muddle in the victim, without the victim necessarily perceiving the muddle he is in. In this sense they are mystifying.

I have suggested (Laing, 1961, pp. 132–136) that the schizogenic potential of such maneuvers lies not so much in the activation of various areas of the personality in opposition to one another, the activation, that is, of conflict, but in the generation of confusion or muddle or doubt, often unrecognized as such.

This emphasis on unconscious or unconscious confusion or doubt about one's self, the other(s), and the shared situation, this emphasis, that is, on a state of mystification, has much in common with Haley's (1959b) hypothesis that the control of the definition of relationships is a central problem in the origin of schizophrenia. The mystified person is operating in terms that have been misdefined for him. This definition is such that, without realizing it or without understanding why he may perhaps intensely but vaguely feel it to be so, he is in an untenable position (Laing, 1961, p. 135). He may then attempt to escape from his untenable position in the mystified situation by in turn deepening the mystifications.

The concept of mystification overlaps, but is not synonymous with, the double-bind concept (Bateson, Jackson, Haley, and Weakland, 1956). The double-bind would appear to be necessarily mystifying, but mystification need not be a complete double-bind. The essential distinction is that the mystified person, in contrast to the double-bound person, may be left with a relatively unequivocal "right" way to experience and to act. This right thing to experience or right way to act may entail, from our viewpoint as investigators and therapists, a betrayal of the person's potentialities for self-fulfillment, but this may by no means be felt by the person himself.

However, the right and wrong things to do in the mystified situation can be only *relatively* unequivocal. The tourniquet is always liable to be tightened by a further twist, and this is all that is necessary for the mystified situation to become a double-bind in the full sense.

In the example given earlier of the boy for whom happy equaled grateful and unhappy equaled selfish and ungrateful, the conflict and confusion would have been much intensified if strong prohibitions had been put on dishonesty. In such circumstances, to express unhappiness would be to be bad, since to be unhappy was to be selfish and ungrateful, while to put on an act of happiness would be equally bad because this would be dishonest.

In the case of the boy who put a berry up his nose, his parents could well be imagined saying: "But we *asked* you if your nose was all right and you told us it was and that you had made the whole thing up." This turns the situation into one that is at once double-binding and mystifying.

Case Descriptions

The following examples are from the families of three female schizophrenics, Maya, Ruby, and Ruth.[4]

MAYA

Maya (aged 28) thinks she started to imagine "sexual things" at about the age of 14 when she returned to live with her parents after a six-year separation during World War II. She would lie in her bedroom and wonder whether her parents had sexual intercourse. She began to

---

[4] For extended phenomenologic descriptions of these and other families of schizophrenics, see Laing and Esterson (1964).

get sexually excited, and at about that time she began to masturbate. She was very shy, however, and kept away from boys. She felt increasingly irritated at the physical presence of her father. She objected to him shaving in the same room while she had breakfast. She was frightened that her parents knew that she had sexual thoughts about them. She tried to tell them about this, but they told her *she did not have any thoughts of that kind.* She told them she masturbated *and they told her that she did not.* As for what happened in 1945 or 1946, we have, of course, only Maya's story to go on. However, when she told her parents in the presence of the interviewer that she still masturbated, her parents simply told her that she did not!

Maya's mother does not say: "How bad of you to masturbate," or "I can hardly believe that you could do *that.*" She does not tell Maya not to masturbate. She simply tells her that she does not.

Her mother repeatedly tried to induce Maya to forget various episodes that she (mother) did not want remembered. She did not, however, say: "I don't want you to mention this, much less remember it." She said, instead: "I want you to help the doctor by remembering, but of course you can't remember because you are ill."

Mrs. Abbott persistently questioned Maya about her memory in general, in order (one gathers, from the mother's point of view) to help her to get insight into the fact that she was ill by showing her either (1) that she was amnesic, or (2) that she had got some facts wrong, or (3) that she imagined she remembered because she had heard about it from her mother or father at a later date.

This "false" but "imaginary" memory was regarded by Mrs. Abbott with great concern. It was also a point on which Maya was most confused.

Mrs. Abbott finally told us (not in Maya's presence) that she prayed that Maya would never remember her "illness" because she (mother) thought it would upset her (daughter) to do so. In fact, she (mother) felt this so strongly that she said that it would be kindest even if it meant she had to remain in a hospital!

Both her parents thus not only contradicted Maya's memory, feelings, perceptions, motives, intentions, but their own attributions are curiously self-contradictory. And, further, while they spoke and acted as though they knew better than Maya what she remembered, what she did, what she imagined, what she wanted, what she felt, whether she was enjoying herself or whether she was tired, this "one-upsmanship" was often maintained in a way which was further mystifying. For instance, on one occasion Maya said that she wanted to leave the hospital and that she thought her mother was trying to keep her in the hospital even though there was no need for her to be an in-patient any more. Her mother replied: "I think Maya is . . . I think Maya recognizes that whatever she wanted really for her good, I'd do . . . wouldn't I . . . Hmm? (no answer) No reservations in any way . . . I mean if there were any changes to be made I'd gladly make them . . . unless it was absolutely impossible." Nothing could have been further from what

Maya recognized at that moment. But one notes the mystification in the statement. Whatever Maya wanted is qualified most decisively by "really" and "for her own good." Mrs. Abbott, of course, was arbiter (1) of what Maya "really" wanted, in contrast to what *she* might *think* she wanted, (2) of what was for her own good, (3) of what was possible.

Maya sometimes reacted to such mystifications by lucid perceptions of them. But this was much more difficult for her to achieve than for us. Her difficulty was that she could not herself tell when she could or could not trust her own memory, her mother and father, her own perspective and metaperspective, and her parents' statements of their perspective and metaperspectives.[5]

Close investigation of this family in fact revealed that her parents' statements to her about her, about themselves, about what they felt she felt they felt, etc., and even about what factually had happened could not be trusted. Maya *suspected* this, but she was told by her parents that such suspicions were her illness. She often therefore doubted the validity of her own suspicions; often she denied what they said (delusionally) or invented some story that she clung to temporarily. For instance, she once insisted she had been in the hospital when she was eight, the occasion of her first separation from her parents.

This girl was an only child, born when her mother was 24, her father 30 years of age. Mother and father agreed that she had been her daddy's girl. She would wake him up at 4:30 in the morning when she was 3 to 6, and they would go swimming together. She was always hand in hand with him. They sat close together at table, and he said prayers with her last thing at night. Until she was evacuated at the age of 8 they went for frequent long walks together. Apart from brief visits home, she lived away from her parents until the age of 14.

Mrs. Abbott expressed nothing so simple as jealousy in and through her account of Maya's early intimacy with her father. She seemed to identify herself so much with Maya that she was living through her a re-vision of her relationship with her own father, which had been, according to her, one of rapid, unpredictable switches from acceptance to rejection and back.

When Maya at 14 came back to live permanently at home, she was changed. She wanted to study. She did not want to go swimming or for long walks with her father anymore. She no longer wanted to pray with him. She wanted to read the Bible by herself, for herself. She objected to her father expressing his affection for her by sitting close to her at meals. She wanted to sit further away from him. Nor did she want to go to the cinema with her mother. She wanted to handle things in the house and wanted to do things for herself. For instance (mother's example), she washed a mirror without telling her mother she was going to do it. Her parents complained to us also that she did not want to

---

[5] By perspective is denoted p's point of view in a situation. By metaperspective is denoted p's viewpoint on o's point of view (see Laing, 1961, appendix).

understand her mother or her father and that she could not tell them anything about herself.

Her parents' response to this changed state of affairs, which was evidently a great blow to them, was interesting. Both of them felt that Maya had exceptional mental powers, so much so that both the mother and the father became convinced *that she could read their thoughts*. Father attempted to confirm this by consulting a medium. They began to put this to the test in different ways.

FATHER: "If I was downstairs and somebody came in and asked how Maya was, if I immediately went upstairs, Maya would say to me, 'What have you been saying about me?' I said, 'Nothing.' She said, 'Oh, yes, you have, I heard you.' Now it was so extraordinary that unknown to Maya, I experimented with her, you see, and then when I'd proved it, I thought, 'Well, I'll take Mrs. Abbott into my confidence,' so I told her, and she said, 'Oh, don't be silly, it's impossible' I said, 'All right, now when we take Maya in the car tonight, I'll sit beside her and I'll concentrate on her. I'll say something, and you watch what happens.' When I was sitting down, she said, 'Would you mind sitting at the other side of the car. I can't fathom Dad's thoughts.' And that was true. Well, following that, one Sunday I said—it was winter—I said, 'Now Maya will sit in the usual chair, and she'll be reading a book. Now you pick up a paper and I'll pick up a paper, and I'll give you the word and er . . . Maya was busy reading the paper and er . . . I nodded to my wife, then I concentrated on Maya behind the paper. She picked up the paper . . . her . . . em . . . magazine or whatever it was and went to the front room. And her mother said, 'Maya, where are you going? I haven't put the fire on.' Maya said, 'I can't understand . . . No, 'I can't get to the depth of Dad's brain. Can't get to the depth of Dad's mind'!"

Such mystifications have continued from before her first "illness" to the present, coming to light only after this investigation had been underway for over a year.

Maya's irritation, jumpiness, confusion, and occasional accusations that her mother and father were "influencing" her in some way had been, of course, completely "laughed off" by her father and mother in her presence for years, but in the course of the present investigation the father told Maya about this practice.

DAUGHTER: Well, I mean you shouldn't do it, it's not natural.
FATHER: I don't do it . . . I didn't do it . . . I thought . . . 'Well, I'm doing the wrong thing, I won't do it.'
DAUGHTER: I mean, the way I react would show you it's wrong.
FATHER: And there was a case in point a few weeks back, she fancied one of her mother's skirts.
DAUGHTER: I didn't. I tried it on and it fitted.
FATHER: Well, they had to go to a dressmaker . . . the dressmaker was recommended by someone, Mrs. Abbott went for it, and she said,

"How much is that?' The woman said, 'Four shillings.' Mrs. Abbott said, 'Oh, no, it must have cost you more than that,' so she said, 'Oh, well, your husband did me a good turn a few years back and I've never repaid him.' I don't know what it was. Mrs. Abbott gave more, of course. So when Maya came home, she said, 'Have you got the skirt, Mum?' She said, 'Yes, and it cost a lot of money too, Maya.' Maya said, 'Oh, you can't kid me, they tell me it was four shillings.'

DAUGHTER: No, seven I thought it was.

FATHER: No, it was four you said, exactly, and my wife looked at me and I looked at her . . . So if you can account for that, I can't.

Another of Maya's "ideas of reference" was that something was going on between her parents that she could not fathom and that she thought was about her but she could not be sure.

Indeed there was. When mother, father and Maya were interviewed together, mother and father kept up a constant series of knowing smiles, winks, nods, gestures that were so "obvious" to the observer that he commented on them after about twenty minutes of the first triadic interview. From Maya's point of view, the mystification was that her mother and father neither acknowledged this remark from the researcher, nor had they ever, as far as we know, acknowledged the validity of similar perceptions and comments by Maya. As a result, so it seemed to us, she did not know when she was perceiving something to be going on and when she was imagining it. The open, yet secret, nonverbal exchanges between father and mother were in fact quite public and perfectly obvious. Her "paranoid" doubts about what was going on appeared, therefore, to be in part expressions of her lack of trust in the validity of her suspicions. She could not "really" believe that what she thought she saw to be going on was going on. Another consequence to Maya was that she could not discriminate between what (to the researchers) were not intended to be communicative actions (taking off spectacles, blinking, rubbing nose, frowning, and so on) of people generally and what were indeed signals between mother and father. The extraordinary thing was that some of these signals were partly "tests" to see if Maya would pick them up. An essential part of the game the parents played was, however, that if comented on, the rejoinder should be, "What do you mean, what wink?" and so on.

RUBY

When Ruby (aged 18) was admitted to the hospital, she was completely mute, in an inaccessible catatonic stupor. She at first refused to eat, but gradually she was coaxed to do so. After a few days she began to talk. She rambled in a vague way, and she often contradicted herself. At one moment, for instance, she said her mother loved her, and the next she said she was trying to poison her.

In clinical psychiatric terms, there was incongruity of thought and affect, e.g., she laughed when she spoke of her recent pregnancy and miscarriage. She complained of bangings in her head and of voices outside her head calling her "slut," "dirty," "prostitute." She thought that "people" were talking disparagingly about her. She said she was the Virgin Mary, and Elvis Presley's wife. She thought her family disliked her and wanted to get rid of her; she feared she would be abandoned in the hospital by them. "People" did not like her. She feared crowds and "people." When she was in a crowd, she felt the ground would open up under her feet. At night "people" were lying on top of her, having sexual intercourse with her; she had given birth to a rat after she was admitted to the hospital; she believed she saw herself on television.

It was clear that the fabric of this girl's sense of "reality," of what is the case and what is not the case, was in shreds.

The question is: Has what is usually called her "sense of reality" been torn in shreds by others?

Is the way this girl acts and are the things she says the intelligible effluxion of pathologic process?

This girl was confused particularly as to who she was—she oscillated between the Virgin Mary and Elvis Presley's wife—and she was confused as to whether or not her family and "people" in general loved her and in what sense—whether they liked the person she was or desired her sexually while despising her.

How socially intelligible are these areas of confusion?

In order to spare the reader the initial confusion of the investigators, not to say that of the girl, we shall tabulate her family nexus.

BIOLOGICAL STATUS	TITLES RUBY WAS TAUGHT TO USE
father	uncle
mother	mummy
aunt (mother's sister)	mother
uncle (mother's sister's husband)	daddy, later uncle
cousin	brother

Simply, Ruby was an illegitimate child, reared by her mother, her mother's sister, and the sister's husband.

We shall refer to her biological relatives without inverted commas, and as she called them, and/or as they referred to themselves, with inverted commas.

Her mother and she lived with her mother's married sister, this sister's husband ('daddy' and 'uncle'), and their son (her cousin). Her father, who was married and had another family elsewhere, visited them occasionally. She referred to him as 'uncle.'

Her family violently disagreed in an initial interview with us about whether Ruby had grown up knowing "who she was." Her mother ('mummy') and her aunt ('mother') strongly maintained that she had no inkling of the real state of affairs, but her cousin (her 'brother') insisted that she must have known for years. They (mother, aunt, and uncle) argued also that no one in the district knew of this, but they admitted finally that of course everyone knew she was an illegitimate child, but no one would hold it against her. The most intricate splits and denials in her perception of herself and others were simultaneously expected of this girl and practiced by the others.

She got pregnant six months before admission to the hospital (miscarriage at four months).

Like so many of our families, this one was haunted by the specter of scandal and gossip, by the fear of what "people" were saying or thinking, etc. When Ruby was pregnant, all this became intensified. Ruby thought "people" were talking about her (they in fact were) and her family knew they were, but when she told them about this, they tried to reassure her by telling her not to be silly, not to imagine things, that of course no one was talking about her.

This was just one of the many mystifications to which this girl was subjected.

The following are a few of the others.

1) In her distracted, "paranoid" state, she said that she thought her mother, aunt, uncle, and cousin disliked her, picked on her, mocked her, despised her. As she got "well," she felt very remorseful about having thought such terrible things, and she said that her family had been "really good" to her and that she had a "lovely family."

Indeed, they gave her every reason to feel guilty for seeing them in this way, expressing dismay and horror that she should think that they did not love her.

In actuality, they told us that she was a slut and little better than a prostitute—and they told us this with vehemence and intensity.

They tried to make her feel bad or mad for perceiving their real feelings.

2) She guiltily suspected that they did not want her home from the hospital and accused them, in sudden outbursts, of wanting to get rid of her. They asked her how she could think such things, but in fact, they were extremely reluctant to have her at home.

They tried to make her think they wanted her home and to make her feel mad or bad if she perceived that they did not want her home, when, in fact, they did not want her home.

3) Extraordinarily confused attitudes were brought into play when she became pregnant.

As soon as they could after hearing about it from Ruby, 'mummy' and 'mother' got her on the sitting-room divan, and while trying to pump hot soapy water into her uterus, told her with tears, reproaches, sympathy, pityingly and vindictively at once, what a fool she was, what a slut she was, what a terrible plight she was in (just like her 'mummy'), what a bastard the boy was ("just like her father"), what a disgrace, history was repeating itself, how could one expect anything else. . . .

This was the first time her true parentage had ever been explicitly made known to her.

4) Subsequently, Ruby's feeling that people were talking about her began to develop in earnest. As we have noted, she was told this was nonsense, and her family told us that everyone was "very kind" to her

"considering." Her cousin was the most honest. "Yes, most people are kind to her, just as if she were colored."

5) The whole family was choked with the sense of shame and scandal. While emphasizing this to Ruby again and again, they simultaneously told her that she was imagining things when she said she thought that people were talking about her.

6) Her family *accused* her of being spoiled and pampered, but when she tried to reject their pampering, they told her (1) she was ungrateful, and (2) she needed them, she was still a child, etc. (as though being spoiled was something *she* did).

The uncle was represented by the mother and aunt to the researchers also as a very good uncle who loved Ruby and who was like a father to her. They were assured that he was willing to do anything he could to help them elucidate Ruby's problem. Despite this, at no time was it possible to see him for a prearranged interview. Six mutually convenient appointments were made during the period of the investigation, and every one was broken, and broken either without any notice at all or with no more than twenty-four hours' notice. The uncle was seen eventually by the researchers, but only when they called at his house without notice.

According to the testimony of uncle, mother, and aunt to the researchers, this girl was repeatedly told by her uncle that if she did not "mend her ways" she would have to get out of the house. We know that on two occasions she was actually told by him to go and she did. But when she said to him that he had told her to get out, *he denied it to her* (though not to us)!

Her uncle told us tremblingly how she had pawed him, run her hands over his trousers, how he was sickened by it. His wife said rather coolly that he did not give the impression of having been sickened at the time.

Ruby, when questioned later, had apparently no conscious idea that her uncle did not like being cuddled and petted. She thought he liked it, she had done it to please him.

Not just in one area, but in every conceivable way—in respect of her clothes, her speech, her work, her friends—this girl was subject to mystifications, permeating all the interstices of her being.

The members of the families of the schizophrenic patients so far studied use mystification frequently as the preferred means of controlling the experience and action of the schizophrenic patient.

We have never yet seen a preschizophrenic who was not in a highly mystified state before his or her manifest psychotic breakdown.

This mystified state is, of course, unrecognized as such by the actively mystifying other family members, although it is frequently pointed out by a relatively detached member of the family circle (a "normal" sib, an aunt or uncle, a friend). The psychotic episode can sometimes be seen as an unsuccessful attempt to recognize the state of mystification the person is in. Each attempt at recognition is violently opposed by every conceivable mystification by the active mystifiers in the family.

RUTH

The following example of mystification again entails the confusion of praxis with process.

What to the investigators is an expression of the girl's real self, however disjunctive it is with her parents' model of what this is, her parents regard as mere process; that is, they ascribe no motive, agency, responsibility or intention, to such behavior. Behavior that to the investigators seems false and compliant, they regard as healthy, normal, and her true or real self. This paradoxical situation is a constantly repeated one in our data.

Ruth from time to time puts on colored woolen stockings and dresses generally in a way that is quite usual among certain sections of Londoners, but unusual in her parents' circle.

This is seen by her parents as a "symptom" of her illness. Her mother identified Ruth's act of putting on such stockings as the first sign of an-other "attack" coming on. That is, her mother (and father) convert her action (praxis) into a sign of a pathologic process. The same action is seen by the investigators as an assertion of a self that is disjunctive with her parents' rigidly held view both of who Ruth is and what she ought to be.

These acts of self-assertion are met with tremendous violence both from Ruth herself and from her parents. The result is an ensuing period of disturbed experience and behavior that is clinically diag-nosable as a "psychotic episode." It ends with a reconciliation on the basis that Ruth has been ill. While being ill she felt things, did things, said things, that she did not really mean, and which she could not help, because it was all due to her "illness." Now that she is better again she herself realizes this.

When Ruth puts on colored stockings at first, the issues for the parents are: What is making her disgrace us this way? She is a good girl. She is always so sensible and grateful. She is not usually stupid and in-considerate. Even if she wants to wear stockings, etc., like that, she knows it upsets her father and she knows he has a bad heart. How can she upset him like that when she really loves him?

The difficulty in analyzing this girl in her nonpsychotic periods, as is not infrequently the case with schizophrenics in their "mute" phase, is that she completely sides with her parents in their view that she has "attacks" of her "illness" periodically. Only when she is "ill" does she repudiate (and then, of course, only with part of herself) her parents' "axis of orientation."

An approach to the logic of the mystification in this case might be attempted as follows.

X is good. All not-X is bad. Ruth is X. If Ruth were Y she would be bad. But Ruth appears to be Y.

Thus Y must be the equivalent to X, in which case Ruth is not really not-X, but is really X.

Moreover, if Ruth tries to be, or is, Y, she will be bad. But Ruth is person X, that is, she is good, so Ruth cannot be bad, so she must be mad.

Ruth wants to put on colored woolen stockings and go out with boys, but she does not want to be bad or mad. The mystification here is that without being bad or mad she cannot become anything except a dowdy aging spinster living at home with her aging parents. She is persecuted by the "voices" of her own unlived life if she is good and by the "voices" of her parents if she is bad. So she is maddened either way. She is thus in what I have called an *untenable position* (Laing, 1961, p. 135).

The therapist's task is to help such a person to become *demystified*. The first phase of therapy, in such a case, consists largely in efforts at demystification, of untangling the knot that he or she is tied in, or raising issues that may never have been questioned or even thought of except when the person was "ill," namely, is it bad or is it a disgrace, or is it selfish, inconsiderate, ungrateful, etc., to be or to do not-X and is it necessarily good to be X, etc.?

But the *practice* of therapy is another story.

References

BATESON, G., JACKSON, D. D., HALEY, J., AND WEAKLAND, J. (1956). Toward a theory of schizophrenia. *Behav. Sci.* 1, 251–264.

BRODEY, W. M. (1959). Some family operations and schizophrenia. *A.M.A. Arch. gen. Psychiat.* 1, 379–402.

HALEY, J. (1959a). The family of the schizophrenic: a model system. *J. nerv. ment. Dis.* 129, 357–374.

HALEY, J. (1959b). An interactional description of schizophrenia. *Psychiatry* 22, 321–332.

LAING, R. D. (1960). *The divided self.* London: Tavistock. Chicago: Quadrangle Press, 1961.

LAING, R. D. (1961). *The self and other.* London: Tavistock. Chicago: Quadrangle Press, 1962.

LAING, R. D. (1962). Series and nexus in the family. *New Left Rev. 15*, May–June.

LAING, R. D., AND COOPER, R. D. (1964). *Reason and violence. A decade of Sartre's philosophy—1950–1960.* London: Tavistock. New York: Humanities Press.

LAING, R. D., AND ESTERSON, A. (1964). *Sanity, madness and the family,* vol. 1. *Families of schizophrenics.* London: Tavistock. New York: Basic Books.

LIDZ, T., CORNELISON, A., TERRY, D., AND FLECK, S. (1958). Intrafamilial environment of the schizophrenic patient: VI The transmission of irrationality. *A.M.A. Arch. Neurol. Psychiat. 79*, 305–316.

LOMAS, P. (1961). Family role and identity formation. *Int. J. Psycho-Anal. 42*, July–Oct.

RYCKOFF, I., DAY, J., AND WYNNE, L. C. (1959). Maintenance of stereotyped roles in the families of schizophrenics. *A.M.A. Arch. gen. Psychiat. 1*, 93–98.

SARTRE, J. P. (1960). *Critique de la raison dialectique.* Paris: Gallimard.

SEARLES, H. F. (1959). The effort to drive the other person crazy—an element in the etiology and psychotherapy of schizophrenia. *Brit. J. med. Psychol. 32*, 1–18.

WYNNE, L. C., RYCKOFF, I. M., DAY, J., AND HIRSCH, S. I. (1958). Pseudo-mutuality in the family relations of schizophrenics. *Psychiatry 21*, 205–220.

10

ANTHONY F. C. WALLACE

RAYMOND D. FOGELSON

The Identity Struggle

In the fall of 1960, the writers were invited by Dr. Ivan Boszormenyi-Nagy and his associates to participate as anthropological observers in their family therapy program at the Eastern Pennsylvania
Psychiatric Institute.[1] In the first meetings with Dr. Boszormenyi-
Nagy, we were impressed by his group's interest in the styles of interpersonal conflict in which their treatment families were chronically
engaged. These struggles seemed to center in obstinate, and verbally
manifest, efforts by the participants to coerce each other into simple
and culturally conventional, but mutually incompatible, nurturant
roles, basically by the crude device of calling each other names,
and they often persisted for long periods of time, even in the face
of resolute efforts by the therapeutic team to intervene on occasion
and divert the several strivings into more healthy channels.

[1] We wish to acknowledge our gratitude for the expert aid provided by the following members of the anthropology section, who served as secretaries, research
assistants, and collaborators in various phase of the project: Dr. Robert Ackerman,
Mrs. Nina Balis, Miss Connie Davidejt, Mrs. Josephine Dixon, Mrs. H. Pollard
Dow, Miss Virginia Tovey.

365

The label *identity struggle* seemed an appropriate one because, in brief, we found that the manifest content of the verbal conflicts in family therapy often took the form of an argument over what kind of person each of the participants was. Each party alternately played the role of aggressor and defender, at times accusing the other of having one undesirable characteristic or another, and at times stoutly defending his own character from criticism. Such struggles appeared, once launched, to be more than simple, symptomatic expressions of libidinal needs (although certainly they depended on such needs for their origin) and to be, in fact, quasi-autonomous transactional processes with a "life" of their own.

This chapter is, therefore, a description of representative instances of identity struggle and a report of some theoretical formulations which, at the present time, we feel to be useful and even necessary, even if not all-sufficient, in any explanation of the phenomena we observed.

The chapter contains three sections. In the first, case materials are presented, for, at this stage of work, it is not possible to give controlled experimental data. Nevertheless, in order to communicate the concepts more clearly, to demonstrate that the identity struggle as a phenomenon does occur, and to illustrate some of the methods, and difficulties of observation, we shall present some "natural history" descriptions based on clinical observations of families in treatment. In the second section, theoretical formulations are presented. In the course of thinking over and discussing the family conflicts under our observation, we have gradually formulated a theoretical position which has, increasingly, determined the choice of phenomena to which we have paid attention. We shall state this formulation, and some of its social contexts beyond the family therapy situation, as precisely as we can.

And, finally, in the third section, we shall consider the identity struggle in family therapy of schizophrenia. Although we have made no special effort to relate our work to the literature on family therapy, we cannot avoid making certain inferences from our observations. These inferences concern the conditions under which either therapeutic or antitherapeutic processes may be promoted by identity struggle in the situation of psychotherapy, both individual and familial.

Throughout the chapter, we maintain (as well as one can in dealing with subject matter so highly charged with social, medical, and personal values) the role of *anthropological* investigators, impartially observing both patients and therapists in a system of interaction whose rules constitute just one more of the various ways in which human behavior can be structured. In so doing, we deliberately avoid the routine interpretation of behavior in psychiatric terms; thus, for instance, we only occasionally introduce the concept of unconscious psychodynamics, and we emphasize the manifest content of verbal communication rather than the sometimes more libidinally revealing nonverbal communication. We are well aware that by so restricting our attention, we leave out many important phenomena. On the other hand, various ego-controlled processes, conscious, cognitive, and verbal, are also important parts of human behavior, and are indeed the most characteristically human behavior of all. And in this work we are concerned with the manifest form of a type of interpersonal interaction which needs to be described first on the level of overt verbal behavior and of conscious cognitive process. Only after this description is reasonably complete can a meaningful explanation in terms of psychodynamics be essayed.

Case Materials

Our case materials are drawn from visual observations and tape-recordings of family therapy sessions in Dr. Ivan Boszormenyi-Nagy's unit at the Eastern Pennsylvania Psychiatric Institute. (The routine of these meetings is described in the companion chapters by Ivan Boszormenyi-Nagy and James L. Framo in this volume.) The anthropologists observed the sessions through one-way windows, never entered the treatment situation, and, as far as we are aware, were personally unknown to the subjects (although the subjects were informed that research personnel might be observing and recording any session). During the course of about six months, from January to June, 1961, we observed four families in weekly treatment sessions over periods of several months each; one of these families, whom we shall call by the fictitious name of Smith, we followed throughout the six months' observation period. It is certain material from the Smith family sessions which we shall be discussing in some detail.

Initially, we devoted considerable effort to developing a system for coding the transcripts of the tapes and picking out the images of self and others presented by the participants. Our hope was to delineate the stochastic structure of the identity conflict characteristic of each individual family. Although in principle this approach has merit, the technical difficulties of establishing interobserver reliability in coding proved to be discouraging. An even more serious drawback of such an approach was the superficiality of the semantic interpretation of the participants' statements. Reducing each utterance, rich in imagery and illusion, to a small number of symbols (twenty-seven), each signifying a category defining the type of image, its valence, and its vector, eliminated so much of its meaning from the analysis of what was happening in the communication that we abandoned the procedure and turned to a less rigorous, but more appreciative, method. This method placed reliance on the observers' abilities, as speakers of the same general language as the subjects, to "understand" a good deal of what they were saying to each other. This more intuitive procedure made it possible to recognize tactical gambits, to delineate the structure of conflict, and to relate interpersonal communication to psychodynamics not much less reliably, and a good deal more validly, than had the more austere coding procedure.

The Smith household consisted of the patient, a 17-year-old girl, and her father and mother. The parents faithfully attended the weekly sessions along with the patient's therapist (who was concurrently seeing her in individual therapy) and another therapist from Dr. Boszormenyi-Nagy's group. The parents were a middle-class, middle-aged, middle-income couple, without college education but reasonably well aware of the purposes of modern dynamic psychiatry and accepting of the principle that they themselves might be harboring emotional difficulties whose resolution could contribute to their daughter's recovery and later successful adjustment to life on the "outside." The daughter, Mary, had entered treatment at the Institute after a nearly successful suicide attempt. When she first entered the hospital, some two months before the family treatment program began, she had been mute, withdrawn, dishevelled, and prone to sit on the floor for hours staring at the wall. At the time of her initial involvement in the family treatment program, some improvement in her condition had occurred, presumably partly as a result of her work in individual therapy.

Throughout the series of sessions which we observed, despite manifest oscillations in the patient's condition, despite a change in her therapist midway through the process, and despite the variety of particular topics discussed, one feature of the interview remained virtually constant. This was the tendency for every conversation, whatever its subject, to spiral rapidly into an identity struggle. The therapists, of course, aided and abetted this process, since their standard tactic was to diagnose the identity implications of any utterance and then work to make implicit images explicit. Thus, if the father said he had felt uneasy about some specific event, one of the therapists would be apt to suggest that perhaps he was liable to be a little uneasy in a large class of situations of which that event was only a single instance; the mother would confirm this; a therapist would ask the patient what she thought; and the struggle was on, father on the defensive, the pack closing in, the father accusing the mother of having a characteristic which made him uneasy, mother defending herself, daughter defending mother, father accusing daughter of partiality, therapist generalizing this comment, and so on. The therapists, we believe, played this incendiary role deliberately in the interests, first, of making the conscious emotional issues among the family explicit and available for conversation, and, second, of bringing to conscious attention the internal conflicts of the individual participants, particularly the patient, who could then, both in the family session and in private sessions with her therapist, work out the dilemmas thus presented.

A recurrent dialogue in these sessions, particularly involving Mary and her mother, concerned their complementary images of themselves and each other as more or less understanding, and more or less friendly, persons. This struggle was apparently an old one, going back for several years. The mother wished Mary to be more friendly, outgoing, and confidential with her; the mother's tactic was to force Mary to act in a more friendly way by accusing her of being unfriendly, thus challenging her to prove that she was friendly. Mary would counter this by saying that her mother was not an understanding person and that she herself was not unfriendly in any hostile or antagonistic way but was simply honestly and actually cold, withdrawn, and indifferent. The mother would then say that Mary was basically not really indifferent, or cold, or withdrawn; if she would just behave in a more friendly way, as she could if she wished, then she would be rewarded by kindness, warmth, and release from the hospital. Mary would point out that this proved that her mother didn't understand; she really wasn't capable of warm interaction with people; she was too sick; this was her illness; and for anyone to say that she was "really" a lively person underneath was just a coy way of demanding that she display a warmth that wasn't there. Let us now allow the transcripts to speak for themselves.

1. First Excerpt

February, 1961. Present: Mary, father, mother, Dr. A. (family therapist), and Dr. B. (Mary's private therapist).

MOTHER: Well, I have tried to, I try to talk to Mary even if it is just about certain things. I do try . . . to get some spark even if it is about everyday occurrences. I just can't sit there. I'm not that kind. I have to ask her questions and I . . . sometimes she shows a little interest, sometimes she doesn't. She's just like a piece of wood . . . sayin' words. But if . . . she . . . er . . . I sometimes see a little, little spark of response which I see, a little spark and I feel better. I'm happier and I'm glad for any sort of response that I get.

MARY: (laughs)

MOTHER: That's the way *I* feel.

DR. B.: This puts your entire disposition, in a way, if she gives just a little spark, then you can be happy.

MARY: (laughs)

MOTHER: I feel I (unintelligible) but she doesn't; she has a lot of life, and she has a lot of feelin'.

DR. B.: We just saw that now with the laughter. She thought a piece of wood was exciting, somehow.

MARY: No.

DR. B.: No?

MARY: Struck me funny (low voice).

DR. B: Funny?

MARY: Not that . . . the whole thing . . .

FATHER: But don't you feel that . . . our visits could be a great deal more pleasant . . . if you'd, er, try to share them a little bit more? But you retreat . . . in other words, I feel that it doesn't really make too much difference to you whether we come or not, or when we go . . . or not. Of course, I may be wrong and I stand to be corrected, but that's what my impression is. Of course, like I said, you can comment on it.

MARY: This place is blooming . . . life . . . bubbling underneath me . . . (laughs) (pause). Ah, ah, I don't know really what, what you're requiring of me . . . (laughs) . . . to be frank.

FATHER: Very little. We haven't asked you for anything.

MARY: Oh. (laughs)

FATHER: Outside of a little bit of friendliness and I don't think that's a great deal. After all, if it was strangers that meet, they act friendly, and I assure you I don't believe that we're strangers.

MARY: (small laugh) I wouldn't be too sure.

FATHER: Why? Why do you say you wouldn't be too sure. Do ya mean that after all these years we're . . . I'm a stranger to you?

MARY: Well, (pause) you're overlooking something . . . I mean . . . I don't think that I communicated with you or for that matter anybody else for the past two years . . . and you seem to overlook that and that small matter, you know . . .

FATHER: Well, I admitted that I was negligent, but purely it was through . . . er . . .

MARY: (excited) I didn't say anything . . . about your neglect . . . un, ah . . . I didn't say that. I just said that I haven't communicated with you or other people . . . or on my part . . . I didn't say anything to do with you . . . so ah . . . I mean its not . . . ah . . . something I so abruptly, oh assumed, ya know, since I arrived here . . . or anything . . . and I didn't really, ah . . .

FATHER: But I feel that you retreated even further since you've been here . . .

MARY: I don't communicate with that many people or say that much to them that means very much. Ah . . . don't feel . . . ah . . . as if I

. . . y'know . . . I just simply do this . . . when you, when you come to visit me . . . (laughs). Oh . . . and der I ah . . . don't really understand what you want me to talk about.

DR. B.: I think that's true.

MARY: I don't know what you want me to say (laughs). I mean I don't have too . . . ah . . . too much to say.

FATHER: Well, possibly I don't want you to be bubbling over with enthusiasm, but I do expect you to show a little bit more feeling and joy at our coming.

MARY: I can't (high voice) you always . . . all you . . . want me to do something that I can't.

FATHER: Well, that at least is a little bit of explanation that I've never heard before.

MARY: You would like me to . . . oh, I, I suppose I could . . . play something there (laugh) which wouldn't be there. If you'd really like me to do that, I suppose I could manage (laugh) . . .

DR. A.: I have somehow the feeling that Mary is in the position of some-one who can give or withhold and, ah, both her parents are asking for something from her, Mary, that should give friendliness, and thereby make them feel happy.

FATHER: Well, let's put it this way: not only in our case—'course we are possibly more personally involved than anybody else at the present time—but it's a theory that you must carry through with everybody. You expect friendliness, then you have to extend something. You cannot be cold, and expect friendliness. It's an impossibility. You wouldn't get that from anybody.

DR. A: It is very true—I am not disagreeing, I am not questioning that— all I'm saying is that this situation as it is now, you see her sick-ness, and your coming in visiting her as parents, creates, as it looks like, as though, the way you are talking, both of you, that, now, if you could be only a little nicer, you could make us happy, and this is the kind of thing . . .

FATHER: Well, na, er, uh, uh, possibly maybe you're right when you say that of course being so deeply concerned and coming as we do, it's very hard. After all, this is a three hour visit. In three hours, er uh, to try to hold interest in the conversation . . . with a someone who's very unfriendly . . .

MARY: I am not unfriendly } [at the same time]
FATHER: . . . seems to be unhappy

MARY: Wha' do I do? I argue with you occasionally.

FATHER: Well, that's something!

MARY: Twice I argued with you.

FATHER: Yes, I believe that an argument is better than nothing at all.

MARY: Twice I argued with you and ah . . . I don't really know what you want me to extend. I, ah, can't extend something that . . . that's simply not there. That would be difficult. And I really don't think it would make you so very much happier (laughs).

FATHER: Well, how do you know if you don't try?

MARY: There's nothing to try. You're . . . as far as I'm concerned, I ah, I can't instill something there that's not there. Ah, (laughs) I don't know what you want from me.

MOTHER: I have seen all sorts of interests . . . ah, Tuesday . . . I haven't been coming every Tuesday, but sometimes when I have, ah, can get out of the house, I do try, and this Tuesday I had a strong feeling that I wanted to see Mary, and my daughter-in-law helped me and we rushed and we got out of the house. And, ah, Mary shows some interests, sometimes. She asked her father if he had a brand new shirt and some days she asked me if I had a new bag. These are signs of some interest in her parents. I honestly don't expect the friendliness that my husband is talking about . . . knowing some of the things she feels right now.

MARY: I'm not unfriendly toward you. I don't see where you get the feeling that I'm, I mean I don't think that I'm unfriendly.

FATHER: Well, I said it could have been the wrong word. Let's say not overly friendly.

MARY: Well, I'm not especially an overly friendly person anyway, so its kind of hard to expect from me. I think sometimes you expect something to be there that isn't any longer there . . . might possibly have been there (laughs), but a, ah, I'm sorry but, but, not anymore. I can't help that.

DR. A: Do you also feel, Mary, that this is sort of a demand on you that sort of drains your energy, that you have to not only think of your own troubles, but you have to consider not to disappoint your parents?

MARY: I think sometimes that when my parents come, I have to be required to keep up a conversation and that a, to appear . . . I don't know . . .

DR. A: Cheerful, or . . . ?

MARY: Well, like when my sister comes, I mean, and knew my sister came a long way to see me, and I know well, ya know, if ah . . . she comes to see me and everything, and I don't say anything to her . . .

DR. A: You have to reward her?

MARY: Then she'll go back feeling perhaps bad, worried, I mean, I am her sister . . . and I don't think she'd come to see me unless she really wanted to, so I'm required to (sigh) huh, say something or two, be something which I'm not to . . . a certain extent.

DR. A: Do you ever feel that you have already went, gone to the end of your attempts to try to keep this good front even though you don't feel it, or that you just can't pretend any more when you don't feel it?

MARY: That I think would be very hard to do for me now. I mean, I can make conversation sometimes, but . . .

DR. B: In relation to Mary's own self and some connection that we know to be existing between you and her, ah, I want to point out that Mary has been neglecting her hair very much lately. Now, I don't know whether it was that way at the other hospital, but I have a feeling somehow that, ah, although I do not understand why, it started lately.

DR. A: Few days after she's been here. I do have the feeling it is connected with the incident we have talked about, not the incident itself as much as the importance of Mary's hair in relation with you.

MARY: (laughs)

DR. B: It, ah, it does impress me very much that Mary should neglect her hair that much, you know, Mary is not, ah, the type of patient who has really given up to the point where they are regressed, ah, even their body is not, ah, constantly present to themselves, and yet with the hair it is striking. There's also the lipstick which might have some connection with it all. I don't know, but I have, ah, asked Mary to consider this, and to comb herself, and this is something she wouldn't do at any cost, and I wonder what, whether you had noticed that yourself, and what had been your impression, how do you explain that?

MOTHER: I certainly do notice it.

2. Second Excerpt

March, 1961. Present: Mary, father, mother, Dr. A. (family therapist), and Dr. B. (Mary's private therapist).

MARY: I don't know. Anything you say practically. (laughs) You, you say that I never confided in you. Well, if you knew how . . .

MOTHER: I didn't say you *never* confided in me.

MARY: You said that I didn't *come* to you, or something like that, that I didn't come to you with much of anything. Well, if I didn't come to you, I didn't even think you'd be hardly aware of what, what I really was feeling or, or what my problems *were*, practically at all.

MOTHER: Well, you did come to me sometimes, Mary, but the day . . .

MARY: I came to you about the religion. About that, uh . . .

MOTHER: Well, you had also told me that you didn't *want* to feel.

MARY: I didn't!

MOTHER: That it hurt you too much to feel, that's why you didn't want to feel.

MARY: I didn't feel, that, that's just the point. You mean . . . the time you thought I was depressed? I'd long since passed that stage (laughs) where people get depressed (laughs). Oh, I don't know. It's not important.

DR. A: Yes, it is, because you feel that your mother is not seriously interested in you and she doesn't even know your problems.

MARY: She doesn't.

DR. A: But yet she feels that . . .

MARY: Well, I don't know you give me the feeling, ah, I don't know sometimes that, uh, you, the way you talk to me, you talk about the other people here and you say to me, Mary, when *she* came here, she was very sick and this one was very sick and that one was very sick, you know, as if sometimes you know, not that I say I'm very sick—I, I really, I couldn't estimate anymore at this point, I really couldn't estimate—but you, like what you said to me, Sunday, "Well, Mary," you know . . . I don't remember what you said to me. You said something about that I could be finished being, that you . . . All you said was, I remember now, all you said was, you didn't say anything about if I *tried* or anything like that. You said, that you'd been thinking about it and that you thought that, ah, yeah, you did say something about trying (laughs) that's right. You said that if I tried that I could be done being an out-patient [in-patient] by July.

MOTHER: No, I said it was not an impossibility.

MARY: Well, you said, well, I can't remember the exact word, that is all I remember what you said. I'm just telling you what I think you said.

MOTHER: Well, you remember some things I say to you, don't you?

MARY: Yes, well, I'm not, you know, I can't remember *everything* people say to me or, you know, *exactly* what they say to me.

DR. A: Now, and here your mother meant to tell you, you hope to get out in a few months and you took it as an underestimation of how sick you are?

MARY: Well, she does underestimate it because she doesn't know.

DR. A: Because you are sick enough not to get well in a few months?

MARY: No, I get the feeling, not that I say it's impossible, I simply get the feeling, you know, that my mother thinks that, well, if Mary puts just a little effort forward, everything will come out in some kind of a miracle, you know. In a couple of months, I'm, I get the feeling that I'm really supposed to bloom, you know, and I'll come out and I, you know, I mean really get the feeling that she expects something very great to happen and that I'll be so different and everything, and to me this *is* an impossibility, that I would be so very changed. I mean, it's not that it's a question of being *well* or anything I, I just get the feeling sometimes that she expects me with just very small little effort, you know, put forward that every-thing's going to be very fine, and you know and I, to me it's just that this is quite impossible.

DR. A: 'Cause you can't do it by yourself?

MARY: No, it's just impossible (laughs).

DR. A: Who should do it?

MARY: Well, it's not a question of people doing it. It's just a question that even if I did put a certain amount of effort into it, I don't think I'd be that so very, very changed as I get the feeling that she expects from me.

DR. A: Well, what could change you? What could change you and what *way* could it be done and what is the best plan for it? If your own effort is not enough, then what else will be needed?

MARY: Oh, I don't know.

DR. A: To change her attitude, is that it?

MARY: Well, I don't know. I, I don't even think I understand what she thinks. I think sometimes that she expects this something great from me and perhaps this gives me the feeling that she underestimates me and to the extent that she doesn't know really . . . Oh, I don't know. I can't explain it.

MOTHER: I don't understand, Mary, when you say *I* expect you to change. What do you mean by that?

MARY: Well, you do expect me to change, don't you?

MOTHER: Well, then do you know in what way?

MARY: Looking at the practical side of it, you know in order to get well I'd have to change. Wouldn't I to some extent?

MOTHER: Is that what you don't want to do?

MARY: You know people don't like change in other people and they don't like change in themselves, Mother. It's not something entirely personal to myself.

DR. A: What should be changed . . . we are talking about change . . . what should be changed?

MARY: Oh, I don't know . . .

DR. A: You must have an idea what changes should be . . .

MARY: What should be changed?

DR. A: Because you say you can't change in that length of time, so what would be the change that is expected of you? How would you know?

MARY: The change that *she* expects from me that I, I think . . . I think would be, I don't know. I, I just simply get the feeling she expects me to be very, with a very small amount, you know, just put this, put an effort forward and (laughs) you know and I'm, I'm simply going to blossom, which, uh, and just like she says, I'll be finished being an out-patient [in-patient] by July with really, ah, to me I don't know. I, ah, which seems like something really impossible for me to accomplish even if I really did want to accomplish, accomplish it . . . I, I think it would be impossible. It's not a question of my getting well or . . . anything like that.

DR. A: What's missing then that you possibly can't blossom, why not?

MARY: (laughs) Because I can't.

DR. A: What is missing?

MARY: I don't know (laughs).

DR. A: There on, see there's a very interesting thing because, on the one hand, many people would say that this is a very well-meaning support from your mother, but apparently it doesn't sound like this to you. A mother telling a sick daughter: you see, you put in all your best effort and maybe in a few months you will be out and come home and yet you find this as a . . .

MARY: She doesn't say get out and come home. She says, I'll be completely finished with all therapy, I'll have nothing to do, you know, I'll be finished, finished, finished, you know.

DR. A: I see.

MARY: Well, I don't think, I don't know . . .

MOTHER: Isn't that what you want, Mary?

MARY: I wanted, I, I don't want to go into it at all. I, I just said that before to you. We don't have to go through all this, I mean to begin with. But let's say that we were going to go through all this. If we did, I doubt very much if by July, we, er, I'd be blossoming all over the place so much.

Despite the absence of visual and a good deal of auditory material, the foregoing excerpts from family therapy sessions can be usefully evaluated from several standpoints. One can, for instance, say something about the libidinal wishes of several members of the group, particularly the demands on the part of each of the three principals that the others accept and love him for what he is, without placing impossible conditions of health, wisdom, or tolerance. And one can observe the aggressive and even self-destructive responses of the several family members to each other's fancied or actual refusal to play the nurturant role. But we wish to draw attention to another feature of these passages: their content of imagery. The argument about who is, or can, or should be doing what for whom is rapidly converted into *an argument over what kind of people they are.* This currency in which identity struggle is carried on is a set of adjectives, metaphors, comparisons, and other expressions which describe a person, either the speaker or the person spoken to.

Let us consider the first passage. It begins with the mother saying that when she visits Mary, although most of the time Mary is "just like a piece of wood," she sometimes shows "a little spark of response" that makes her mother feel better. Although the manifest content of the mother's utterance concerns Mary's withdrawal, the introduction of the mother's feelings (she is "happier" when Mary responds) implies that Mary is able to make her mother happy or sad. The father then accuses his daughter of being indifferent to her parents and of making the visits to the hospital unpleasant for them. This adds up to an explicit charge that Mary is hostile to her parents.

Mary in the meantime has been fending off these gambits with giggles; the father's charge forces her, however, to accuse them in turn of being demanding, of "requiring" some behavior from her which she claims she does not understand.

The father denies that they are demanding: all they want is "a little bit of friendliness," which isn't much to ask, not any more than he would expect from a stranger, and certainly the parents are not strangers to her. The father demands to know if she really thinks this. (If she were to agree, it would imply that she *was* hostile after all, since openly to accuse one's parents of failing to be closer to their child than strangers could only be done in anger:

in this culture, at least, such a parental failure would not only justify, but would virtually require, anger in the neglected child.) Mary backs away, explaining that she meant that *she* has been too sick, too withdrawn to communicate with her parents for the past two years. The father, seeing that the daughter is on the defensive, presses his advantage, even admitting apologetically that he has been negligent.

Mary has now been worked into a corner: the parents have built up a case against her, in front of two psychiatrists (and perhaps, she may feel, in the presence of other observers), based on her indifference during visits and her supposed charge of negligence against them (although this was largely manufactured by the father), that she is hostile to her parents. But she tries to defend herself. She denies having said her parents were negligent and insists that her failures to communicate were and are not personal or purposive but are general aspects of her sickness; because of this sickness, she isn't able to communicate with anyone. The father and daughter now engage in brief face-to-face argument, father demanding that she abandon her hostility and show "feeling and joy" at their visits, and she retreating into the explanation that she is sick and withdrawn, and implying that the parents are demanding that she be hypocritical in pretending feelings which are not there.

The therapist now adds fuel to the fire by suggesting that Mary's parents are emotionally dependent on her and that she has the power to make them happy or unhappy. The statement implies a slightly sadistic quality in Mary's employment of the opportunity. The father, missing the point, interprets this as a criticism of himself and justifies *his* hostility by pointing to hers; finally, he states flatly that she is "very unfriendly."

Mary jumps to her own defense at this and says, equally flatly, "I am not unfriendly." She admits that sometimes she argues. Father says, "At least that is something." But she goes on to cite her illness as the reason for her emotional indifference, and asks him if he really wants her to be a hypocrite. He says she won't even try to be friendly. The mother now enters the argument, saying that Mary actually is capable of *some* emotional response, but that she has feelings now that make friendliness impossible for her.

Mary now repeats her claim that she is *not* unfriendly in the sense of being hostile; she is just not naturally a warm, outgoing kind of person, at least "not any more." She is sorry; she has nothing personal against her parents; she is just sick and "she can't help that."

The family therapist, who has been working on the premise that the parents actually depend on Mary for emotional support and that she resents this, especially now that she is sick, suggests this to her as an explanation for her hostility. Mary admits that her relatives, including her sister, *do* want to see her give signs of health, by chatting with them when they visit. She agrees with the doctor to the extent of admitting that keeping up a front of interested conversation is "very hard to do for me now."

The patient's therapist and the family therapist now break in, and temporarily divert the struggle by a long disquisition on Mary's disheveled hair.

The second episode largely concerns the degree of illness of the patient, Mary. It begins with a disagreement over the extent to which Mary confides in her mother. The implication here is that the mother sees her daughter as secretive and nonrelating, an image that both Mary and her mother soon come to repudiate. This leads to the mother's citation of a specific instance in which Mary confided that she didn't want to "feel" because it was too painful. The patient accuses the mother of misunderstanding this confidence, saying that she *didn't* feel, that she was well past the stage of depression at that point. The therapist intervenes and interprets the patient's re-action to mean that she feels her mother lacks interest in her and doesn't even know her problems. Mary accepts the latter part of this interpretation and launches into a description of her mother's image of her condition. She seems to accuse her mother of simpli-fying her sickness, of maximizing potential degrees of therapeutic progress, and of giving false hope that a little bit of effort is all that is required to improve her condition sufficiently to gain release from the hospital. Also in this passage, Mary claims to be unable to evaluate how sick she really is. After some qualifications of this image of both parties, the therapist again steps in and tries to sum-marize the structure of the dispute. He suggests that when the mother tries to offer encouragement, the daughter interprets it as an underestimation of the severity of her sickness. Mary agrees with the second part of the therapist's interpretation. She goes on to amplify what she takes to be her mother's naive view of her condition: that with a little effort miraculous change will occur. Mary considers this prediction improbable, if not impossible.

The therapist asks Mary about her ideas concerning the mecha-nisms of personality change. Mary seems to feel that such change as her mother expects of her would require something beyond mere effort. When the therapist suggests that perhaps the mother's attitude is the crucial element that has to be changed, Mary avoids the question and merely points again to the mother's underestimation of her illness. Next, the mother begins questioning her daughter about the nature of the change required. Mary admits that some change is a prerequisite to getting well (by which she seems to mean getting out of the hospital), but, on the other hand, she states incisively, ". . . people don't like change in other people and they don't like change in themselves . . ."

The therapist then asks the patient for a clearer description of what this required change constitutes. Mary reiterates her contention that her mother expects a miraculous change with a small amount of effort but that such an expectation is unrealistic, even if she might be willing to expend such effort. The therapist tries to make the patient verbalize the essential ingredient necessary to make her well but Mary does not comply. The therapist again poses a seeming paradox to the patient: the mother appears to be offering her encouragement to get well, but the patient doesn't regard this offer as well-meaning support. Mary responds with her own rendering of her mother's attitude ". . . she (her mother) says I'll be completely finished with all therapy, I'll have nothing to do, you know I'll be finished, finished, finished . . ." The mother assumes that Mary is talking about the usually desirable goal of getting well and asks her daughter if that isn't what she wants. But Mary cuts off discussion of the topic with a final hypothetical example to the effect that even if she were willing to put forth maximum effort to get well, the magnitude of change expected by her mother would not be forthcoming in the specified time. As the patient so picturesquely describes the matter, ". . . I doubt very much if by July . . . I'd be blossoming all over the place so much."

In sum, then, the manifest content of the sample of conversations which we have quoted (and which are, we believe, representative of the bulk of the interviews) is very largely devoted to *ad hominem* arguments. The purpose, initially, of these arguments presumably is manipulative: the libidinal needs of the speakers lead them to use this kind of harassment to force their kinsmen to act in compliance with their own wishes. A functional consequence is no doubt also cathartic: the struggle affords an opportunity for ventilation of feelings of frustration and hostility. But we feel that there is another consequence of these arguments: the tendency for the participants to become preoccupied with the tactical problem of defending themselves against accusations of unworthiness. This latter tendency contributes heavily to the maintenance of the argument as an *identity struggle*. What begins as it were, as an open forum for the declaration of mutual needs is transformed into an arena of identity combat wherein, if he does not protect himself, the unwary participant may find his self-esteem destroyed.

Let us now consider in more detail the concept of identity, which is crucial to the analysis of the phenomenon, and then proceed to formalize the structure of the identity struggle.

Theoretical Formulations

1) THE CONCEPT OF IDENTITY

By an *identity* we mean any image, or set of images, either conscious or unconscious, which an individual has of himself.[2] An image, in this sense, may be recognized introspectively as an internal "visual" or "verbal" representation, but it is observed in others as an external assertion in words, deeds, or gesture which is assumed to reflect in some way an internal representation. The full set of images of self (or *total identity*) refers to many aspects of the person, on a number of levels of generality: his appetites, his strengths and capabilities, his fears, his vulnerabilities and weaknesses, his past experience, his moral qualities, his social status and role, his physical appearance, and so on. There is no requirement that the several images which compose this total identity be noncontradictory; thus, identity may, in some of its domains, be ambiguous or inconsistent. Not infrequently, and perhaps generally, the total identity, or full set of images, can be divided into two or more subsets, each more or less internally consistent and all more or less mutually interrelated in a complex pattern of conflicts and alliances. A minimal fourfold division, which is used throughout this study, recognizes *real identity, ideal identity, feared identity* and *claimed identity* as analytically separable aspects of one individual's total identity. Real identity is a subset of images which the person believes, privately, to be a true present description of himself as he "really" is. Ideal identity is a subset of images which the person would like to be able to say was true but which he does not necessarily believe is true at present; the ideal subset of images often includes morally ideal components, but may also incorporate amoral or even, in relation to local conventions, immoral or "negative," in Erikson's sense, identities. (Ideal identity thus

---

[2] The term "identity" (as well as the related term "self") has been used in a number of different senses in the psychological and psychiatric literature. Our definition does not correspond precisely to any of the several major usages but has been influenced primarily by Erikson (1959), Goffman (1959), and Rogers (1942, 1947, 1951, 1954, 1959), who have made distinguished contributions in, respectively, the psychoanalytic, the sociocultural, and the psychological tradition. Some of the bibliographic resources available in the literature are cited in the bibliography.

embraces both id-determined and superego-determined fantasies, and often is not internally consistent.) Feared identity is a subset of images which the person would not like to have to say was true of himself at present and which he does not necessarily believe is true; the feared subset of images may include socially disvalued components, but it may also include identities which are, by some public convention, positive in value. Claimed identity is a subset of images which the person would like another party to believe is his real identity. Sometimes, with respect to a given dimension of variation, the real, ideal, feared, and claimed identities can be construed as points on a linear continuum, such as a scale, or a discrete or continuous variable.

For example, a man's real identity might be an image of self as five feet five inches tall; his ideal identity, an image of self as six feet tall; his feared identity, an image of self as a midget of four feet; and his claimed identity (claimed by the use of specially built shoes, high-topped haircut, and militant posture) as five feet seven inches. Other dimensions, however, are nonordered except by affective value: a woman's real identity may be an image of self as a mental patient consigned by her family to the impersonal but potentially therapeutic care of a hospital staff; her ideal identity, an image of self as a beloved daughter at home with her family; her feared identity, an image of self as an evil, hostile, despised back-ward psychotic; and her claimed identity, the Queen of France. It may be useful to visualize the four aspects of identity as arranged, with respect to any given dimension of variation, on a scale of value, meaningful to the person himself, usually in the following order:

| Feared | Real | Claimed | Ideal |
Identity	Identity	Identity	Identity
Negative		Positive	

The location of real and claimed identity on the value continuum is especially subject to rapid change in response to personal experience, the communications of others, and the pressures of psychological forces on fantasies about the self. It may be noted that this scale implies a correspondence between similarity and value relationships among the components.

There is, of course, no reason for any observer to agree *a priori* that any component of identity is a valid description of its subject. Even "real" identity, in the sense used here, is not necessarily more valid than any other description of a subject. And commonly enough the individual himself may be uncertain about the validity of his real identity, seeing it now closer to the ideal, now farther away, on the value-ordered scale.

As we have suggested, an identity has value; that is to say, a particular set of images of self can be invested with positive or negative affect. The individual works to achieve a real identity that is positive in affective value and to avoid the experience of negative affect in connection with his real identity. Since he strives to keep his real identity reasonably close to the ideal, and reasonably far away from the feared identity, by definition the ideal identity is relatively more positive, and the feared identity more negative, in affective value than the real identity. Thus, there is generally a motivation, more or less pressing, to change the real identity into something closer in affective value to the ideal identity, or, if this is not successful, to change the ideal identity into something closer in affective value to the real identity,[3] and, *pari passu*, to increase the distance between the real and the feared identity. The process of identity change is, of course, closely, but not completely, dependent upon social interaction. To the extent that real, ideal, and feared identities are internalization of the implicit or explicit commentaries and values of others, they are built upon, and require, repeated validation in social communication. But the individual also privately monitors and evaluates his own behavior and thus both refines his concept of ideal identity by the requirements of experience and also estimates for himself any discrepancy between real and ideal and between real and feared identity. Identity formation thus is dependent upon both self-evaluation and interpersonal communication.

We do not minimize the complexity and variety of the ways in which identity is formed and defended and in which it constantly changes. Hence, we avoid here touching upon the subjects of identity formation in childhood and adolescence, which depends upon the use of many processes (only some of which are the various forms of "identification," and the operation of the traditional mechanisms of defense in other phases of identity dynamics). We shall consider in detail, however, certain techniques of interpersonal communication which individuals employ to reduce the dissonance (what Erikson terms identity conflicts in an intrapsychic sense) between real and ideal identity and to maximize the dissonance between

---

[3] The process by which rapprochement between the real and ideal identity are achieved follow closely some of the postulates contained within Festinger's theory of cognitive dissonance (1957). The Q-sort studies reported by Rogers (1959) in which increased congruence between real and ideal self-concepts accompany positive therapeutic movement also have relevance to the statements made above.

feared and real identity, because there is a certain social consequence of the employment of these techniques: the identity struggle.

2) THE IDENTITY STRUGGLE

Two kinds of related personal motives, in varying combinations, may prompt a person to initiate an identity struggle.

First, there is the simple manipulative motive to persuade or influence another person to act in a certain way toward one's self by convincing him that one's identity, and his identity, make such a role on his part reasonable and in the mutual interest of both parties. Such a motive is, at least at the outset of the transaction, a simple and straightforward effort to satisfy a felt need and is to be observed in such everyday encounters as requests for favors (e.g., "Be a good fellow and lend me five bucks"); it can also, at the more extreme end of the continuum, be unashamedly exploitive ("Brother, can you spare a dime?"). This kind of simple maneuver does not generally set in motion an identity struggle because, on the part of the initiator, it is not so much an effort to resolve problems of personal identity as to satisfy needs, both practical and libidinal, which are already acceptable within his existing identity structure. But, occasionally, an identity struggle can be precipitated by a trivial challenge of this kind if the object of manipulation refuses to be "conned" and responds instead by attacking the other's identity (if, for instance, he refuses to make the loan and replies instead, "I can't afford to lend any more money to deadbeats").

Second, there is the psychodynamically more complex motive of maintaining or restoring a favorable identity in one's self. It is this second motive, arising from identity dynamics, that is of principal interest to us in this paper. Identity maintenance or restoration involves a minimizing of dissonance between the values associated with the real and ideal identities, and a maximizing of dissonance between real and feared identities. The problem of dissonance control can, of course, be met in many ways. One avenue of action is principally internal and consists of either exploiting certain mechanisms of defense, such as denial, repression, projection, rationalization, and so forth, or of "reforming" the self by means of a personality resynthesis achieved by such devices as religious conversion, prophetic inspiration, psychotherapy, or the seemingly perverse assumption of a "negative identity" (Erikson, 1959). To the extent that neither inner defense mechanisms nor internal resyntheses are adequate (for any one of a number of reasons) to the task of maintaining the dissonance at a tolerable level, the individual must act outwardly to secure dissonance-reducing (or dissonance-increasing) communication from others. Rarely are the two types of dissonance-controlling tactics found in isolation, but one or the other may predominate in a given instance.

When the individual turns to another party for help to control identity dissonance, his fundamental strategy is typically twofold. First, A attempts to secure from B testimonials, overtly stated or implicit in the roles which B assumes toward A, that, in B's eyes, A's identity is what A wishes it to be; and, at the same time, A tries to avoid hearing, or even to prevent B from expressing, explicitly or implicitly, descriptions of A which are in A's identity structure unfavorable. Second, A attributes to B an identity which will be so negative in value that B will attempt to modify B's real identity in a direction less antagonizing to A. In effect, A says, "I want you to treat me as such-and-such kind of person; the reason why you won't do this for me is that you are a so-and-so." Furthermore, the wish is in these instances not for the treatment itself so much as for the identity-reinforcement which this treatment connotes. Typically, in self-defense, if not in response to his own identity needs, B will begin to apply the same strategy to the aggressor. A, and an identity struggle emerges. In time, such a struggle can involve a group, such as a family, in a complex net of mutual identity struggles, with various temporary coalitions arising in the course of combat.

In analysis of an identity struggle, we deal only with the *images* exchanged verbally in the communication network within the group. We must distinguish between these images and the affective states, and libidinal drives, which motivate both the struggle and also the other transactions simultaneously taking place. Thus, although the images in the previous excerpt concern love and affection, and the parties' demands for warm response from each other, we do not consider directly the communication of these wishes but only the exchange of images. The content of the images which constitute identity, when they are put into words, are most easily thought of as descriptive terms and phrases, sometimes simply adjectival, like "honest," "pretty," "oafish," "cruel," etc., and sometimes more complex, like, "He is always putting things off," or "She nags her husband." In verbal form they are easily conceived as attributes or predicates, denoting some more or less enduring characteristic of the object.

But images are, of course, not always communicated in clear and simple descriptive language. They may be conveyed by subtle, indirect, or elaborate verbal content, such as orders and instructions, questions, jokes, "double talk," parables and allegories, stories, abstract discussions, and even by the choice of topic; furthermore, images of self or others can be conveyed by tone of voice, dress, personal adornment, posture and stance, gesture, the gamut of kinesic communication, and even by relatively involuntary, but perceptible, physiologic responses, such as sweating, flushing, or pallor, respiratory pattern, etc. And, as Bateson *et al.* (1956) have pointed out, the images conveyed simultaneously or successively in these various modalities need not be consistent.

If the images are viewed more dynamically, however, they seem to imply an element of relevance to some class of plans or intentions and to express some evaluation of the competence of the object to succeed in enterprises of this kind. Thus, the images which a person has of himself generally have to do with some goal and his confidence in his ability to reach this goal. Viewed from this standpoint, then, the images which the person has of another are significant (at least in terms of interpersonal relations) in their promise, or lack of promise, of that other's performing some instrumental act, or class of acts, which are necessary to the success of ego's plan. Thus, for example, a young woman may have, as her libidinal goal, a clinging, childlike dependency relationship with her mother. Her ideal image of herself, and the image which she claims, is of a warm, friendly, lovable, and devoted daughter who is capable of eliciting the desired maternal behavior. The mother, however, has been behaving in a way which the daughter regards as rejecting, and although the mother denies that she is being cold to her daughter, she confesses to her friends that she *does* feel cold. The daughter wants the mother to accept her plea and give her motherly love, but she is unsure whether the rejection which she is now suffering is owing to a discrepancy between her own real and ideal identities (maybe, she thinks, she herself is not really warm, friendly, and lovable enough) or to her mother's coldness.

This leads to a consideration of the basic strategy of the game. Ego has intentions, a plan, and an identity (or rather, identities) related to that plan, which attest to his possession, or nonpossession of the qualities requisite to the completion of the plan. Other parties (either individuals or a group, such as the rest of the family) are important, partly in order to reinforce (by accepting a claimed identity) a real identity which is not too divergent from an ideal identity, and (sometimes) partly in order to play an instrumental role as well. Where the other party has an instrumental role to play, ego must endeavor to ensure that alter's identity is appropriate to that role, if alter's identity is not already appropriate; this he does by attempting to induce him to accept an attributed identity and to abandon his present (claimed) identity. Thus, to pursue the illustration given in the preceding paragraph, the daughter wants to secure two things from the mother: first, reassurance that she regards her daughter as being warm, lovable, and devoted; and, second, acceptance of the daughter's "request" that she once again play the role, and maintain the real identity, of the loving mother. In order to accomplish all this, the daughter schemes first to induce the mother to admit publicly that she now has a "cold" real identity; once such an admission has been secured, the daughter believes, the mother will be shamed or driven by guilt into redevelopment of the "motherly" real identity (because the daughter well knows, from past experience, that the mother's claimed identity is motherly).

The identity struggle, in a social sense, can be classified as a form of negotiation between parties (whether individuals or groups) whose interests and characteristics are mutually perceived as being in certain respects presently antithetical but potentially complementary. It has the form of conflict, but its proper outcome is an agreement or contract on mutual rights and duties (with their necessary identity concomitants) such that the two parties can interact to mutual satisfaction in an equivalence structure (see Wallace, 1961). But an identity struggle is a hazardous negotiating procedure, partly because it invokes powerful and irrational internal motives and partly because of the unreliability of human communication. Other outcomes, less desirable than an equitable agreement leading to an equivalence structure, are possible: excessive stress, resulting in psychosomatic disorders, in one or both participants; cognitive and emotional damage, to one or both participants, in the form of an internalization of negatively valued images of self (see Searles, 1959); mutual social withdrawal; violence leading to physical damage to, or destruction of, the participants and/or of material apparatus. Hence, a number of rules of behavior either emerge into consensus from the experience of the participants or are formally stated as expectations of the culture. The purpose of these rules or ethics is to prevent the conflict from becoming so bitter that the probability of a successful outcome is low. Indeed, overt identity struggles may in some cultural domains be regarded as so pernicious that they are proscribed in all but the most carefully regulated situations, such as the courtroom, the political arena, or the dueling ground. Too frequent participation even in these licit struggles, or participation outside the formally permitted contexts, may be regarded as a sign of personal inadequacy or of membership in a "lower" status group which permits such behavior; analogies to (if not homologies with) the mutual smelling and bristling behavior of dogs, and the mutual identity establishment procedures of other lower animals, may be pointed out with disdain. The nature of such rules varies, of course, from culture to culture and from subject matter to subject matter, but in general they would seem universally to involve a prohibition of open rage, physical violence, or excessive cruelty in nonphysical coercion; some confinement of allusion to matters both conventionally permissible and relevant to the subject of negotiation; the avoidance, if possible, of the involvement of others than the principal parties to the conflict; and the requirement that neither party ruthlessly seek a unilaterally acceptable solution.

It would take us too far afield in this preliminary paper to attempt to explore the range of logical complexities and special tactical maneuvers, involving such special problems as identity concealment, alliances, falsely claimed and attributed identities, ambivalent or even contradictory real identities, promises of mutual identity transformation, and the like, as well as the more straightforward assertions, counterassertions, and defenses (some of which, however, have been illustrated in the case materials earlier). Indeed, we are led to suspect that a full exploration of the internal dynamics and external tactics of identity struggles would contribute significantly to a truly social psychiatry, and to psychodynamic theory as well. But we move on now to examine some of the nonpathologic ways in which identity struggles have been institutionalized in various cultures.

3) INTRODUCTORY CROSS-CULTURAL OBSERVATIONS

We have suggested that a process as fundamental as the identity struggle, growing as it does out of generic human (if not phyletic) characteristics, should not only be discoverable in any human society, but should also be institutionalized in various forms within different cultural traditions. There should be reflections of the process in the myths and legends of nonliterate peoples and in the formal literature of civilizations; it should raise issues to be dealt with by codes of etiquette and ethics and law; it should generate sanctions intended to restrain and limit the ramifications of conflict in order to reduce damage both to the immediate participants and to the society more generally.

Let us consider first the simpler societies, the so-called "primitive" or "nonliterate" tribal peoples who have been of special interest to anthropologists. In these simpler cultures, as in the advanced, minimum socially relevant aspects of an individual's identity, and the rights and duties pertaining thereto, are generally defined by the individual's status as a member of several publicly recognized groups: a kinship unit (such as a moiety, clan, or extended family), a community or band, an age grade, a sex, an occupational specialty, a secret religious society, etc. (see Goodenough, 1961). But the prevailing concepts of identity in a society are more complex than a bundle of half a dozen statuses and may more easily be regarded in anthropological jargon as aspects of the national character, modal personality structure, or ethos of that group. Primitive communities differ markedly in ethos, as well as in particular customs, of course, and such variation implies variation in the forms and spirit of courtesy. In at least some primitive communities, however, and probably in most, the ethos opposes the sort of direct confrontation of opposing identities which we have been denoting as an identity struggle. Thus, among the Indians of northeastern North America, identity struggles between individuals of any community, except in clearly sanctioned situations, often ceremonial, are avoided. If a person openly impugns the identity of a member of another community, either by physical injury or insult, the offended party has available the resources of his community in a physical (and/or magical) assault on the other group to gain an appropriate revenge, and may proceed directly to retaliate in kind or, in many instances, to terminate the issue by killing the offender. Such retaliation would not be desirable within the small community, however; and perhaps in consequence tribal peoples of this area show noteworthy courtesy and discretion in their face-to-face interactions (even though there may be much malicious gossip, suspicion, and fear of witchcraft). In other culture areas, a preoccupation with reciprocal taboo and avoidance systems among members of different status positions in the same community—for instance, the taboos on male contacts with menstruating women—may work to the same end. In social structures of this kind, however, latent identity struggles may require ceremonial expression as a cathartic device to prevent the accumulation of hostility; this function is often performed through organized games, reinforcing ritual role reversal, and other devices. If a non-ritualized intergroup struggle emerges within the society, the consequence is likely to be social disorganization or radical change.

Sometimes, however, and particularly among members of the same status group in a society, formalized identity struggles with a highly ritualized etiquette are permitted to occur over certain issues. For instance, formal struggles are apt to happen within elite groups where recognition of high rank by an individual must be earned by a demonstration of pre-eminence in some relevant characteristic. One familiar example of this was the potlatch of the Kwakiutl and other Indians of the northwest coast of North America. In the potlatch, leading men vied among themselves for dignity at public feasts at which vast quantities of goods were consumed or given away; the victor in a series of feasts was the man who could give away or destroy the most blankets, oil, slaves, and other items of worth in the society.

Another context in which identity struggles may be precipitated by intention is that of illness. Here, where the object is to remove the suspected supernatural cause of the affliction, the sufferer may be ritually harassed by accusations of taboo violation and be encouraged to confess, lest he, and perhaps others, suffer death or chronic illness in punishment. Somewhat similarly, adolescent males and sometimes females are often subjected to severe humiliation, deprivation, and even physical mutilation, in order to induce an abandonment of a childish identity in favor of an adult one.

Sometimes ritual is designed explicitly and consciously to resolve identity struggles. For example, among the Tangu, a Melanesian tribal group resident in New Guinea, the ideal in social relations is a state of neutral amity and moral (or, in our terms, identity) equivalence. But the circumstances of life, and the vagaries of impulse and opportunity, frequently bring about breaches in amity or equivalence, arousing anger and raising the ugly specter of sorcery or murder if someone suffers intolerable moral damage. For instance, as Burridge relates:

An exchange which is not regarded as precisely equivalent, or which remains not honoured in full too long, is taken to indicate a lack of moral equivalence. A sense of grievance cannot imply either amity or equivalence. One or another party to the exchange is thought to be attempting a dominance or moral superiority. He who produces more is suspected of endeavouring to assume a loftier moral status in virtue of what may be a simple physical competence: which is deplorable. Brute strength may help towards attaining a higher social standing, but it can only reflect degrees of moral perfection when used in particular ways for certain ends. He who produces less may be suspected of contumely, of behavior which is essentially contemptuous and therefore not in conformity with amity. And either may be suspected by the other, or by members of the community, to be resorting to a technique which is meant to shroud the other in obloquy. The ideal is equivalence, neither more nor less, neither 'one-up' nor 'one-down.' To be 'one-up' is to offend and therefore to invite mystical retaliation. To be 'one-down' and remain content is almost unforgivable: it implies a complete retreat into sorcery, a resolve to maintain equivalence by doing evil only [Burridge, 1960, p. 82].

The proper way of handling such potentially explosive conflicts is to bring them to public forum where the contestants may engage in a delicate exchange of insults, so balanced that both can quit at some precise moment when neither is winning. The name for this ritual is *br'ngun'guni*. It begins with a redefining, if that is possible, of the issue into terms of food:

All transgressions in Tangu may be seen as attacks on equivalence: and where possible the wrongdoing is related to an individual's potential for producing foodstuffs in an exchange. In this way public equivalence may be reached through *br'ngun'guni* and a series of feasting exchanges. Theft and trespass, the most frequent offences, are automatically regarded as attacks on food producing potential; those emotionally at odds can always take the opportunity to find fault with a food exchange; if adultery is not to slide into sorcery, or plain killing, it must be reduced to a matter of food production. Food is the conventional pretext for a quarrel; and *br'ngun'guni* is the accepted procedure for returning to amity. Just as a denial of equivalence can be formulated in terms of behavior relating to food, so is it re-established through activities directly connected with the production of foodstuffs: *br'ngun'-guni* and a series of feasting and dancing exchanges. Moral relationships, therefore, are reflected in the way people behave over food; food is economic wealth; the amount produced and the way in which it is distributed yield political power; and each is geared to equivalence, the primary expression of amity . . . .

The *br'ngun'guni* is a talk between two antagonists in the dancing space of the village with other villagers as audience. Ideally, the debate is noisy but carefully kept within the bounds of possible return to amity.
. . . The seemingly careless remark strikes home: and a riposte is immediate. Does the cap fit? One man probes to find a weakness; then thrusts, retreating for the parry. The language flickers to sting and annoy; it should not draw blood. There should be just enough room for one to advance, just enough room to fall back. To press an opponent into a corner leaves him with little alternative but to take refuge, later, in sorcery. If a man appears to be going 'one-up' by so hurting another he is only hurting himself. Sensibly, support falls away. By retiring a little, by parrying the consequent onslaught with a whoop and thump on the buttocks, the ball comes back into play. The victory is never to the dominant; it goes to the man who knows when to sit down, to the man who can look through his audience and know that nobody is certain who is 'one-up' [Burridge, 1960, p. 83].

In this type of combat, the winner of an identity struggle is, in a sense, the loser, since he has made it impossible for his opponent to return to amity or equivalence without resorting to sorcery.

In addition to establishing rules of superficial decorum which obviate manifest identity struggles, and in addition to providing a means for combatants in an identity struggle, once it has become manifest, to carry out the battle in a forum which permits a bounded resolution of the issue, societies generally recognize certain ethical principles which, however phrased and rationalized, have the function of inhibiting the proliferation of identity struggles. Nowhere is it desirable for a group to permit its own members to suffer identity damage; and those who, whether maliciously or self-righteously, wreak unnecessary and unprovoked damage upon the identity of their fellows are violating moral principle. The precise issues upon which identity depends are, of course, highly variable cross-culturally. But those who persistently treat sport or other forms of competition (in which the loser need not lose face or honor[4]) as identity conflicts; those who patronize; those who violate the identity of others by demanding that they assume roles incompatible with self-respect; such people are, we suspect, in all cultures regarded as dangerous, as committing the sin of pride, of risking the anger, not only of men, but of the gods (as the widely distributed trickster myths point out vividly and as is so well exemplified by the Greek notion of *hubris*). Sometimes this principle is applied even to the relations of men to animals; among the Algonkian and Iroquoian hunters of eastern North America, for instance, the good hunter was always careful to indicate, by ritual, his respect for the animals whom it was his duty to kill. And corresponding to the ethical commitment to respect one's fellows, there is the ethical commitment to an appropriate honesty (but not necessarily to modesty) in claiming only that identity which in its objective particulars is "true." Thus, if the society values bravery in war, the warrior must not boast unless his claim to valor has been confirmed by the test of battle; if it values chastity in women, the bride must not claim a virtue which is not hers. The possible intricacies of the interaction of respect and contempt, honesty and deceit, pride and shame are inherently interesting to human beings, it would seem; even the simplest peoples are entertained by tales, such as trickster stories (*vide* Radin, 1956), which explore the many moral and emotional combinations of these stances, which are possible in any human culture.

4) IDENTITY STRUGGLES IN AMERICAN SOCIETY

The implications of the foregoing discussion are not only that identity struggles are well-nigh ubiquitous phenomena but also that they are regarded with some disfavor in most, if not all, societies, on the ground that they are potentially damaging to the relations of cooperation and mutual interdependency upon which any society is based. We have also seen, however, that identity struggles are often permitted in certain bounded situations in which the participants are restrained by formal or informal rules of decorum. It

---

[4] The "good sportsmanship" ethic in American athletic contests would seem to be a device, *par excellence*, for minimizing the possible identity damage inflicted upon "losers."

has been further suggested that in a few of these contexts, such as illness and status change, identity struggles are exploited in a rather formal way in order to force individuals to abandon socially inappropriate identities for appropriate ones and to negotiate amicable equivalence structures with their fellows.

In our society, there seem to be relatively few situations in which serious identity struggles are sanctioned by all segments of the community. In most circumstances they are regarded as unfortunate accidents, breaches of etiquette, or even violations of equity or law for which blame can be assessed and penalties assigned by the courts. Thus, for instance, a long-continued identity struggle between husband and wife can not only lead to unhappiness in marriage; it can also, for non-Catholics in many states, lead to divorce actions based on grounds of mental cruelty and humiliation. Three of the principal relationships in which serious identity struggles are explicitly licensed in our culture are: first, the relationship of ad-man and potential customer either in direct face-to-face interaction or through advertising media; second, the relation between contending parties, or their counsel, in adversary proceedings in a court; and third (and in a special sense), the relation between psychotherapist and patient. It may be noted that the second and third situations may overlap or be connected in sequence. We shall, in the next section, discuss the psychiatric (and thus some aspects of the legal) identity struggle in connection with the psychotherapy of schizophrenia.

It has been suggested by the editors, Dr. Boszormenyi-Nagy and Dr. Framo, that a fourth locus of sanctioned identity struggles is the nuclear family. We do not hesitate to agree that identity struggles do in fact occur at one time or another among the members of many, if not most, American families. We do hesitate, however, to accept the suggestion that serious identity struggles (as we have described them in this paper) are *culturally* defined as a *desirable* aspect of family living even though they may be accepted by many as inevitable. It seems more plausible to construe the prevailing cultural attitude as one of wary tolerance: spouses are advised to expect identity issues to develop as the marriage partners work out their relationship, and parents are warned that issues of identity occur among children and between children and their parents; but everyone is on notice that these matters should be resolved by friendly accommodation, and that if an outright struggle develops, it is to be regarded as "dirty linen," not to be aired in public, and to be resolved as quickly as possible, albeit as honestly as possible, within the family, lest it erupt in the courts or the doctor's office. The issue has a bearing on the strategy of family therapy in schizophrenia for, as we shall point out later, if the psychiatrist believes that such struggles are not only frequent but culturally sanctioned, then he may regard it as his responsibility to encourage latent struggles to find free and regular expression in his patient family as an aspect of normal family living; whereas, if he feels that open struggles are not culturally normal, then he may consider the struggles he observes in the patient family as symptoms, if not a cause, of illness, to be lanced when found but not nourished or cultivated.

Let us consider for a moment American popular fiction. In the works to which we refer, the identity struggle is conceived as a chronic, grinding war between two unhappy people who are bound together, like stags with locked horns, in a deadly embrace which even the death of one partner cannot end. This formulation is integral to some of the work of such popular writers as F. Scott Fitzgerald—*vide,* for instance, his novel, *Tender is the Night* (1934), in which a recently psychotic heiress and a conscientious psychiatrist marry and drive each other to near-destruction with catatonic outbursts and adultery on the wife's part and professional abdication and alcoholism on the husband's. The only solution offered is the husband's leaving his wife in command of the field of battle (the Riviera) and retiring, alone, to the general practice of medicine in a small town. John O'Hara's *Appointment in Samarra* (1954) explores a similar type of cyclical identity struggle. An even more direct delineation of the theme is given in a recent popular movie, starring Alec Guiness, entitled *Tunes of Glory*. The story concerns a drunken, vulgar but heroic acting regimental commander, who rose from the ranks during the African desert campaigns of World War II, and an old-school-tie career officer, son of a former commanding officer, who is ordered to replace the acting commander in peacetime. The two men battle desperately to preserve their somewhat different conceptions of self-respect; in the end the tricked and shamed new man commits suicide, and the older man, humiliated by the circumstances of his own victory, disintegrates in a welter of hallucinations. These themes are presaged, in a limited way, by Hemingway's elegant exercises on the subject of manhood. In Hemingway's stories the opponent (whether man, woman, bull, lion, fish, or mountain) does not do much more than present a moral dilemma to the hero, who must work out for himself what it is to be a man under various trying circumstances (which, however contrived they may be for literary effect, are in a general sense types of situational traps into which any man may fall). The Hemingway story thus presents in sharp outline the identity struggle from one person's point of view. Hemingway, however, generally attempts to provide an ideal solution: a model of optimum fortitude, of doing the best one can under impossible circumstances, of failing nobly without destroying the identity of the opponent (for, in identity struggles, as the Tangu emphasized, sometimes the only way to win is not to win, especially if the opponent has the dignity of Hemingway's animals).

It must be pointed out, however, that in the United States not everyone reads Hemingway and F. Scott Fitzgerald and that some Americans did not see and enjoy *Tunes of Glory*. In other words, the ethos which we are attempting to delineate cannot be prescribed as valid for all citizens of the country, partly because of individual variability and partly because of differences among groups defined by ethnic, religious, occupational, regional, and other characteristics. Indeed, differences in attitude toward identity struggles probably constitute a profoundly important source of friction between groups who in many other respects share a common culture. Thus, one may suspect that some of the antagonism felt by Anglo-Saxon Protestants against Jews may grow out of differences in customary attitude toward identity struggles. The ideal-type Protestant, we suggest, has a lower threshold of tolerance for identity struggles, and perceives as unacceptable "pushing" and as ill-mannered squabbling patterns of interaction involving manifest commentary, however trivial the issue, on the partner's identity, which are tolerable and even desirable to the Jew. The Protestant in response tends to freeze and withdraw. The ideal-type Jew, in complementary fashion, regards mutual identity commentary as an acceptable and even necessary component of social interaction and regards the Protestant's manner as aloof, two-faced, and unfriendly. He responds at first by intensifying the commentary and then by a complementary withdrawal. Inasmuch as issues of identity, for the reasons which we have given earlier, involve self-esteem, such a cultural discordance, even with respect to "superficial" decorum in identity commentary, can be profoundly alienating.

In American society, identity struggles, or situations possessing the formal properties of the identity struggle, are frequently "denatured" by redefining them as "play" or "entertainment" and thereby rendering them less dangerous. Thus, hazing or initiation rituals, which in many simpler societies are taken as deadly serious mechanisms for status transformation, are publicly defined by Americans as tradition, as "innocent fun." Parlor games, friendly chit-chat, comedian's jokes, and public entertainments supervised by wisecracking masters of ceremony derive their spice in large part from the use of playful mutual insult; what is said in jest would be intolerable if said seriously: as the saying goes, "Smile when you say that."

Among American adolescents, especially lower-class Negro youth, a common game or verbal play involves mutual insults with semi-standardized responses which serve to neutralize the insult, transform the insult into a compliment, or turn the insult back upon the sender. The game goes under various names in different parts of the country. The oldest and most widely used name for the contest is "Dozens," although it is also sometimes referred to as "Sounding (down)," "Cuts" (or "Cutting each other up"), "Playing," "Slipping," "Screaming," or "Mocking."[5] The game has been described in the scholarly literature by Dollard (1939) and Abrahams (1962). The latter authority provides a concise description of the structure of the game:

. . . One insults a member of another's family; others in the group make disapproving sounds to spur on the coming exchange. The one who has been insulted feels at this point that he must reply with a slur on the protagonist's family which is clever enough to defend his honor (and therefore that of his family). This, of course, leads the other (once again, due more to pressure from the crowd than actual insult) to make further jabs. This can proceed until everyone is bored with the whole affair, until one hits the other (fairly rare), or until some other subject comes up that interrupts the proceedings (the usual state of affairs) (1962, pp. 209–210).

Abrahams also notes that the game contains an implicit set of rules or ethics: "The rules seem to say, 'You can insult my family, but don't exceed the rules because we are dealing with something perilously close to real life'" (1962, p. 211). In lower-class Negro culture the game is most appropriate to adolescent boys. Among pre-pubertal boys the game tends to be less intricate owing to incompletely developed verbal facility and an unfamiliarity with the semantic complexities of erotic slang, while later ages, between 16 and 26, the game becomes less acceptable and in those settings where it does occur, as in military service, poolrooms, or bars, it quite frequently results in physical violence (Abrahams, 1962, p. 210–211). This violence usually arises when one of the parties "goes too far" or oversteps the bounds of good form. If the game of "Dozens" is kept within reasonable bounds with no intent to do serious damage to the identity of the opponent, no violence is likely to occur, and the game may be enjoyed as a humorous interlude or innocent "letting off of steam" by both spectators and participants alike. From the example of "Dozens" and similar forms of verbal play, we can see that among adults, as well as children, one of

[5] We are indebted to Miss Pamela Dixon and Mr. Mark Davis for sharing with us some of their first-hand knowledge of the game.

the standard techniques of diverting an incipient identity struggle from erupting into an open feud is for one of the participants, or a third party, to twist the issues into a joke; thus what might have been an explosive conflict is by common consent transformed, by the fiction of humor, into "kidding around."

Many observers have remarked that contemporary society appears to contain an increasing number of persons who suffer from "character disorders," and particularly, in language closer to our own, "problems of identity." It can be argued that the incidence of persons suffering from identity problems is increasing in Western society as the technology makes human beings increasingly dispensable, and that our social problems are decreasingly the result of economic want and increasingly the result of efforts to resolve identity problems by means which lead to identity struggles between individuals and groups.

One of the semi-institutionalized mechanisms for resolving identity conflict (and in many ways the least threatening) is the assumption of a socially devalued identity. It is as if the person, after trying and failing to convince himself (with the help of others) that his "ideal" identity is his "real" identity, says, "To hell with it," and claims (and acts out) a "bad" identity with, literally, a vengeance. This process is, we believe, involved in those forms of deviation, delinquency, or criminality (as they are culturally defined, of course) which seem to be better explained as a revolt against society than as a means of securing needed goods and services, personal respect, or affection absolutely unavailable through other means. It is a kind of impulsive ritual of rebellion, highly social in character, in which a group of people agree to renounce "good" identities (as being "square" or "nowhere") and to accept fully the "bad" ones (as being "hip" or "cool"). It does not seem accidental that this value inversion is most common among precisely those groups (minority or majority) who happen, at any one time, to be classified as "inferior," or "immature," by those who operate the technology, control mass communication, or are otherwise influential in molding popular sentiment. The consequence of this process is, of course, an identity struggle between the rebellious person and his family, teachers, employers, or others whom he regards as his enemies.

Another kind of semi-institutionalized mechanism for resolving identity conflict is, in many ways, much more dangerous because it leads to massive intergroup identity struggles. This mechanism is the projection by an individual of his own feared identity onto another whole group. Inasmuch as many individuals in each group (e.g., whites and Negroes) may be employing this mechanism to resolve internal conflicts, the system of complementary negative projections can lead to extensive intergroup fear and hostility. This process is, we feel, in large part responsible for those extremes of racial prejudice, religious antagonism, and national chauvinism which seem to be particularly prevalent in technologic societies. It appears to us that these three phenomena, particularly racial prejudice, have not (despite the cross-cultural ubiquity of ethnocentrism) been in any degree as savagely and indiscriminately destructive in nonindustrial societies as they have been in the technologic societies of the past four hundred years. The anti-Semitism of Nazi Germany, the ethnic conflicts of Algeria, the racism of the white South Africans and, to a somewhat lesser degree, of many white Americans, and of organized minorities of American Negroes (*vide* the Black Muslims), and similar phenomena elsewhere, are not really matched to our knowledge either among nonliterate peoples or in the ancient classical civilizations. To be sure, slavery was a common feature in many of these earlier and non-Western societies, but it was generally maintained with impartiality toward the racial and ethnic characteristics of its victims. Wars were conducted with more obvious economic or cultural issues at stake than has been the case in modern times. Preoccupation with the idea of subordinating, segregating, or exterminating a racial or ethnic group *on the grounds of its alleged inherent and inborn inferiority in moral or intellectual spheres*, rather than simply on account of its perversity in refusing to behave properly or to follow orders, appears to be a unique product of technologic societies, and this idea arises, we suggest, precisely out of identity conflicts which this type of society induces to such a high degree in its members. If our suppositions concerning the nature of the identity conflict in technologic societies are correct, then it is no accident that the group against which prejudice is directed is always accused of having precisely the properties which the accuser fears may characterize himself: namely, worthlessness, infantilism, laziness, cupidity, dishonesty, incompetence for civilized living, and other "bad" qualities associated with the accuser's own sense of being expendable within the technologic society. The ruthless, bitter, vengeful nature of this kind of hostility, its frequent independence of actual experience with members of the hated group, and its immunity both to personal knowledge and to rational scientific thinking, are corroborative evidence of its origin in intrapersonal identity conflict rather than in any history of actual intergroup relations.

It is, of course, one of the tragedies of this type of situation that once many of the members of one group have begun to project their own feared identities onto another group, members of the second group, whether or not they had previously suffered from severe identity conflict, are likely to begin to experience complementary identity conflicts, and an identity struggle between the two groups will ensue. In the long run, at least in technologic societies, there are only three stable solutions for intergroup identity struggles: mutual withdrawal; the annihilation of one group by the other; or the abandonment of the struggle by both and the sanctioning of contractual relations, devoid of invidious distinctions, between individuals and institutions of both groups. Only the latter solution is conducive to the continued success of the technologic society, because intranationally it eliminates an important source of waste effort and psychological damage to the citizenry. Although it is hazardous to generalize a phenomenon discovered in dyadic relations between individuals to such complex entities as social classes, ethnic groups, nations, and coalitions of nations, it seems that some of the dynamics of the identity struggle may be applicable to events taking place on an international scale, as in the continued discussions between East and West over such matters as disarmament, colonialism, and the relative merits of "capitalist imperialism" and "communist totalitarianism."

The Identity Struggle in Family Therapy in Schizophrenia

In our discussion so far, we have illustrated and described the identity struggle as a phenomenon, and have shown how not only our own culture but also others attempt to prevent or to canalize by ritual such struggles in the interest of social stability. But we have avoided as much as possible introducing the familiar psychiatric concepts appropriate to the analysis of the individual motivations.

Our model of psychodynamics has principally utilized those conscious cognitive states, and their associated affects and verbalizations, which are directed toward identity maintenance. We have furthermore employed our own definitions of identity processes and have not explicitly discussed their relationship to the rich existing literature on identity or to the writings on family therapy. We took this position not because we felt that psychiatric concepts were of no explanatory value but because we believed that the first task was to describe the social phenomenon, and that psychiatric explanation and application had to be directed toward an accurately described type of event.

But now we turn to the psychodynamic and psychotherapeutic implications of the identity struggle, and the first order of business is to recognize that what we have described, under the rubric "identity struggle," is a manifest, overt, conscious process which presumably succeeds another phenomenon. This other phenomenon is less grossly manifest, and often less conscious, but it involves similar attitudes; we may refer to it as the latent identity struggle, in contrast to the manifest identity struggle which we have been describing. In the latent identity struggle, the participants do not overtly claim and challenge in an explicit, verbal way; rather, they cherish private claims for their own identities and nourish private contempts for their partners', and take considerable pains not to reveal their attitudes in a form sufficiently explicit to arouse manifest responses from one another. It is from a situation of latent struggle that manifest struggles undoubtedly arise.

Now what we have been calling the latent identity struggle is, in effect, a type of interpersonal and intrapersonal conflict that is presumed in psychiatric theory to be pathogenic if not pathologic, if it is permitted to continue indefinitely without resolution. It constitutes the setting of the double-bind; it is exemplified in the silent conflicts of transference and countertransference which the analyst endeavors, with his patient, to "work through." And the latent identity struggle is a form of family combat which, if it has not already developed into a manifest identity struggle, becomes manifest in the course of family therapy in schizophrenia, most conspicuously in the effort by members of a family to blame the family's problems on the sick member. The aim, in regard to treatment, is therefore the management of the latent identity struggle in such a manner that it is resolved; and the tactical question is the proper handling of the manifest identity struggle which seems inevitably to develop as soon as the latent struggle is probed.

Here we must reintroduce one of our cultural observations. It is difficult for the participants in an identity struggle to resolve their own conflict; hence many cultures surround such struggles with rituals designed to obviate or canalize them. Merely offering to a family a license for open conflict, in place of a silent struggle, will probably contribute nothing to the resolution of the latent struggle and may permit not only a rapid deterioration of morale but also irreparable damage to the structure of the group; it may well contribute to the progressive psychopathology of one or more members of the family. Yet, it is also probably impossible to deal with the real issues of the latent identity struggle without, in the process, transforming it into a manifest identity struggle. The tactical problem in family psychotherapy is thus to make the latent identity struggle manifest, and then, once it is manifest, to resolve it before the struggle itself destroys the family and damages one or more of its members.

Can we, in contemporary Western civilization, find models for this therapeutic process? I think we can in at least two settings:

the conference method, and the method of psychoanalysis. In psychoanalysis, the patient is permitted, indeed he is encouraged, to enter into intimate communication with a doctor. He reveals to him, as well as he can, important thoughts and feelings, and depends heavily upon the doctor to relieve him of a burden of emotional, and sometimes physical, illness. As the relationship develops, the patient begins to look more and more to the doctor for the satisfaction of powerful, and hitherto repressed, needs, and because the doctor refuses to satisfy some of these needs, he also develops resentments. So a latent identity struggle develops between the two: the patient claims an identity (as child) which the doctor resolutely denies, and he attributes to the doctor an identity (as father) which the doctor refuses; the doctor, likewise, claims an identity (as doctor) which the patient denies, and attributes an identity (as mature and independent person) which the patient refuses. The explanatory concept for the origin of this process is the well-known process of transference; it is the analysis of the transference, by making its elements and history conscious, which constitutes both the manifestation of the identity struggle and the means of its resolution in psychoanalysis. In our language, then, psychoanalysis is a technique for the resolution of the identity struggle between two people. But, it must be emphasized, the success of this technique depends upon surrounding it with restrictions which, however reasonable they may be, are comparable to the rituals which surround any culturally canalized identity struggle. The patient must remain upon the couch; the interview must be terminated at the end of the hour; the analysis must be performed in a specified place, in privacy; the analytic interaction between doctor and patient must be confined to the analytic situation, and therefore acting out the struggle in other contexts (such as job or social gathering) is prohibited; the patient should commit himself to the task of getting well.

Assuming that similar transference psychodynamics are responsible for the positions of the participants in a familial identity struggle, it is reasonable to suppose that analytic treatment (or analytically oriented psychotherapy) of all the family members would lead to a resolution of the identity struggle. In this sense, we can say that the hitherto unexplained intransigence of the struggle, its chronicity and immunity to rational intervention, is the result of the mutual transference (and fixation) problems of the family members and their lack of an analyst to resolve them.

But psychoanalysis is too expensive a procedure to permit its application to all of the members of a family simultaneously at the hands of the same, or different, therapists. Can family therapy, as a form of conjoint therapy, do the same work, and if so, under what conditions? Here we may look to the conference method for the resolution of manifest identity struggles. In various situations, such as labor-management conflict, racial strife, the cold war, etc., the participants, after a period of fruitless and frustrating confrontation of more or less rational demands according to the dictates of self-interest, fall into a phase of manifest identity struggle.[6] In this phase, names are called, characters are impugned, and progress toward settlement is nil. Only after representatives of the participants have come together (often under the chairmanship of a neutral moderator) with assigned and accepted responsibility to bargain continuously about the several needs of the contending parties, can a settlement be reached. Such a settlement has to take into account, not only the obvious economic and political needs of the parties, but also at least some of their emotional needs for such intangible, but important, values as "dignity," "self-respect," "honor," "good faith," and so on.

These considerations lead directly to the following propositions:

1) That in family therapy in schizophrenia (and in any other conjoint therapy process) it is necessary that the latent identity struggle be made manifest.

2) That the manifest identity struggle must be resolved as quickly as possible in order to minimize emotional damage to the participants and structural damage to the group.

3) That a principal role of the family (or group) therapist must be to interpret the identity struggle to the group: i.e., to point out the nature and structure of the conflicting claimed, real, feared, and ideal identities of the several participants. He should also set the rules which bound the conflict and define the permissible channels of expression.

4) That the group itself must consciously and openly accept the responsibility for achieving a settlement of the struggle which is agreeable to all parties. The therapist cannot prescribe a solution for a family any more than he can for an individual.

Theoretically, at least, in this culture such a procedure should permit the struggle to be resolved either by mutual agreement on identities or, if this is impossible, by an agreement to dissolve the group. This latter possibility should not be denied the group any more than the privilege of the patient in therapy to leave his family, or his job, or his therapist can be denied, provided the motives for the action have been brought to consciousness and analyzed and the "reality factors" have been faced.

---

[6] R. R. Blake and J. S. Mouton (Group Dynamics: Key to decision making. Houston: Gulf, 1961) have referred to this process in union-management disputes as the onset of Win-Lose dynamics and consider the process "pathologic" in intergroup relations.

If we were to evaluate the performance of the therapeutic group in the family therapy program which we have observed, it would seem to us that the therapeutic team was probably highly successful in making manifest struggles out of latent ones; at least we were struck, and sometimes shocked, by the directness with which the therapists, in the sessions we observed, brought such material into the verbal arena. Less activity, however, we felt, was shown in interpreting the manifest identity struggle to the family itself; and the level of family commitment to achieving a settlement appeared to be very low. One reason for this was a tendency, remarked on by the staff itself, to shift back and forth, on the part of both the therapists and the family (and of these observers too, for that matter), between primary concern for the patient's psychiatric status and primary concern for the emotional structure of the family. Another reason, of course, is that the identity struggle formulation was not developed until after the observations had been made, and, even if it had been, could not be communicated to the therapists without risk of changing the nature of the phenomenon being observed. A third reason, perhaps, may be a reluctance to concede that the motive of identity maintenance and enhancement can be regarded by itself as a "deep motivation," quite comparable, in its psychodynamic importance, to sexual and aggressive motives.

The patient's own identity problems have a dimension not shared by the other members of the family (although each of the individual members can and does have more or less severe identity problems). Not only does he bring with him the difficulties he experienced before he became a psychiatric patient, he has the additional burdens of being ill and of being publicly classified as incompetent. Considering that a schizophrenic illness means, for the victim, a painful decrement in self-esteem, we may assume that the schizophrenic's real identity is very sharply discrepant and highly negative in value in relation to his ideal identity. Inasmuch as we assume that the organism strives to achieve (although, no doubt, it never succeeds) a total identity in which the value of the real identity is no less than some optimal finite quantity in relation to the value of the ideal identity, we can expect the schizophrenic to work to reduce the dissonance. The kind of work he undertakes can be guided, fundamentally, by either of two strategies: first, to reduce the value of the ideal identity and increase the value of the feared identity; second, to increase the value of the real identity. The aim may, but need not, imply a congruence of content in the two identities. The two strategies may be labeled the withdrawal strategy and the paranoid strategy, respectively. In the withdrawal strategy, the victim says, in effect, "I give up, not only am I worthless, incompetent and crazy, but there is no point in aspiring to be anything better, all I want is to be left alone." His claimed identity is therefore his feared identity. In the paranoid strategy, the victim says, in effect, "It is not I, but someone else, who is worthless and incompetent, and perhaps even evil; I am good and pure and well able to take care of myself." His claimed identity is therefore his ideal identity; he attributes his real identity to others by the paranoid defensive process of projection. These strategies may, of course, be mingled by a single person, who will be withdrawn at one time with regard to a particular component of identity, and paranoid at another time with regard to another identity component. Inasmuch as the issue is of extreme importance to the schizophrenic, who will suffer from intolerable tension unless the dissonance is reduced, his efforts will be both desperate and stubborn and also more or less bizarre and crude because of the cognitive damage associated with the illness. Furthermore, there will, because of the intensity of the internal conflict, and because of the schizophrenic constriction of semantic range, be a tendency for the schizophrenic to feel that his total identity is at stake in issues which, to an observer, would seem to involve only one or a few components and relatively trivial plans.

It is too much to hope that the resolution of the identity struggle will, in the case of the psychiatric patient, bring about by itself a remission or cure of the psychosis. In addition to the possibility that the psychosis is dependent on a physiologic or biochemical disorder, the analysis of the struggle will not necessarily resolve all psychodynamic issues in either patient or family. But the resolution of the struggle should terminate the imputation of identities which the patient fears and, to the extent that this has been pathogenic, contribute to the patient's welfare. Furthermore, the resolution of the identity struggle should, theoretically, be accompanied by a minimizing of the "psychotic neurosis" (the neurosis *about* the psychosis; see Wallace, 1960). These two changes in the patient's situation should facilitate the establishment of a milieu in which the program of individual therapy can proceed more efficiently, unimpeded by the patient's need to defend himself against multiple and chronic assaults upon an already damaged confidence in self, and not delayed by unnecessarily prolonged repetitions of a stalemated identity struggle.

References

ABRAHAMS, R. (1962). Playing the dozens. *J. Amer. Folklore* 75, 209–220.
ALLPORT, G. (1943). Ego in contemporary psychology. *Psychol. Rev. 50*, 451–478.

BATESON, G., JACKSON, D. D., HALEY, J., AND WEAKLAND, J. (1956). Toward a theory of schizophrenia. *Behav. Sci. 1*, 251–264.

BUHLER, C. (1962). Genetic aspects of the self. In E. Harms (Ed.) *Fundamentals of psychology: psychology of the self. Ann. N.Y. Acad. Sci. 96*, 730–764.

BURRIDGE, K. O. L. (1960). *Mambu, A Melanesian millenium*. New York: Humanities Press.

COOLEY, C. H. (1902). *Human nature and the social order*. New York: Scribner's.

DES LAURIERS, A. (1960). The psychological experience of reality in schizophrenia: therapeutic implications. In L. Appelby, J. M. Scher, and J. Cumming (Eds.) *Chronic schizophrenia*. Glencoe, Ill.: Free Press.

DOLLARD, J. (1939). The dozens: the dialect of insult. *Amer. Imago 1*, 3–24.

ERIKSON, E. (1950). *Childhood and society*. New York: Norton.

ERIKSON, E. (1959). Identity and the life cycle. *Psychol. Issues 1* (whole no.).

FESTINGER, L. (1957). *A theory of cognitive dissonance*. Evanston, Ill.: Row, Peterson.

FISHER, S., AND CLEVELAND, S. E. (1958). *Body image and personality*. Princeton, N.J.: Van Nostrand.

FITZGERALD, F. S. (1934). *Tender is the night*. New York: Scribner.

FREUD, A. (1946, originally published 1936). *The ego and the mechanisms of defense*. New York: Int. Univer. Press.

FREUD, S. (1959, originally published 1914). On narcissism: an introduction. In E. Jones (Ed.) *Sigmund Freud, Collected Papers*, vol. 4. New York: Basic Books, pp. 30–59.

GOFFMAN, E. (1959). *Presentation of self in everyday life*. Garden City, N.Y.: Doubleday Anchor.

GOFFMAN, E. (1961a). *Asylums: Essays on the social situation of mental patients and other inmates*. Garden City, N.Y.: Doubleday Anchor.

GOFFMAN, E. (1961b). *Encounters: Two studies in the sociology of interaction*. Indianapolis: Bobbs-Merrill.

GOODENOUGH, W. H. (1961). *Formal properties of status relationships*. Paper read at Amer. Anthropological Ass. Ann. Meeting, Phila., November.

GOODENOUGH, W. H. (1963). *Cooperation in change*. New York: Russell Sage Found.

HALLOWELL, A. I. (1955). *Culture and experience*. Phila.: Univer. of Penn. Press.

HARMS, E. (Ed.) (1962). *Fundamentals of psychology: psychology of the self. Ann. N.Y. Acad. Sci. 96*, 681–894.

HILGARD, E. R. (1949). Human motives and the concept of the self. *Amer. Psychologist 4*, 374–382.

JAMES, W. (1890). *Principles of psychology*, 2 vols. New York: Holt.

LECKY, P. (1945). *Self-consistency*. New York: Island Press.

LEE, D. (1950). Notes on the conception of the self among the Wintu Indians. *J. abnorm. soc. Psychol. 45*, 538–543.

LEWIN, K. (1936). *Principles of topographical psychology.* New York: McGraw-Hill.

LOWE, C. M. (1961). The self-concept: fact or artifact? *Psychol. Bull. 58*, 325–336.

LYND, H. M. (1958). *On shame and the search for identity.* New York: Harcourt, Brace.

MASLOW, A. H. (1954). *Motivation and personality.* New York: Harper.

MEAD, G. H. (1934). *Mind, self and society.* Chicago: Univer. Chicago Press.

MURPHY, G. (1947). *Personality. A biosocial approach to origins and structure.* New York: Harper.

NEWCOMB, T. M. (1954). *Social psychology.* New York: Dryden Press.

O'HARA, J. (1954). *Appointment in Samarra.* New York: New American Library.

PIAGET, J. (1926). *Language and thought of the child.* London: Kegan Paul.

RADIN, P. (1927). *Primitive man as philosopher.* New York: D. Appleton.

RADIN, P. (1956). *The trickster, a study in American Indian mythology.* New York: Philosophical Library.

ROGERS, C. R. (19.42). *Counseling and psychotherapy; Newer concepts in practice.* Boston: Houghton Mifflin.

ROGERS, C. R. (1951). *Client-centered therapy; its current practice, implications, and theory.* Boston: Houghton Mifflin.

ROGERS, C. R. (1959). A theory of therapy, personality, and interpersonal relationships, as developed in the client-centered framework. In S. Koch (Ed.) *Psychology: a study of a science*, vol. 3. New York: McGraw-Hill, pp. 184–256.

ROGERS, C. R., AND DYMOND, R. F. (Eds.) (1954). *Psychotherapy and personality change; co-ordinated studies in the client-centered approach.* Chicago: Univer. Chicago Press.

SARBIN, T. R. (1954). Role theory. In G. Lindzey (Ed.) *Handbook of social psychology*, vol. 1. Cambridge, Mass.: Addison-Wesley, pp. 223–258.

SCHILDER, P. (1950, originally published in 1934). *The image and appearance of the human body.* New York: Int. Univer. Press.

SEARLES, H. F. (1959). The effort to drive the other person crazy—an element in the aetiology and psychotherapy of schizophrenia. *Brit. J. med. Psychol. 32*, 1–18.

SHERIF, M., AND CANTRIL, H. (1947). *Psychology of ego-involvements.* New York: Wiley.

SMITH, M. W. (1952). Different cultural concepts of past, present, and future. A study of ego extension. *Psychiatry 15*, 395–400.

SNYGG, D., AND COMBS, A. W. (1949). *Individual behavior.* New York: Harper.

SYMONDS, P. M. (1951). *The ego and the self.* New York: Appleton-Century-Crofts.

WALLACE, A. F. C. (1960). The biocultural theory of schizophrenia. *Int. Rec. Med. 173*, 700–714.

WALLACE, A. F. C. (1961). *Culture and personality* (Anthro. Series #1). New York: Random House.

WENKART, A. (1962). The self in existentialism. In E. Harms (Ed.) *Fundamentals of psychology: psychology of the self. Ann. N.Y. Acad. Sci. 96*, 814–822.

WHEELIS, A. (1958). *The quest for identity.* New York: Norton.

WORLD FEDERATION FOR MENTAL HEALTH. (1957). *Identity.* Introductory study no. 1.

WYLIE, R. C. (1961). *The self concept. A critical survey of pertinent research literature.* Lincoln, Nebraska: Univer. Nebraska Press.

11

JAMES L. FRAMO

Systematic Research on Family Dynamics

From time to time in the course of our family therapy project at the Eastern Pennsylvania Psychiatric Institute, outside professional workers observe the treatment sessions through one-way mirrors. These observers are from various professions, such as psychiatry, psychoanalysis, anthropology, research psychology, etc., and family treatment is usually quite new to them. Almost invariably their reaction is the same: they all use the word "fascinating" as they describe how caught up in the process they became. It is not clear to us why people get so involved; I have speculated that the strong emotional interchanges among the family members somehow transport observers back into the emotional atmospheres of their own childhood families. The two-party individual psychotherapy situation, from the standpoint of either a participant or an observer, is not nearly so evocative of memories of one's own family feelings.

Gratitude is expressed to friends and colleagues who have read this chapter, offered suggestions for revision, and given support: Drs. Ivan Boszormenyi-Nagy, Robert S. Davidon, James R. Frakes, David Rubinstein, Albert S. Scheflen, and Oscar R. Weiner, and Mrs. Geraldine Lincoln. The responsibility for the ideas in this paper rests, of course, with me.

407

Everyone talks at once after sessions: "How can you stand that mother? What did she *really* mean when she said her own childhood was idyllic? Why does that father take it from her? Did you notice how the father had to keep his eyes averted when his daughter kept crossing her legs? Did you see the patient making that sucking motion with her lips whenever her father got her mother's attention? Doesn't it seem to you that they all want to possess each other but yet they have to push each other away because it's so devouring? If you didn't know better, you'd think all that arguing meant that they hated each other. Mother there thinks of herself as the perfect breast. That quiet father is potentially a murderer. Did you see the patient coming to the protection of her mother by talking crazy every time you explored her relationship with her other daughter? It's hard to believe what I see: that patient, who is practically mute on the ward, spent all her time screaming at her parents. The boy is really father's wife; he is the only person in the family who means anything to him. This family keeps shooting up SOS flares. They're eating each other up. Why did the patient begin to laugh at certain crucial points in the session? I feel that this family is just absorbing the therapists. The way that patient criticizes her parents it's as if she is saying, 'You won't let me live, so I will stop you from living.' Why don't you forget about these parents and concentrate on the patient? The parents are bankrupt. Notice how the patient and her parents maneuver each other into shifting active and passive roles, as if they're very unclear who is woman and who is man, who is parent and who is child? Isn't it appalling the way that father keeps asking the patient what *she* can give to the family? Did you hear that normal sibling make that marvelous statement that her mother does 'rotten little things'?"

During a lull, I occasionally ask the question, "Tell me—I know it's difficult—but do you have any idea how one would go about doing systematic research on these family dynamics?" An awkward silence follows. I am met with bewildered looks, and the conversation soon moves on to more comfortable grounds.

Science, of course, requires us to systematize our knowledge and follow a set of ground rules as we search for the truth, namely, laws that can be generalized beyond the individual instance. But what are the scientific facts, objective and subjective, about the human experience of family living? What are the main dimensions of family life?

The literature on the family is vast and has had an extended and respectable history long before the relatively recent psychodynamic, clinical emphasis upon the family exemplified by the writings in this volume and the new journal, *Family Process.* A number of disciplines (e.g., sociology, social psychology, anthropology, clinical psychology, social work, home economics, marriage counseling, etc.) have brought to bear on family study the particular orientation of their profession, dealing with problem areas ranging through many levels of substantive and methodological purpose: family theory and conceptual frames, socialization and personality-forming aspects of the family, the family as a social institution and its relationship to other institutions, mate selection and courtship, marital roles and marriage adjustment, parent-child relationships, the family in different cultures, the study of subcultures, child and family development, family disorganization (mental illness, crime, divorce), etc. The methods used in studying the foregoing have varied considerably in level, scope, sophistication, and rigor, some utilizing large-scale census data, others longitudinal methods; some stating formal hypotheses and making use of control groups and significance tests, still others being simple surveys or clinically impressionistic. The data yielded by family researches of all types are so voluminous as to defy classification; the reader is referred to the following family research reviews and bibliographies: Burgess, 1947; Cottrell, 1948; Dager, 1959; Ehrmann, 1957; Hill, 1951; Hill, et al., 1957; Hill, 1958; Nimkoff, 1948; Nye, 1963; Walters, 1962. Hill and Hanson (1960) have performed a valuable function by attempting the onerous task of making an inventory and codifying the mass of family research into a systematic arrangement of various conceptual frameworks that have been utilized in family study. Five conceptual frameworks have been posited by these authors as follows: Interactional, Structure-Function, Situational, Institutional, and Developmental. The reading of Hill and Hanson's article is recommended to all those planning to do family research.

The present chapter does not fit in with, nor is it to be considered a part of, the tradition of the kind of family research just cited. The focus of this chapter is on systematic research approaches to the inner dynamics of family life, with particular emphasis on transactional phenomena directly observed and measured when the family members interact together as a unit. An attempt will be made to resist isolating systematic research from the deeply human problems of family life. The interest is not in schizophrenia, nor even in families of schizophrenics as such, but in family dynamics in general. It needs to be emphasized at the outset that, despite the prodigious literature on the family, there is no body of formalized literature on *systematic research on family dynamics* with clearcut stands taken on issues and specified limits from which departures can be made. While the material for this chapter was being gathered, certain issues and problems emerged as being central, and these are discussed in some detail: e.g., the advantages and disadvantages of direct and indirect report of the family members about themselves; how to gain access to the emotional heart of the family process; the private vs. public aspects of the family; the problem of the family's resistance against exposing its inner workings to outsiders; the problems of direct observation and sampling and measuring of family interaction; the influence of an observer on spontaneity; some problems involved in experiments with families; the issue of manifest vs. latent content in communication; the problem of meta-messages; and, perhaps most important of all, some of the difficulties involved in penetrating and revealing the unconscious and transactional aspects of the system of the family. Some of these problem areas have been considered by the small-group discipline, and consequently a selected portion of the small-group field is surveyed, although it needs to be stressed that the small-group discipline is not considered to be the experimental foundation of family dynamic research.

Practically everything the behavioral sciences know about families is derived from questionnaires and interviews obtained from family members seen alone, not in the presence of other members of the family. The shortcomings of individually oriented family research should be apparent; most studies yield data based on conscious report and judgment and are subject to the memory distortions and conscious and unconscious biases and falsifications which always creep into this type of indirect research. A host of vitally important data about families escaped detection until the family members were observed interacting together: e.g., the family's emotional organization, its communication patterns, its overt and covert role assignments, its forms of influence, etc., most of which the family is unaware of. Family researchers are coming to realize, or should realize, that it is much more valid to observe directly what people's behaviors (and inferred attitudes) are and what they actually do or don't do rather than what they say they do or feel. Bowman (1956) made an eloquent plea for the abandonment of the questionnaire approach by sociologists in the study of family dynamics and marital adjustment. Congruent with the thesis of this chapter, he pointed out the superficiality of getting simple responses to questions which cannot circumvent the unconscious defensiveness of respondents, however honest they try to be. Bowman suggested, further, as does this chapter, that only long-term intimate knowledge of the family, based on first-hand clinical observation, combined with theory building and systematic research, would lead to really meaningful findings about family dynamics. One example from our own work may suffice: After one of the mothers from our treatment unit had been in family treatment for some time, she blurted forth about her own mother: "Do you want to know how I *really* felt about that woman? She was a disgusting, cold, selfish witch who never really gave me anything." This same mother, prior to family exploration, had checked the following adjectives on the Leary Interpersonal Checklist (1957) as being true of her mother: warm, helpful, friendly, affectionate, understanding, etc.

Family investigators are so aware of the distortion that can result from seeing each family member privately (like the story of the three blind men describing an elephant after each touching a different part of its body) that one of them, by design, deliberately capitalized on this phenomenon by interviewing family members separately, telling each they could be assured of confidentiality, and then bringing them together for discussion after telling them that there were gross discrepancies in the different stories of the family (Watzlawick, 1963a). For many years we have had to rely on information at secondhand, *about* relationships in the family. This chapter, therefore, will contain no discussion of family research based on approaches to a single family member or self-administered inventories.

This chapter is divided into four sections: (1) the contribution of the small-group discipline to family dynamics; (2) a critical evaluation of the few scattered studies in which the family or parts of the family, in interaction, were used as the experimental unit; (3) methodological problems connected with measuring family interaction; and (4) the development of a point of view about research on family dynamics.

The Contribution from Small-Group Research

The most formal attempt to establish an objective science of the properties of groups of people in face-to-face relationships has been undertaken in the area known as small-group research. Sociologists, social psychologists, clinical and consulting psychologists, social anthropologists, and members of other disciplines, basic and applied, have contributed to what has come to be a rather voluminous literature. Hare (1962) cites over thirteen hundred relatively recent references pertinent to the study of small groups. Among the reference sources consulted in the present analysis are the following: Hare, Borgatta, and Bales *Small Groups: Studies in Social Interaction* (1955), Cartwright and Zander's *Group Dynamics* (1962), Strodtbeck and Hare's "Bibliography of Small Group Research: from 1900 through 1953" (1954), Hare's *Handbook of Small Group Re-*

search (1962), and Roseborough's "Experimental Studies of Small Groups" (1953).

No attempt is made in this present section to profer any comprehensive survey or interpretation of the small-group literature; many issues in the small-group field itself are not dealt with at all. The purpose is to highlight selected issues and findings from the small-group discipline that appear to have relevance to family dynamics, particularly to the kind of intimate knowledge about families revealed in the course of family therapy work. In this connection, the first curious fact discovered in surveying the small-group literature is that although all workers in this field would agree that the family, the most elemental of the primary groups, falls within the purview of small-group research, almost no studies have utilized the family group as the unit of study, either in the laboratory or in the field. If, as Hare, *et al.* (1955) have said, the study of small groups is a microscopic study of small cultures which has implications for the study of social systems, of culture at large, and of personality, the virtual omission of the family as an object of systematic small-group investigation is singular indeed.[1]

Some of the research on groups has been oriented toward basic research questions such as the developing of conceptual theories of groups and the intrinsic dimensions of group dynamics (Borgatta, Cottrell, and Meyer, 1956; Hemphill and Westie, 1950). Other research has been motivated by the seeking of answers to social problems such as increased efficiency or morale, the modification of attitudes, diminishing of intragroup conflict, enhancing of the learning process, propagating leadership, etc., in such settings as business, industry, the military, government, the classroom, and the clinic. The emergence of more refined observational techniques and measuring instruments has led to more precise examination of such empirical problems as cooperation vs. conflict, decision-making, group pressures on the individual, sociometric choice patterns, communication networks, clique memberships, status and power in the group, group cohesiveness, the individual in the group, interaction patterns, personality factors affecting group behavior, etc.

Practically all systematic investigations have been based on *ad hoc* groups, those without a history as a group and no expectation of future relationships. The most likely reason for this state of affairs is that temporary groups were more readily available (especially

---

[1] On some occasions small-group workers have attempted to evaluate the significance of particular small-group findings for the family, at times searching for structural similarities between *ad hoc* groups and the nuclear family (e.g., Bales and Slater, 1955, ch. 5), but the family itself as an object of small-group experiment has been virtually ignored.

the overused university student), although it is suspected that even behavioral scientists have felt a certain amount of compunction about examining the private and personal aspects of family life. Without intending to detract in any way from the great value and contribution of *ad hoc* group research, and keeping in mind that everyone must bring at least part of his unique personality *sui generis* to any situation, nonetheless we must point out that a group of strangers is not a mother, father, mate, brother, and sister. Different rules, feelings, and behavior patterns obtain when one is with members of one's own family. Although, on one hand, people are more "open" when with family members (you can do things in your home which you cannot do in public with outsiders), there is, on another level, more need for concealment, which is often the reason one can talk more easily about personal things with relative strangers who are uninvolved (e.g., adolescents getting sex information). It is true that some small-group research has been based on groups with a short history of association (e.g., bomber crews, college fraternities, industrial groups, therapy groups, etc.), and here one would expect less polite, "experimental" behavior, greater familiarity, and intensification of family feeling, but the behavior in these groups, too, is largely "as if" insofar as relationship bonds are concerned. There are crucial differences between *ad hoc* groups and the family; it is much easier to dissociate oneself from secondary groups. One's parents and siblings will always be one's parents and siblings —nothing can change that. It is part of the thesis of this paper that, although feelings of guilt, disloyalty, anger, jealousy, love, and so forth, probably develop in all groups, they do have a special, real rather than symbolic quality in the family group. Subjects in a group study who know they are not going to see each other again after the experiment will have a drastically different set during the experiment than those who know they are going to have to live with the group afterwards. The possible consequences or after-effects of an experiment with temporary groups are radically dissimilar (e.g., after an experimental session the family on the way home in an automobile may recapitulate the session or bring to bear recriminations against those members who were disloyal to the system). The social psychology of experimental behavior is pertinent in this connection (Orne, 1962).

What follows is an attempt to deal with some leading issues of, and results from, small-group research that are pertinent to research with the family. Probably the most imperishable topic in the small-group literature is that of leadership. Cartwright and Zander (1962, p. 496) say that: "It is unfortunate that most of the carefully controlled studies of leader behavior have been conducted with temporarily organized groups where, almost of necessity, members are not concerned with the preservation of the group." In defining leadership functions, they state that: "Nearly every conception of leadership contains the notion that a true leader exerts more influence on the group and its activities than does the average member" (p. 493). Viewed from the standpoint of influence, which is a neutral concept, the effect of the leader can be either positive or negative with respect to group goals, although almost all studies of leadership, obviously, deal with positive influence. Applied to the family, the concept of leadership and power becomes not only much more complicated but also ambiguous and confusing. If members of intact American families were to be asked who is the boss at home, undoubtedly almost all would respond, "father," reflecting the desired cultural stereotype. But those who have observed families intensively have independently commented on the shifting role of leadership in families; because of their deep emotional investment in each other, every family member exerts a silent, potent influence on the others. The idea that there has to be *a* leader is a cultural-bound myth; in a system what element is the leader? As is well known, in many families the father assumes a subordinate role to the mother, and, what is less widely realized, the leadership, parental role is sometimes taken over by the children (Schmideberg, 1948). Parsons (1955, ch. 2) suggested that the structure of the nuclear family can be differentiated on two axes, that of power, on the one hand, and instrumental vs. expressive functions (goal-directed, working behavior vs. integrative, social-emotional), on the other. When mother takes over the instrumental role in the family and father the expressive, definite implications occur for the sexual identity of the children, but when the children assume the superior instrumental-expressive functions the consequences are even more foreboding. Parentification of the child is one of the most damaging forms of rejection, not only because it is a deterrent to development, but because it may lead to later regression: after growing up, the child often feels compelled to go back and get what he missed in the early years.

Even observing the family in a controlled experimental situation, using standard criteria of leadership (e.g., "directs the conversation," "evaluates progress," "arbitrates disagreements," etc.), can contribute misleading findings if one attends primarily to the overt interaction, content of the words, or extent of participation and apparent decision-winning. The whole question of disguised or concealed influences is an intriguing problem which has largely escaped systematic investigation thus far. What is meant here, for example, is the passive member who controls by quiet means (e.g., by warning glances or even no observable signals at all). The active participant is readily identifiable and can be opposed or undermined; how does one resist the effects of passive mastery when the group members are hardly aware of it? Rosenthal and Cofer (1948) made some attempt to highlight the effect on the group of an indifferent and neglectful attitude shown by one of the group members, although they did not deal directly with passive mastery effects. Another problem, even more subtle, is that passive mastery can be practiced by the apparent group leader. In many families, for example, the apparently strong member is actually drawing strength and dependency gratification from the other family members, all the while convincing himself and others that he only provides for the needs of the others (e.g., when everyone caters to the autocratic father, he is really getting sustenance from the rest of the family). The extremely complex, hidden, nonverbal cues, the signalling systems, the subtle ways members of a group influence each other assuredly escape detection by any large-mesh observational technique yet devised. The work of Birdwhistell and Scheflen, who make very detailed, microscopic analyses of interactional behavior by drastically slowing down film recordings, is very promising in this regard (Birdwhistell, 1961, in press; Scheflen, 1963; Scheflen, et al., in press).

A concept closely connected to that of leadership in the small-group literature is that of power or status. One of the classical experiments in this area was done by Mills (1953), who confirmed Simmel's observation that a three-person group tends to break up into a coalition and a third party in structuring the power relations. He found that the third party can become a scapegoat, a common enemy, or one who may strengthen the twosome as much as he menaces it. Mills suggested that this study be repeated using the family as the experimental unit, a proposal followed through by Strodtbeck (1954) in one of the very rare small-group studies in which a family group was used. Strodtbeck used what has come to be known as the "Revealed Differences Technique" (1951), which required the family to arrive at common agreement on problem situations about which they independently disagreed. Varied combinations of coalitions in a three-person family were experimentally manipulated. Strodtbeck, in the main, did not confirm Mills' findings and suggested that the division of a trio into two and one is attenuated in families as compared with *ad hoc* groups. One can contrast this finding from the small-group frame of reference with that of family therapy experience, where alliances and splits are seen as the very essence of maintaining family equilibrium (Haley, 1962; Wynne, 1961).

Coalitions in families are of a much more complex order than such a simplistic formula as "Mother favors Johnny and Father favors Suzie." The alliances are intricate phenomena; each family member at one time or other allies himself with each other family member, depending on the stakes involved and the strategic intrafamilial advantage being sought. When coalitional maneuvering occurs within a context of close relationships, it is carried out surreptitiously, usually behind camouflaging, more superficial alliances (e.g., father and mother may appear to be in open disagreement; yet they may be allied against the child by wanting the same thing—to possess the child—and they may be pursuing this goal via different routes). Strodtbeck's finding that alliances occur with less frequency and force in families as compared with temporary groups is based upon a single observational session of a family who knew they were being observed. One can almost guarantee that in this public (i.e., experimental) situation the deeper, more meaningful alliances within the family would be the least observable. The son in the Strodtbeck situation just cited, for example, not wanting his mother to know he was in secret sympathy with the father, might have lent support to mother by overtly siding with her on issues. Reluctance to exhibit family dissension before an outsider, on the other hand, may make the son temporize any display of disloyalty to a parent. Each of the three family members has his own gambits, ploys, and strategies. The Bales system of interaction analysis (Bales, 1950), which Strodtbeck used to measure the support which determined a coalition, relies heavily on the kind of face value, manifest statement which seems not especially adapted to the deeper levels of motivation. Mills pursued the study of coalitions in three-person groups in a subsequent paper (1954) and suggested that even in temporary groups the subjective, emotional allegiances are of central importance. One of his conclusions was: "In a role structure of some stability, the structure of personal, emotional attachments (positive or negative) is stronger than the structure of common values and beliefs that are relevant to the purpose of the group, and these structures are stronger than the pattern of manifest interaction between members" (p. 667). Joel and Shapiro (1949) used a notational system of evaluating feelings in group interaction and ignored content, and Thelan and Withall (1949) attempted to describe the same event by experimentally varying three different social-emotional climates, thus suggesting several promising approaches toward eventual measurement of emotional organization in all types of groups, including the family.

The conditions under which groups have appeal, maintain loyalty, work toward common goals, and are united against external attack or criticism have been explored under the rubric "group cohesiveness." Various aspects of the concept of group cohesiveness have been studied in groups whose members were superficially related (see, for example, Back, 1951; Festinger, Schachter and Back, 1950; Gross and Martin, 1952). Jansen (1952) has explored the problem of family solidarity within a sociologic frame of reference, using a questionnaire method to elucidate the extent to which there is in the family concern with each other's welfare, enjoyment of association with each other, cooperation, trust in each other, etc. Cartwright and Zander (1962) postulate that the valence of a group or its attractiveness depends on the extent to which it is need-satisfying, although some evidence indicates that when social interaction in *ad hoc* groups is characterized by high self-oriented need, there is more conflict in the group, less unification, and the group is considered less need-satisfactory to its members (Fouriezos, Hutt, and Guetzkow, 1950). This latter study is pertinent to family interaction because it is one of the few which have attempted to evaluate deeper motivational factors in social interaction by focusing on the affect behind the communication rather than its content. Within the family there are extremely high degrees of "self-oriented" needs which, because of the members' long association with each other, are communicated in highly condensed and cryptic fashion. It is quite understandable that these self-oriented needs (as measured by Fouriezes *et al.*, 1950: dependency, dominance, aggression, and catharsis) operate as a disruptive force in groups in business and industry, whereas in the family deep needs constitute the essence of interactional involvement, even though they may seem to lead to rupture. Gross (1956) found that groups characterized by symbiosis (defined in sociologic, not psychiatric, terms as people cohering as a group when each has something needed to offer the other) as contrasted with consensus (relationships in which persons are held together by agreement to a set of values) have greater cohesive strength because they are based on needs rather than the unstable ties of positive feelings on which consensual groups are based. Gross says: "As long as those needs persist, and so long as each has no easy alternative of satisfying those needs, then the two will be linked. This does not mean they will necessarily like each other; it does mean that they will remain united *whether they like each other or not*. And therein lies the strength of the symbiotic tie." Although Gross does not mention either the family or the psychiatric implications of symbiosis, he has indirectly provided some evidence for the basis of the adhering power of family groups.

A particularly ingenious small-group study done by Festinger,

Pepitone, and Newcomb (1952) provides experimental support for the idea that when de-individuation occurs in a group (where members do not notice other individuals *as* individuals), inner restraints are reduced, members feel more free to indulge in behavior from which they are usually restrained, and the members find this a satisfactory state of affairs which increases the attractiveness of the group. Though the de-individuation quality in a family group is of a different order than that which occurs with artificially formed groups, we are here provided with some clue as to what makes the family valence so compelling, namely, that this is the one group where inner restraints of certain kinds can be most loosened. Though it is true that certain behaviors are permitted in some families which would not be permitted in other group-living situations (e.g., walking around in one's underclothing or talking back to parents), some behavior can be expressed more freely outside the home (e.g., smoking, drinking, telling shady stories).

French (1941) has provided some evidence to indicate that organized groups with a longer history of a relationship develop more We-feeling and are less likely to split up than unorganized groups. Applying this principle to family living, few would question that the family provides a cohesive force of great power. In secondary groups (job, clubs, organizations), when there is too much competition, too much disagreement, too many unpleasant experiences, one can withdraw from the group without disastrous consequences. These same disappointing experiences take place in all families to some degree, but the effect can work in reverse, that is, the more frustrating the experiences in the family during the process of growing up, the less free is the person, psychologically, to leave the family. Non-violent separation from the family seems to be able to occur only when the life experiences have been relatively favorable, when conflicts have been settled to some extent.

Family loyalties, based on blood ties and early personality-formative influences, supersede all other allegiances, even when the family members do not like or have much to do with each other. As Robert Frost put it, "Home is the place where, when you have to go there, they have to take you in!" Killian (1952) described how when people were forced to choose between various allegiance groups during a disaster, the family commanded by far the greatest loyalty. Only a few unusual group situations can approximate this intensity of group feeling (e.g., a veteran combat infantry squad whose very lives depend on each other). Insofar as defense against external criticism is concerned, it is interesting to observe the special quality of offense which creeps into a person's voice when he feels his family is being criticized ("Now just a minute, Buster, this is my *family* you're talking about!"). Witness, for example, the mass outrage when personal attacks are made on the families of men in public life. You can work beside another person for many years and even though you may share many experiences and feelings with this person, if he has never talked about his personal family difficulties, it is maintained, you do not really know him. When certain kinds of slurs are made in prison (intimations of sexual relations with one's mother), inmates frequently feel it necessary to murder the offender.

Asch (1951) and Sherif and Cantril (1947) have investigated in laboratory experiments the persuasive effects upon individuals of group pressures to conform to standards of the group even when these standards are perceived by the individual to be contrary to fact. The group pressure in these situations was the effect of staged majority opinion in getting a naive subject to question his own sensory impressions and go along with the group. Pressures and forces in the family are much more subtle yet much more powerful than those which occur in outside groups. In the family, what choice does the child have but to conform to the unrealities of the parent? The individual family member has pressure of the most powerful kind exerted upon him to conform to the family rules which maintain the family system. Family persuasive techniques can be obvious ones, ranging all the way from threats of physical punishment to withdrawal of love. The most effective influences, however, rely on inherent family relationship needs and utilize threats of love withdrawal, the forceful, yet subtle effects of guilt provocation, as well as parentification of the child (e.g., parental admonitions such as: "You'll be the death of me yet" and "How can you hurt your mother?" or "You'll be sorry after I'm gone" or "You are the ruination of my life." Take a situation in which a mother with an ulcer ostentatiously "cheats" on her diet, forcing her children to worry about her health more than she'll worry about it herself. Consider, further, the situation when children are pressured to take sides in a parental argument). Haley (1959) gives a fascinating account of an interchange in the family of a schizophrenic in which the parents, cloaking their guilt-inducing with the most innocent of remarks, impel their son not only to yield from his previous position but to deny and distort reality in the most extravagant way.

Small-group studies of formal communication patterns have emphasized the power-and-status dimension as being most crucial in the establishment of communication channels and networks (Bavelas, 1950; Kelley, 1951; Leavitt, 1951; Ruesch, Block and Bennett, 1953). The structure of communication linkages in families is undoubtedly different than in those organizations studied thus far. Every family has its own special rules, channels, and styles of patterns of communication. (See Epstein and Westley, 1959, for a preliminary study of patterns of communication in the family.) The family is a well-oiled machine with many years of practice in communicating; an outsider can get the feeling that the meaningful signals are communicated by a kind of subliminal ESP. The communication system in the family accommodates not only to the inherent status dimension (e.g., sex and age) but also to the field of forces surrounding the various family constellations *within* families (the sibling world, mother-father-child, grandmother-children, mother-father, etc.) (Henry and Warson, 1951). (When parents wish to protect the child from certain family happenings, they will often speak in intellectualized phrases or in a foreign language in order to talk over the heads of the children. Note the adult talk which ceases when a child enters the room and the distortion in the child's mind on the basis of the few words he does pick up.) In our work with families we have learned that each family has its own unwritten laws regarding the exclusiveness of certain information which is reserved for special members of the family; there are large areas of information, secrets really, that do not get passed around (sometimes put into words like, "We better not tell this to Dad, you know; it will only upset him and he has enough to worry about"). Ordinarily, when a family member needs to discuss something emotionally important, he chooses one other particular family member or someone outside the family to discuss it with (e.g., brother with sister, husband with wife, wife with friend, etc.). As far as we know, the family treatment situation is the only one in which all family members are forced to discuss their secrets in the presence of all other members. One of the reasons family-treatment is perceived by the family as such a great demand and as so threatening is that the existing channels of communication become exposed. A recurring clinical finding about family communication, particularly in some disturbed or poorly differentiated families, is that meaningful communication between husband and wife is almost nonexistent; it is all funneled through and monitored by the children, usually through one selected child, who becomes the presenting symptom of the family. (In the early stages of family treatment, for example, whenever the therapist tries to discuss something with the parents about themselves or their marriage, they almost invariably try to divert the discussion back to their sick child.) In these families, not only is information routed in this way, but also the all-important communication of affect. Those who do family treatment of schizophrenia have come to entertain a different view about the origin of schizophrenic omnipotence, seeing it as arising not so much from regression to an earlier infantile state of omnipotence or as reaction to inferiority, but as actually representing a real state of affairs in which the primary patient has the exalted position, power, and privileges accorded a super-parent (e.g., sleeping with one of the parents, "making" decisions, measuring the flow of affect, etc.). Of course, for such omnipotence a price must be paid in a burden of guilt so overwhelming as to help bring about ego disruption. A great deal of work remains to be done in the area of family communication, begun so well by the recently discontinued Project for the Study of Schizophrenic Communication under the direction of Gregory Bateson. For an example of a family experiment based on communication theory, see Haley (1962). Haley has performed a useful service by pointing out for the first time some of the unique problems involved in conducting experiments with families and suggesting criteria for their resolution (e.g., the experiment should deal with responses of the family members to each other rather than their individual responses to stimuli from the experimenter). The by-now classical double-bind formulation, which has had an enormous impact on psychiatry and has become a part of everyday psychiatric language, was derived from the studies of this group (Bateson, *et al.*, 1956; Bateson, *et al.*, 1963; Watzlawick, 1963b).

The present review of those parts of the small-group literature which appear to have pertinence to family dynamics certainly reflects the bias of the author by virtue of his selection of articles. It is necessary to keep in mind that the goal of most small-group research is the development of methods for increasing efficiency of some type in group interaction (how much got learned, whether the problem got solved etc.), whereas the goal in family treatment research is more likely to be along the subjective line of, say, greater individuated, yet collective human and emotional integration. Though the clinical investigator has the advantage of evaluating many levels in depth and over a longer period of time, his work, of course, lacks the control and precision of the experimental approach. It probably comes as no small surprise to learn that the small-group discipline has more intensively investigated the kinds of relevant problems having to do with family research, even though done within a different structure, than has anyone working within the family framework. Although, too often, small-group studies have achieved preciseness at the expense of relevancy, nonetheless the small-group discipline has a most respectable history of scientific methodology, which can be of inestimable value to family researchers. It is curious that more small-group workers have not followed the lead of Strodtbeck (1954) in replicating classical small-group experiments utilizing the family group as the experimental unit; in this area, indeed, lie rich resources for future doctoral dissertations.

Review and Evaluation of Systematic
Family Interaction Studies

In this section an attempt will be made to review and evaluate, with major emphasis on method and lesser emphasis on results, the few existing systematic or potentially systematic studies based on direct observation of family interaction which the writer has been able to find in the literature. These studies, done within the context of different disciplines with varying research goals, will occasionally be examined from the standpoint, too, of the kind of knowledge about family dynamics gained from extended family treatment.

The earliest work in the area of family interaction centered on child-oriented home and laboratory observations. Extensive work was done with the Fels Parent Behavior Rating Scales devised by Champney (1941) and elaborated by Baldwin (1949). The studies by Bishop (1951) and Moustakas, Sigel, and Schalock (1956) are also representative of direct-observation investigations of parent-child interaction. Insofar as the study of family interaction process is concerned, these studies, though they have contributed carefully worked out schedules for categorizing observations of mother-child interactions, fall short of capturing the transactional meaning of the interchanges; further, the observations were not conducted over a long enough period of time, and the resonating effect of the marriage relationship and of other family members upon the mother-child relationship was not taken into account.

Drechsler and Shapiro (1961) described a procedure for direct observation of family interaction in a child-guidance clinic. After a psychiatric interview was conducted with the family in which the presenting problem was identified, the family was presented with a family task to be completed without the presence of the investigators. The family was asked to discuss together a Family Questionnaire of twenty items, containing factual as well as fantasy items (for example: "Draw a diagram of the home with all the rooms. What sort of things does the family argue about? Describe how one special holiday is celebrated by the family. What was the worst nightmare that each of you has ever had? If each of you could change one thing about yourself and the other members of the family, what would you change?"). The purpose of the family task was to provide a medium upon which the family could act out their characteristic relationships and thereby reveal interactive patterns of which they were unaware. Drechsler and Shapiro (1963) have since reported further details of how they sampled and analyzed the data from the family interaction resulting under the aforementioned conditions. A twenty-minute clinical sample was arbitrarily selected to present in capsule form the family's characteristic pathology. In addition, from each family session twenty one-minute segments were extracted at equal intervals and independently scored for the number of times each person spoke to each other person. The authors' intention was to illustrate a method of comparing clinical and statistical analysis of the same data in order to test hypotheses about a given family and to compare different families.

The study of husband-wife interaction was pioneered by Strodtbeck (1951), whose development of the "Revealed Differences Technique," referred to earlier, has provided the impetus for a number of family interaction studies. The rationale of this procedure was based on an attempt to present a married couple with a structured stimulus situation designed to reveal differences between the two partners. His original purpose was to determine the balance of power in dyadic teams in different cultures (Navaho, Texan, and Mormon). The technique as used originally consisted of each couple's being asked to select three families with whom they were familiar; the husband and wife were then separated and asked to specify which of the three families best met a series of 26 conditions: for example, which family had the happiest children, which family was the most ambitious, etc. The couple were than brought together, asked to reconcile their differences, and decide on a final combined choice. The discussion, for the first ten of 34 couples seen, was conducted in the absence of the experimenter and under such conditions that the couple did not know they were being observed or that the discussion was being recorded. Strodtbeck, using Bales' categories, found that the spouse who talked most tended to win out on decisions, and also that the most talkative spouse tended more frequently to ask questions, give opinions and analyses, and make rewarding remarks, whereas the least talkative participant tended to agree passively but became frustrated and aggressive at times. From a clinical point of view the question can be asked: does the most vociferous participant *really* win the decision?

A number of investigations have used the basic idea of the Revealed Differences Technique to study a variety of problems. March (1953), for instance, used it to examine husband and wife interaction over political issues. Kenkel and Hoffman (1956) asked couples to predict how each would behave in a session at which they would decide together how to spend three hundred dollars; they found, parenthetically, that the husbands and wives not only were poor judges of the roles they themselves would play in the interaction but that even after the session was over they could not recognize the parts they had played.

A modification of the Strodtbeck technique was attempted by Vidich (1956), in which husbands and wives, together, were presented with family problem situations requiring discussion and final agreement. Whereas Strodtbeck presented the couples with *ipso facto* disagreements from the start, Vidich's design was calculated to reveal differences in the course of discussion. A further departure from the Strodtbeck method was that the experimenters stayed with the couples during the discourse, a situation that greatly affected the findings inasmuch as most of his couples directed their statements at the experimenters and the tape recorder rather than toward each other. Because this paper raises some interesting problems about interaction research, it will be discussed in detail later.

The precursor to later systematic *family* interaction studies, mentioned previously, was again introduced by Strodtbeck (1954) when he applied the Revealed Differences Technique to a three-person family group consisting of mothers, fathers, and adolescent sons. The experimenters went to the homes of forty-eight families and asked the three family members to check independently one of two alternatives to problem situations inferentially related to parent-son relationships. Three items were selected in which mother and father were paired against son, three in which mother and son were in coalition against father, and three in which father and son were paired against mother. The family was then presented with the nine disagreements, in which the isolate role was rotated, and were instructed to talk them over and select the one alternative in each set that best represented the thinking of the family as a whole. The experimenters left the family alone but recorded the discussions. Interaction process was again analyzed by Bales' categories. Strodtbeck's purpose was to examine power relations in the family as contrasted with those in *ad hoc* groups. In a later paper, in which he attempted to relate his findings to cultural factors and achievement, he noted that the families, even when the disagreements were "squarely joined," needed to give the impression that they "never really disagreed" in the first place (1958, p. 176). This finding is congruent with Wynne's (1958) concept of pseudomutuality based on the clinical experience of treating families. The need to present family solidarity to the outside world is a fact of family life which has to be dealt with in any design for a family interaction experiment which attempts to get at a truer state of affairs.

The theme of power in the family appears to have been a stimulus to other studies of family interaction. One of the earliest systematic interactional studies utilizing families with a schizophrenic member was reported by Garmezy, Farina, and Rodnick (1960). Based on preliminary evidence by Rodnick and Garmezy (1957) that maternal dominance was associated with poor premorbid adjustment of the schizophrenic son, and father dominance with good premorbid adjustment, Farina (1960) subjected this finding to further experimental test. He studied 36 pairs of parents, divided into three groups of 12 parents each: one group of parents had sons whose adjustment prior to the psychosis was characterized by isolation and asexuality; one group's sons had mostly been married and had had numerous friends; and the last group, the controls, had sons who were hospitalized for tuberculosis. All the parents were initially interviewed separately, were given the Parental Attitude Research Inventory (PARI), and were then asked to state how they would handle a series of problem situations between parent and child (e.g., "Your husband [wife] has punished your ten-year-old son for something he did. As he walks by now, you hear him mumble a nasty description about his father [mother]"). Subsequently, each set of parents, together, were requested to agree about what they would do if they had to deal with the problems as a team. The investigators were present during the discussions, and their activity was standardized for each family, being limited to occasional eliciting of scorable responses. Interaction between the parents was evaluated by various indices of dominance and conflict (e.g., who spoke first and last, length of speaking time, "yielding" behavior, interruptions, disagreements and aggressions). Farina confirmed with statistical evidence that the "good" patients had more assertive fathers than did the "poors" and the "poor" group parents' interaction was more conflictful. In line with the thesis being developed in this chapter, Farina further found that when the parents were asked to report directly about dominance patterns in the family (the PARI and direct questioning), none of these reports differentiated between the groups; all groups reported the cultural stereotype of father dominance. The interactional situational test, then, revealed a more valid picture of dominance and conflict. These studies have gone beyond the questionnaire approach, have displayed a high degree of sophistication, and were among the first to develop fairly reliable indices of interaction behavior. Nonetheless, the results can be misleading if they are contrasted with a clinical finding which, although lacking statistical confirmation, does need to be explained. What is being referred to here is the kind of family treatment situation, observed repeatedly, in which a father blusters and talks a great deal trying to establish his position as head of the household, and his wife, at the end of the hour, by an almost imperceptible gesture or phrase, negates the thousands of words of her husband, reduces him to raging or quiet impotence, and quickly re-establishes her power. If such a session were to be analyzed by content or total talking time or number of interruptions, by, indeed, almost any objective measure, the father would clearly be labeled dominant. Admittedly, however, the techniques for objectively revealing the truly critical interactional events, which reside largely in the nonverbal area—tone of speech, sighs, hesitations, slips, as well as in grosser behavior—are hardly even on the horizon.

The superiority of direct observation of interaction over a paper and pencil test was demonstrated anew by Caputo (1963) in his attempt to investigate the dominant-mother, passive-father notion in families with a schizophrenic member. In this study the parents of 20 male schizophrenic patients were compared to 20 pairs of parents of "normal" males on Osgood's Semantic Differential (1957). In addition, each pair of parents were asked to discuss ten items of the Parent Attitude Inventory which they had previously answered in divergent fashion. The discussions of the pairs of parents were assessed by the Bales' method. Relatively benign pictures of parental interrelationships of the parents of the schizophrenics were derived from the Semantic Differential data, whereas analysis of the overt interaction revealed considerable antagonism and bilateral hostility between the parents. Caputo's findings questioned the validity of the maternal-dominance, paternal-passivity, and role-reversal theory in families with a schizophrenic member. He found that the discriminating factor between the schizophrenic and "normal" family groups was not with whom the authority rested, but whether it would be shared without conflict. The parent pairs of the schizophrenic group were largely unable to come to agreement or compromise on Parent Attitude Inventory items even though they were explicitly instructed to do so, whereas the control group pairs ultimately disagreed rarely. It is consistent with family treatment experience that some families are so orally hungry that they are in a perpetual state of anger, thereby being unable to agree about anything. As far as Caputo's main findings are concerned, it is unfortunate that only verbal behavior in the interaction sessions was assayed. Words are only one minor channel through which forces like dominance and passivity have their effect on other people.

Garmezy, et al. report (1960) that what was missing in their previous research was the patient; they hesitated about bringing patients and parents together for experimentation in a nontherapeutic setting. In a recent study Farina and Dunham (1963) replicated Farina's earlier study and included the schizophrenic son as a third member of the interacting group. Weakland (1960) has stressed the importance of examining three-party interaction rather than dyadic relationships in studying the dynamics of family life.

Bachove and Zubaly (1959) evaluated role differentiation in nineteen normal families by comparing overt interaction patterns (analyzed by Bales's system) and perceptual data (Leary's Interpersonal Check List, 1957). Each of the families, composed of mother, father, and male six-grader, was exposed to the same standardized tasks consisting of problem situations and joint TAT stories, all of which the families were requested to come to agreement about. When the authors compared Bales's category findings from their families to those established by Bales from 24 different *peer* groups (Bales, 1958), they found that the peer groups tended to agree and disagree far more than the families. They suggested that the disagreement scores of the families may have been funneled into the tension category; the low agreement scores suggested more of a tendency to hold to one's own opinion in a family. The emergence of a task leader (father in most cases) and of a social-emotional leader (mother) was confirmed, with the children expressing most of the negative behavior, mostly because parents prodded them to perform. Whereas father was generally the dominant figure in the interaction, the investigators noted that mother's dominance was of a subtle, manipulative nature whereby she asserted control by delaying decisions rather than persuading other members into a decision.

Levinger (1959), who supervised the Bachove and Zubale study and used some of the same data and design but added clinic families to the normal ones, found that in the clinic families the mother participated most often and also showed the largest amount of negative emotional behavior. This study added support to the contention that reversal of male-female roles leads to disturbing influences on the children, although Levinger rightly points out that this construction is oversimplified. He found also that marital satisfaction, measured as the sum of the difference between each partner's "real" and "ideal" Leary Interpersonal Check List descriptions of his spouse, was positively correlated with the partner's satisfaction with himself, a finding which endorses Harry Stack Sullivan's dictum that: "It is not that as ye judge so shall ye be judged, but as you judge yourself so shall you judge others . . ." (1947, p. 7). Levinger (1963) has recently reported on different aspects of his research on families, comparing in particular the correspondence between three sources of data: standardized behavioral observation, parental descriptions of family members, and outside judges' descriptions.

Although Mitchell's work (1961) was not based on direct observation of families, interactional concepts were used. Family members, before and after family therapy, were asked to rate themselves and other family members on Leary's Interpersonal Check List. He suggested that there should be a reduction in discrepancies between self and ego-ideal and between self-image and the modal picture of the individual held by other family members. Graphic representations, in the form of profiles, were expected to reflect changes taking place within the family as a function of the treatment. This research, done as part of a project of family treatment in the home (Friedman, 1962), will be reported in detail in a forthcoming book. Mitchell (1963) has recently reported on his application of the Leary system to marital pairs of alcoholic husbands and their wives.

One recent, carefully controlled study comparing decision-making in normal and pathologic families, done in the style of small-group research, was executed by Ferreira (1963a). Ferreira used fifty families, divided into 25 normal and 25 abnormal families (containing a psychiatric patient), each family being defined as a mother, father, and a child, male or female, over the age of ten. There were two phases to the testing situation. In the first phase each family member, separately, was requested to make a decision about three comparable, neutral items (e.g., "If you were to take a trip to Alaska next month, would you rather go by (a) train (b) car (c) boat?") and to order them in terms of individual preference. In the second phase the whole family was brought together and requested to make a decision about those very same items but with the awareness that the new ordering of the items, representing a family decision, would have to take into account the wishes of the other family members and that everyone would be affected by and have to abide by the family choice. The family members were left alone by the experimenter for these procedures; the normal families were tested in their own homes and the abnormal families in the hospital or in the tester's private office. Several kinds of family decisions were distinguished: unanimous decisions (when the family choice corresponded with the individual choices of every one of its members), majority decisions (when the family choice corresponded with the individual choices of two of its members), dictatorial decisions (when the family decision corresponded with the individual choice of only one of its members), and chaotic decisions (when the family decision did not correspond with the preference of any one of its members). Ferreira found that all the families were spontaneously in greater agreement than a chance expectation, but also that there was significantly greater agreement between individual preferences and family preferences in the normal families. One intriguing finding, seen frequently clinically, was that in the abnormal families the child had more (or the parents less) to say on what the family decided *not* to want; in the pathologic families the child decided what the family was against rather than what the family was for. Sex differences were found for the normal group but not for the abnormal group of families: in regard to the number of dictatorial decisions made, it was found that father exceeded the mother if the child was a boy, and the mother exceeded the father if the child was a girl. In another inventive study Ferreira (1963b) investigated patterns of rejection and expectancy of rejection in families, and postulated on the basis of his findings that in healthy families a kind of talionic law obtains in that in a given relationship an individual tends to expect rejection in an amount commensurate with the amount of rejection he tends to display. In the pathologic families, rather than an "eye for an eye" attitude being displayed, the attitudes of "two eyes for an eye" or "no tooth for a tooth" are more prevalent.

A particularly appropriate experiment, comparing the value of the interaction approach to that of the individual approach, was done by Fisher, Boyd, Walker, and Sheer (1959). These investigators compared the parents of 20 normal men, 20 neurotic men, and 20 schizophrenic men, using a battery of measures, not only of individual functioning, but also of spouse-interaction patterns. As anticipated, they found that the parents of the normal men were individually less maladjusted than parents of neurotics and parents of schizophrenics. The only measure that differentiated the parents of the neurotics from the parents of schizophrenics, however, was an interactional one, measures derived from the formulating of a joint TAT story: parents of neurotics proved to be less in definite disagreement, less ambiguous in exchange of opinion, more definite in agreement, and more in total communication than the parents of schizophrenics. Foreshadowing a clinical hypothesis developed by those treating the families of schizophrenics, their findings suggested that schizophrenia is a resultant of the combined individual maladjustment of each parent plus a particularly pathologic mode of interaction between them. The data concerning the parents of neurotics indicated that if a husband-wife pair were able to combine forces in a relatively congruent manner, they could compensate to some degree for their individual pathologies, thus sparing the children to some extent. It is likely, in this writer's judgment, that the *lack of clarity* of communication between parents and between each parent and the child is more pertinent to the development of the process type of schizophrenia in the child than is open disagreement and conflict; indeed, in some of the "sickest" families we have seen there was very little open conflict (until much later in the family treatment).

Important work in the area of family research has been begun by Titchener and Emerson (1958). Using as their general orientation the study of the interactional relationships in the family and their influence upon individual personality dynamics, they attempted to associate individual traits with family types according to the following parameters: (1) role allocation and role behavior, (2) identification processes, (3) closeness and remoteness of association, (4) communication, and (5) solution of family conflict by the establishment of family standards. They suggested these variables as the ones that an individual in the early years of his life has to integrate. Methods of investigation consisted of conducting family-oriented individual interviews with all family members, having the family fill out a Family Relations Inventory (200 statements about family life which were judged as more or less true on a six-point continuum), and tape-recorded family-interaction sessions in which one investigator conducted a nondirective interview of the family and the other observed through a one-way mirror. Verbal (who speaks, content of communication, affect, to whom message is directed) and nonverbal behavior was evaluated with interaction categories based on Bales' categories. Mangus (1958) discussed this paper in the same journal, taking up in great detail its heuristic value and shortcomings.

In a more recent paper, Titchener, D'Zmura, Golden, and Emerson (1963) refined and elaborated some of their former concepts and presented further details of the family-interaction observational technique. Subjected to Strodtbeck's Revealed Differences Technique, each family member independently committed himself to one of two choices on controversial issues of family life (e.g., "Most parents are usually willing to let boys and girls choose their own dates, but some believe they should be obeyed when they feel a date is not good for the boy or girl. Do you think parents should have the final word on dating? Yes or No"). Each family member was then presented with his own responses as well as the responses of all other family members, and, after instructing the family to reconcile their differences by discussion, the investigator retired to the other side of a one-way screen and tape-recorded and observed the discussion. Further, two three-minute samples were filmed of most family discussions. These investigators found that though they learned a great deal about the family by observing a forty-minute session, much more was gleaned by repeatedly listening to the tapes and going over the typewritten transcripts in "semi-microscopic" fashion. Tone of voice, inflection, emphasis, and other qualitative features frequently divulged new meaning upon repeated listening. These minute analyses were necessary, according to the authors, because of the speed with which adjustments in the family system occur, as well as the overlapping, shorthand way family members communicate, a kind of coordinated smoothness acquired by the family over many years. Titchener and his associates have developed some attractive and penetrating conceptualizations about family style and formal properties of the family system.

Another method of evaluation of interaction which has not yet advanced to the stage of the reporting of quantitative results was reported by Goodrich and Boomer (1963). Their method consisted of having married couples match colored paper squares, but with disagreement between them built into the procedure by a "rigged" method. Different coping behaviors among the various couples were presumed to be related to attempts at resolving marital conflicts and problems of intimacy.

Watzlawick (1963a), referred to earlier, has developed an ingenious series of stress situations designed to provide a shortcut in eliciting interaction patterns which are typical for a given family. In a situation dealing with mutual trust each family member is separately asked, "What do you think are the main problems in your family?" after being assured that his answers will not be divulged to the rest of the family. Then, when the entire family are brought together, they are all told that though they are under no obligation to disclose their responses, there were discrepancies in the stories and they should attempt to reach a common conclusion as to their main problems as a family. Other tasks were presented for family discussion, each time the investigator exiting and leaving the family to their own devices: to decide what they could do together as a family; for the parents, alone, to answer the question "How of all the millions of people in this world did the two of you get together?"; to decide the meaning of a proverb; to ask each family member in sequence, "Who is in charge of this family?"; and, finally, to discuss each other's faults. These interesting procedures are being evaluated descriptively and intuitively at the present time, although the author is working on a quantitative scoring system.

Methodological Problems in Family Interaction Research

In this section an attempt will be made to deal with a few selected methodological issues evolving out of the previous review of family interaction studies.

If we assume that one of the primary purposes in bringing a family together and presenting them with some task to perform or some issue to resolve is to see how the family "works," to reveal its interconnected and deeper motivational system, its history and its style as a family, then presumably some method must be used that gets behind the natural family defensiveness, stereotypes, clichés, and the need to present a conventional, proper front of harmony. The need for the family to seem "normal, average, just like every other family" is probably stronger than the need for a single individual to appear that way (except for families and individuals under deep stress).

An assumption exists in the concept of the projective hypothesis and in the idea of presenting a task to a family that the members, when presented with an ambiguous stimulus or a revealed difference to resolve, can do naught else but fall back upon "typical," characteristic patterns of behavior. This assumption has been so unquestioned that it has become an integral part of the lore of clinical practice and research. Yet, is the assumption always valid? Do people have recourse only to characteristic behavior patterns, particularly in a *single experimental session?* Do not certain behaviors require special situational and motivational conditions? Just as a psychodiagnostician can get a guarded, restricted Rorschach of the top layer of defenses of a person, so can a family resist revealing, not only its differences, but its characteristic styles. The studies cited have already indicated that even when disagreements were, by design, cleverly introduced into the experimental task, the distinctive, representative patterns often remained unclear, were denied, or were obscured in some fashion. A number of factors can give a distorted picture. In addition to all of the unconscious resistances, which is a large topic in itself, one individual family member may have a conscious "set" (e.g., a father deliberately keeping quiet so that the observer can find out how his wife handles his son). The experimental situation itself introduces its own artifices: to what extent is the produced behavior a function of a contrived game to be enacted for the benefit of strangers, and to what extent are the real attributes or behaviors exposed? Even when experimental sessions are held in the home, a number of questions arise: To what extent are the investigators being treated like guests? What has been the family's past history in having outsiders in the home? Do people come and go easily, or is the presence of visitors a rare occurrence?

There is some basis for questioning whether the really significant happenings of family life ever occur in public, much less in front of an audience whose approval is desired. Goffman's *Presentation of Self in Everyday Life* (1956) deals extensively with the feature of families having a front to present to the public, all the while concealing their secrets in the inner recesses of the "back room."

Unlike *ad hoc* groups, furthermore, families have to live with each other after the experiment is over, and their responses in the experimental situation are monitored by knowledge of the possible consequences or reprisals once they get home. (How free, for example, would a child feel about revealing the alcoholism or unfaithfulness of one of the parents even though this "secret" determines much of the experimental interaction?) Indeed, if it were possible to obtain, the unguarded, "postmortem" discussion of the family after the experiment is over would probably be more revealing than the experiment itself. There is the likelihood, too, that families who are not in critical situations (the crisis of mental illness in the family, for instance, providing motivation to reveal the inner workings of the family) will deal with the experimental task as an intellectual exercise. They will probably attempt to give the discussion a coherent, reality oriented structure in the fulfillment of the presented task. Of course, in the process of doing so they reveal more than they realize, but less, perhaps, than we would wish them to. People can keep from being themselves for longer periods of time than we realize.

The Revealed Differences Technique has largely been used to study power and dominance, but its potential is still unrealized. Most of the studies reviewed stop at the point of totaling who won decisions, without going into the processes involved in making the decisions. Do we know whether it is better to start with disagreement as an established fact or to allow disagreements to develop? Are disagreements the only way we can inject controversy, and is controversy the only way of revealing more genuine interaction? On the basis of our family treatment experience, it would seem to us that a very special type of controversy has to be introduced into each family, one not usually admitted by the family system. There can be a great deal of nonrevealing pseudo controversy; in some families indulging in certain kinds of controversy is part of their way of life. But even these families have certain topics (e.g., the parent's suppression of autonomy in the child) that will always be excluded from discussion, or, if discussed, will lack the emotional connections. A meaningful experiment would require that each family be presented with the controversies it is inherently struggling with, not with abstract controversies which result in polite play-acting. Preliminary study of the family should reveal its Achilles's heels.

If the foregoing is accurate, it is difficult to see how one can present each family with a standard stimulus and hope that the stimulus is comprehensive enough to appeal to the relevant trends in each family. Closer study of the family task, the issues to be resolved by the family, should be made. No one has yet attempted to draw up a population of task problems and situations from which a sample could be drawn. Most of the issues that have been presented to families are only accidentally likely to be the issues with which the family are really struggling. It is somewhat akin to telling a psychotherapy patient what his problems are.

The presence or absence of the investigator during the experimental sessions is a powerful influence which has not been dealt with systematically. Certainly, the investigator's presence introduces a new factor into the interactional relationships of the family, representing parent figure, society, or projected superego audience; he represents, moreover, values which are alien to those entertained by the family. In this situation the temptation is great to have the children "show off" for the doctor. (Incidentally, it is important, for some experimental purposes, to have even young children included in family interaction studies. Children themselves may benefit when they for the first time see their parents as they interact with another authority figure; for the first time they may become aware of tension between their parents; for the first time they may hear their parents lie or be deceitful or childish. When the children are present they may help open up the family, frequently by making naively penetrating and revealing statements on family affairs.) The experimenter's presence can artificially unite the family against him. Moreover, even when the investigator is absent, he is present, because assuredly all families "know" on some level that they are being observed, else why were they brought there—just to talk among themselves with no purpose?

Vidich (1956), mentioned previously, touches on some of these same points and raises serious methodological questions about interaction research which will have to be reckoned with. He pointed out that his couples, in their attempts to come to common agreement about a problem situation, made constant efforts to draw the interviewers into the discussion by requesting an opinion, approval, or agreement. The presence of the tape recorder, interviewers, and the uniqueness of the situation, according to Vidich, introduced artifacts into the situation such that neither the interaction nor the relationship between husband and wife could be understood in terms of their handling of the issues. He said, "A central feature of the interaction was the attempt made by the couple to preserve the private features of their day-to-day modes of conduct from the public . . . Although the spouses attempted to be moderate and to make concessions which they might not make to each other privately, they were still faced with accommodating the existing outlines of their relationship to the interview situation." (p. 237). He went on to say (p. 238) ". . . the interviewers were 'used' by the informants for private purposes in areas of private meanings. Thus, a third level of meaning is introduced into the responses. In addition to the meaning intended for the tape and the publicly obvious meaning intended for the interviewers was added a loaded meaning intended for the spouse only." Vidich concluded: "It cannot be claimed that the interaction protocol and the meanings represented in it are an accurate representation of the day-to-day interaction of the husband and wife. The protocol merely represents a segment of interaction under circumstances not otherwise duplicated in their lives. The clues to interaction processes and dynamics of social relationships lie beneath the structure of disguises called forth by the situation. Mechanical aids, instructions, interviewers, and the social meanings attached to them define the situation of action for the respondent who, in calculating his situation, responds to its totality. Responses are made at several levels of meaning which range from the publicly admissible to the private. Furthermore, techniques of concealment and standards of admissibility vary from respondent to respondent. An interaction analysis based on standardized categories and made without reference to the totality of this situation would be spurious if any claim were made for generally valid interaction processes, even between husband and wife. To treat the subjects in mechanical terms as only responding to experimental conditions is to distort the data and underestimate the respondent." Vidich has been quoted at length, not only because this writer happens to agree with him, but because it is so refreshing to find an investigator stating publicly the kind of quiet misgivings most research workers have, but keep to themselves, about the flaws in their procedures. Most experimenters, in their eagerness to avoid complexity and present neat findings in stereotyped articles, avoid such candor.

Intuitive observers of the human scene are often aware of the multiple communications between people that occur behind the surface speech. Such a person is the lawyer, Louis Nizer, who wrote in his best-selling book, *My Life In Court* (1961), about his observations of certain kinds of husband-wife interaction: "We think of the skeleton in the closet as some really scandalous secret. But most homes are filled with little skeletons: the ordinary foibles and weaknesses of men and women; the conspiracy of lies to make an impression on others; the hypocritical poses for the outside world, which cannot be hidden between husband and wife, making one of them at least a silent partner in the deception; the dishonesties in word and deed of people who pride themselves on integrity; the crudeness and unsentimentality of the physical relationship, while in public there is the social grace of gallantry and love; the dignity in public contrasted with the contempt in the private relationship . . . One need only sit five minutes at the average dinner table to pierce the disguises, which some married couples believe they are wearing successfully. Across the glowing silver candle lights, shining with formal good will, one hears the hostess laughingly sneer at her husband's representations of himself either as a golfer, or a good mixer of Martinis, or handy man with tools, or any other trifle. Perhaps he begins to tell a story, and she comments charmingly, 'Oh, John, are you going to tell that one again? I've heard it a dozen times.' His conduct may be no less revealing, like a good-humored retort that, 'My wife never thinks I do anything well, do you, dear?' . . . Sometimes the discussions are in general terms, or even addressed to a third person, but no one is fooled. The generalities are about as unspecific as a poisoned arrow shot by a keen marksman. The overwhelming impression is that of mutual contempt. It may take many forms, perhaps a pained silence as if the comment was not worth a reply, or a long angry look that says, 'I'm too much of a lady (or a gentleman) to answer and create a scene,' or an exaggerated attentiveness to and admiration of the stranger in the next seat. The air is charged with corrosive bitterness and lack of respect, but such married couples believe at the end of the evening that they have carried off the masquerade successfully and that no one has learned of the inner strains . . . Similarly insensitive is the talk one hears around many a dinner table, in which husband and wife are so magnificently tolerant of the other's professed hunger for an exciting adultery that one is smothered in super-sophistication. She wishes him good hunting. He hopes she will have a good time on her vacation trip, which she will take without him. Once more the self-revelations are vividly etched, but the participants in the discussions seem as unaware of what they are really saying, as if Freud were a German word meaning joy. Sometimes the drawing-room conversation crackles with outspoken jests by the wife about her husband's relative impotence. Bad taste aside, these are the gnawing revelations of the unsteadiness of so many marriages" (pp. 155–157).

Frank conversation between people usually takes place under certain special, rare conditions (e.g., in the wee, unguarded hours of the morning, sometimes after a few drinks). Artificial behavior usually occurs in the laboratory, despite the best efforts of the researcher to create natural conditions for the revelation of "truths." One wonders how a couple like the one in "Who's Afraid of Virginia Woolf?" (Albee, 1962) would behave if they were placed in an experimental interacting situation; how much of their bittersweet sadomasochism would be exposed? Researchers frequently stop being human observers of the real world and develop a peculiar kind of scotomizing attitude about subjective factors when they take people into the laboratory.

Mr. Nizer has a wide practical background in understanding and dealing with people, but he is not, of course, a behavioral scientist who has to account systematically for his observations. Nonetheless, the average layman "knows" that communciation has double and triple meanings, that, generally speaking, people do not say what they mean or mean what they say. One wonders, too, why the behavioral scientist constantly sacrifices meaning for accuracy, relevancy for precision, and settles for measuring systems that tap only the manifest levels, although, to be sure, the problems of measuring the deeper levels are immense.

Among the methods for quantifying face-to-face, group interactive data, probably the most widely used and comprehensively worked out are the non-content system of Chapple (1949, 1953) and the more exhaustive method of Bales (1950). Many other systems have been proposed for particular purposes, for example, one focusing on leadership (Carter, et al., 1951a), one on the motivational needs of the participants (Fouriezos, et al., 1950), a system for describing group atmosphere (Steinzor, 1949), and a multilevel method of exploring interpersonal dimensions (Freedman, et al., 1951; Leary, 1957). The systems of Chapple and of Bales are selected here for discussion because they represent two contrasting, broadly employed procedures.

Chapple, in his attempt to avoid what he considers to be the clinical error of deducing meaning several steps removed from the raw data, developed a contentless, formal measure by recording the *time* each party acts (both verbally and gesturally). He devised for this purpose the Interaction Chronograph, a device with a moving tape driven at a uniform speed on which lines are drawn by pressing a key to indicate length of activity. The measurements show not only how much each person talked or acted but show interruptions, delays, tempo, spontaneous actions and responses, and such low-inference categories as ability to listen, initiative, dominance, etc. By emphasizing the time dimension, Chapple is dealing with a variable that is certainly objective and possesses the virtue of manageability. Moreover, some very provocative findings have eventuated from his work, such as the finding of characteristic curves for activity and silence for various types of psychiatric diagnoses (Chapple and Lindemann, 1942). Chapple believes that there is a relationship between the number and duration of contacts between people and their emotional relationships. Indeed, there probably is, although the relationships are undoubtedly much more intricate than simply being ordered along the dimension of time. If one takes into account the fantasy system, and it is hard to see how it can be left out if human beings are to be studied, the most intense feelings can exist between people who spend very little time with each other. In other words, intensity of relationship is not in direct ratio to the physical proximity of people. One can seem to be in a close relationship with a marriage mate, but the deeper, more meaningful relationship may be the unresolved one with the parents. Sometimes a silent family member exerts a potent influence on two very active members by playing the role of an audience; as a matter of fact, the activity of the two may not be activated unless the third silent member is present. In addition, A may be intensely interested in B, but because A does not want B to know this, he may direct his activity toward C as a cover or screen. Numerous subtleties of interpersonal ploys and maneuvers cannot even be guessed from examination of a chronograph tape. More to the point, however, the Interaction Chronograph really tells very little about *interaction* processes; it reveals largely a compilation of the activity of separate individuals in a group in rather primitive, stimulus-response fashion. Though there would probably be considerable confusion in an observer, trying to decide about the beginning and end of an act in a family therapy session because of the rapidity of events and the amount of overtalking, nonetheless, it would be interesting to see what patterns would emanate from family sessions analyzed by the Chapple system. It is possible that distinctive, family diagnostic profiles could emerge from such research, e.g., low-action families vs. high-action ones, poorly synchronized vs. highly organized families, etc.

The Bales system, probably the most intensively used general system of categorizing social interaction, requires a higher order of inference since it relies on interpretation of the activity. Based upon the theoretical idea that the basic nature of social interaction is problem-solving, the system, briefly stated, is that groups are instrumentally task-oriented, an orientation which in turn creates strains leading to emotional-integrative problems; the groups then attempt to deal with these expressively positive and negative tensions in order to reintegrate back to the task. The flow back and forth between instrumental and expressive activities constitutes the essence of the Bales system. In the process of devising his system, Bales utilized not only the existing literature but also many different kinds of groups and free observation situations in order to come up with a procedure of general utility. The content of the final twelve categories, their sequential and symmetrical relationships, and their ordering with respect to each other, are empirically and theoretically based. The discussion of the categories' relationship to each other is beyond the scope of this chapter. Just reading a list of Bales' categories (e.g., Shows solidarity, Gives suggestion, Gives orientation, Asks for opinion, Disagrees, Shows antagonism, etc.) hardly does justice to the completeness of the system. The appendix in Bales' book spells out the many different kinds of detailed verbal and nonverbal behaviors under each of the categories. Even a cursory examination of the Bales system reveals the impressive amount of work that went into it. Bales' interaction process analysis comes much closer to the concept of interaction as used in the present chapter than does any other system. For a number of reasons, however, the Bales system is not well adapted to the evaluation of family interaction, particularly of the dynamic type that occurs in family treatment.

Since practically all of Bales' observations have been with temporary groups from the time of their original formation, the observers are able to get the feel of the group culture in making their interpretation and scoring. The cultural overtones, emotional stabilization, and status stratification of a family, however, are likely to be so institutionalized as not to permit the observer to establish a baseline for his interpretations. Private meanings, codes, myths, telegraphic styles exist in all families. In addition, there are certain kinds of families (e.g., those with a schizophrenic member) in which meaning is violated in a most drastic kind of way, which is most upsetting to an observer (see Schaffer, *et al.*, 1962). In *ad hoc* groups the members have to make explicit and overt that which is understood among people with a long history of association and high emotional charge. Some inherent differences between the family and other groups, first of all, make it most difficult to apply any standard system to each. Though it is true that the role one plays in one's family (e.g., "mother's protector," "the stupid one," "the shy one," "the troublemaker," etc.) is likely to appear in some form in whatever group one comes to interact with, nevertheless the role one plays when interacting with one's family is likely to be quite at variance in a special kind of way with the way it is enacted with other groups. There are too many other variables operative in groups to enable one to generalize from one's role in the family; for example, one who is scapegoated in a family is likely, when with an outside group, to join others eagerly in scapegoating someone else; and it is very difficult, for instance, for even a mature, professional adult, let us say, to escape from a childlike role vis-à-vis his parents while in their presence.

The Bales system universally assumes the presence of some shared problem or task or common goal for a group to solve, and although it is true that most groups are task-oriented, does this assumption hold true for family living? Quite different processes and problems are shared by a family from those shared by a group of strangers. The uncertainty and unpredictability about the personality and actions of others in a temporary group are considerably attenuated in the family; part of the problem of the family in conjoint treatment is the dead certainty about the predictability of other family members in the face of a need for change. The Bales system does have the advantage of having been used in a wide variety of group situations for which norms have been developed; observations on families can be compared to these other groups, but the native differences between families and transient groups must be kept in mind.

Although Bales recognizes that given acts have a history and future orientation which transcends the present situation, nonetheless, in order to keep the mass of data to workable proportions, he has the observer consider only the immediate preceding act in his classification of the present one. An undue amount of limitation would be placed upon the natural order of events in family interaction by restricting the unit of judgment to single acts occurring within a limited context. Single acts are often incomprehensible or misinterpreted unless seen as embedded in a larger context of motivational strategy. Bales admits that in scoring interaction by his system, qualitative distinctions are systematically ignored, e.g., whether a given act is motivated to deal instrumentally with the group problem or for some deeper (perhaps unconscious) motive of hostility or dependency; both may be scored under the same category. When Bales (1950) says, " . . the observer should try to go as deep or to utilize as much of the context as the other does" (p. 40), he excludes almost all unconscious phenomena. The farthest he goes in depth of meaning is this addition to the foregoing sentence: "In therapy situations, when the other is the therapist, this may be a cut below the ordinary level of meaning given to social interaction." Under these circumstances, sophistication of interpretation would depend upon the clinical experience of the observer. It is quite likely that clinicians observing any kind of group would impute quite different meanings to the behaviors than would the usual kinds of observers Bales has been using, who are more or less bound to work at the surface meaning of the behavior. It would be interesting to compare the profiles of clinicians trained in his method to those of small-group scientists to see how differently the same behaviors would be interpreted. To give just one example, during one of our family treatment sessions most of the interaction consisted of a father and daughter arguing vehemently while the mother looked out the window. A sociologist observing the session commented that he had never seen such a vitriolic exchange and that the two really hated each other. The clinicians in the group looked at each other, sharing the common interpretation that this daughter and father were very interested in each other and that mother jealously felt excluded from this "love-making." The sociologist said, "How, by your trick of clinical reasoning, do you turn hostile behavior into affectionate behavior?" The point is, how would the Bales system handle this kind of behavior, which appears under the guise of negative? How does it handle nonverbal behavior that belies the words? How does it deal with double-binding statements, like the mother's saying to her daughter, "I understand that you're not really angry at me, dear; it's your sickness that makes you talk this way"? On what level does it handle a question like, "Do you really think I care how you feel about me?"

The Bales method, though of proven worth in evaluating the system aspects of groups in a wide variety of settings, attends largely to the manifest level of interaction and, on this account, appears not too useful for exploration of the kinds of deeper levels necessary for evaluating family dynamics. Family therapy sessions have revealed, for example, how a family may seem to be talking about one thing and then you suddenly realize they are talking about something else. A daughter screaming for independence and saying she wants to live away from home may make irresponsible plans which are really calculated to have her parents thwart her intentions. Mother may outwardly say she wants to let her go, but sabotages her with, "But, of course, honey, I'm afraid you'll never make it because you do have such trouble making friends and you might get sick again." None of the systematic observer systems extant have been devised to deal with a sufficient number of levels of communications so that conflicting messages and innuendoes are revealed.

Heyns and Lippitt (1954, pp. 374–375) have listed a series of dimensions of observer category systems useful in evaluating those already available and those yet to be developed: exhaustiveness (how much of the total behavior the system attempts to capture and classify); the dimension of inference (the level of conceptualization and interpretation required by the observer, e.g., inferring motives of the actor requires high inference, while determining on overt act, such as talking or not talking, requires low inference); the number of aspects of social behavior under scrutiny (short- or long-term processes); discrete vs. continuous categories (whether the categories have a quantifiable relationship to each other); size of the unit (sentences, an act, total behavior sequences, total meetings, etc.); and range of applicability (some category systems being applied to a wide variety of situations and others restricted to particular settings). These dimensions raise a number of purely methodological problems which have to be taken into consideration in planning research on family dynamics: e.g., problems of quantification of psychological process (Haeberle, 1959), categorizing qualitative data (Guetzkow, 1950), the relationship between categorization and ratings in the observation of group behavior (Carter, et al., 1951a), problems of laboratory experiments with small populations (Swanson, 1951), statistical problems involved in small-group research (Bales, 1951), the measurement of family life variables (Hoffman and Lippitt, 1960), and problems of time-sampling (Arrington, 1943).

Whether one utilizes check lists, ratings, coded observation guides, critical incidents, event sampling, category sets, or specimen records in evaluating family process, the problem of time sampling is central. One cannot just observe a family and collect willy-nilly everything that seems important; this approach results in data so massive as to be unwieldy. The researcher needs to select his variables, specified according to an internally consistent theoretical structure, try not to lose too much in translation from concepts to operations, and then attempt to determine how often and when a particular instance of that unit occurs. (Or one can set up structural experimental situations deliberately designed to reveal the planned variables.) Time sampling implies that behavior is distributed regularly and that extracting samples at systematic time intervals will reveal representative instances of that behavior. Is behavior, however, a respecter of time units set up in advance by the observer? Does a behavior or act have to occur repetitively in order to be considered significant? For instance, in one of our families being treated, the mother's characteristic behavior, repeated thousands of times, was that of an aggressive, driving, strong, dominating person. On one occasion, however, following a particularly devastating interpretation that she was trying to drive the therapist crazy (Searles, 1959), she burst into tears, grabbed the therapist's hand, begged his forgiveness, and behaved much like a frightened, dependent, whimpering child. Because this occurred just once, does it mean that it is not important? Trivial events may occur frequently and vital ones rarely: an intellectualizer may ruminate endlessly; yet a moment of truth in psychotherapy may occur but once. Is one slip worth ten thousand words? The nature of the relationship between the significance of an event and its frequency of occurrence is tenuous at best. The context of a behavior changes from moment to moment, and the behavior often assumes new meaning: a scowl evidenced by a mother when she is making the child perplexed has a different meaning than when she is praising the child. Attention only to fixed time intervals prevents focus on the situational meaning, the conditions under which the behavior occurs (Coutu, 1949).

We literally do not know enough about the universe of family dynamics to be able to draw meaningful and representative samples. Sampling implies consistency, and from what we have observed thus far in families seen over a long period of time in family treatment situations, though some aspects remain frustratingly rigid and stable, others are capriciously inconsistent. As one gets from one level to another, along with the softening of family defenses, one seems to be dealing with new family constellations, but, frequently, after much time has gone by, you realize you are back to old family patterns. It would seem that at this stage of development of knowledge, observation procedures should be venturesome and all-encompassing and that questions of sampling should be held in abeyance until there is more empirical data. Time sampling has its uses, however, particularly for events which occur frequently so that normative data can be established. The representativeness of the sample must be taken into consideration in the kinds of cross-sectional studies that aim toward statistical generalization. Haley (1962) has given a lucid exposition of some of the kinds of unique factors which should be taken into account in establishing a sample of family systems (especially those families containing a schizophrenic member) for the purpose of conducting family experiments.

A brief concluding note in this methodology section about instrumentation. A number of mechanical devices have been developed for recording observations. Bales and Gerbrands' interaction recorder (1948), Carter and co-workers' stenotype machine (1951b), Lippitt and Zander's IBM recording cards (1943), Chapple's Interaction Chronograph (1949), and others.

Typewritten transcripts of therapy sessions present a number of problems. Typists generally introduce more orderliness into people's speech than truly was there; in actuality, people talk in half complete thoughts with eliding of words, hesitations, simultaneous speech, etc., so that an accurate typewritten version reads almost like schizophrenic word salad. It makes us realize how little of our communication is verbal. In our experience even a good typist will have 50 errors on each page. Motion pictures with sound probably give the most faithful reproduction of an interaction session.

Ever since the introduction of the tape recorder into clinical practice and research, debate has gone on as to its effect on the process being examined. Some say there is practically no effect, that the subjects or patients soon forget its presence and behave as if it were not there. Another school of thought says that the tape recorder has drastic but unknown effects (e.g., arousing paranoid suspicions or exhibitionistic tendencies, creating an atmosphere of power and finality of the recorded word over evanescent spoken words, etc.). It is interesting that no one has yet subjected this controversy to experimental variation. A number of dimensions would have to be varied: is the microphone obvious or concealed? Are the subjects told about it in advance, or afterwards to get permission? Are the subjects just presented with the microphone and subjected to the implicit pressure that they had better go along with it? Is the time dimension relevant; in other words, does the tape recorder have less effect with the passage of time? Are any attempts made to determine what personal meaning it has to the subjects? How anxious is the experimenter about its use? Does he communicate his concern by apology?

A Point of View about Research on Family Dynamics

The orientation of this chapter thus far has probably appeared to be rather negative. The state of research in this new area of systematic investigation of family dynamics, based on what work has been done, would appear to be indeterminate, with more problems raised than answered. It has been concluded that families are not qualitatively similar to other groups, that individually oriented family research is not likely to be fruitful, that we cannot depend upon the statements of family members about themselves or other family members, that methods other than direct observation are likely to be misleading, and that attending only to manifest levels of interaction reveals little about the pulse and inner workings of family life. Barely touched upon and quite unresolved are such questions as the following: How do we go about getting the family to drop its defensive public behavior? How can we determine the effect of observers and instruments upon the behavior? How long does it take for deeper family systems to be revealed? Have we explored the limits of family-situational test experiments? How can the problem of negating and meta messages be handled in any systematic notational system? And how do we deal with the problem of the distribution of behavior and the significance of the rare event? Although this chapter could only begin to deal with these problems, it is hoped that at least some of the more importunate and pertinent areas have at least been identified. If most of the systematic procedures developed thus far by the behavioral scientist are inadequate in delineating the inherently powerful variables of family interaction, where can the family researcher turn? In this section, following some suggestions as to the usefulness of various psychological testing approaches, an attempt will be made to present a point of view, rather than a detailed prospectus, as to some possibly productive directions that systematic research on family dynamics might take.

Some recent work and thinking, both systematic and speculative, appear to be potentially fruitful for the study of family dynamics. In the area of psychological testing, Sohler and her co-workers (1957) attempted to predict family interaction from a battery of projective tests individually administered to family members. In this study, blind interpretations were made on the resemblances between children and parents in their patterns of needs and conflicts, on whether there were factors that characterized the family as a whole, on whether the test material from an entire family helped in understanding individuals. All these interpretations were compared with knowledge gained by psychiatrists who had seen the family for two years in a semitherapeutic setting. They found that the individual personality descriptions contained the highest proportion of agreement and that attempts to predict family interaction had only limited success.

A more promising development has been proposed by Roman and Bauman (1960) in the approach they call Interaction Testing. They use as a theoretical basis the proposition that a group is a dynamic whole with unique properties which cannot simply be deduced from the characteristics of its members. The method consisted of testing each member of the group separately, using standard psychological tests, such as the Wechsler-Bellevue, Rorschach, and TAT, and then readministering these tests to the group assembled together with instructions that they, as a group, arrive at consentaneous test responses. Three types of interaction categories were described: Reinforcement (in which the group response is the same as that of each member when tested individually), Selection (in which the group response is the same as that of at least one of the individuals), and Emergence (in which the group response is different from all of the individual responses). Each of these interaction categories can be characterized as positive or negative, depending on whether it is healthy or pathological. The authors presented some impressive clinical descriptive data illustrating the kinds of new information which Interaction Testing revealed in the following kinds of cases: a comparison of two marriages, an engaged couple in conflict, a mother and schizophrenic son, a stable homosexual relationship, and a therapy group at two points in treatment. There is insufficient space here to reproduce many of the provocative findings of this paper; mention can be made of only a few results. Their test data revealed joint reality distortions, activation of latent pathology of one of the partners by the other's manifest pathology, one partner expressing the other's deeper disturbance, sadomasochistic connivance, deference of the healthier partner to the sicker, absence of affecting each other's responses, enhancement or regression as a function of combined endeavor, etc. Even such data as intelligence test scores were found to undergo drastic change as a function of interaction. In one conflictful married couple, for example, the joint I.Q. was lower than that of its higher member; in a healthier couple the joint I.Q. was higher than that of either of its members. In other words, the interactional pathology not only sometimes lowered intellectual efficiency but occasionally reduced the level of thinking to that of its lowest common denominator. The authors believe that Interaction Testing not only evaluates the psychological process and product of interaction of two or more people and evaluates the characteristics of a group-as-a-group, but also reveals data about the effects of the group on the intellectual and personality characteristics of the individuals in the group.

More recently, Loveland, Wynne, and Singer (1963) described a psychodiagnostic technique whereby family members interpret the Rorschach inkblots to each other, without the examiner present, and attempt to reach consensus in their responses. They linked this procedure to some of their former work which indicated that thought and communication disorders found in individual psychiatric patients could be related to the forms or styles of communicating in their families (Wynne and Singer, 1963). Changes in verbalized responses and perception due to the impact of family interaction were assessed by comparison with prior individual testing of family members. As might be anticipated, the family production was far from any simple summing of features of individual performance. In general, the more disturbed the family, the more the responses agreed upon were less perceptually appropriate, the reasoning less logical and orderly, and the more the communication with each other was more vague and amorphous than each family member had shown during the individual testing. The Family Rorschach record provided a very useful, directly observable sample of how each person related to every other member of the family (e.g., some members addressed their remarks only to certain people and excluded others). Excerpts from one family Rorschach record showed how the parents aided each other's pathology, with the son being able to cope with one parent but not both. Since the authors were making a preliminary report of this procedure, they did not present any systematic data from numbers of families, but it is clear that the family Rorschach can be most illuminating. As the authors note, Rorschachs obtained in this manner must be evaluated differently from individual Rorschachs. What was not agreed upon or mentioned by the family could be as revealing as the agreed-upon responses, a factor mitigating against traditional scoring summaries. Nonetheless, it will be interesting to see what developments follow from large-scale use of this technique, e.g., how formal Rorschach patterns are affected by the presence of family members, such as, for instance, Rorschach Developmental Level (Phillips, Kaden, and Waldman, 1959). It must be remembered that even though traditional psychological tests were used in ingenious ways in the studies just cited, these psychodiagnostic instruments were originally designed out of an individual, intrapsychic orientation to personality structure and dynamics. As transpersonal and transactional system concepts become better understood, new psychological test instruments may be developed that will perform the same family diagnostic functions that psychological tests presently accomplish for individuals.

Parloff (1961), who reviewed some of the work done on the family in psychotherapy, has said, "The relevant literature is vast, but very little of it would be classed by the rigorous investigator as research. Most of the contributors to the area have been clinician naturalists who, having perhaps a Freudlike vision of themselves, have made saltatory advances from observations to conclusions with a maximum of vigor and a minimum of rigor . . . [practitioners] move about with majestic disregard of our research literature" (pp. 445–451). Though it is hoped that this chapter has not disregarded the research literature, majestically or otherwise, it is necessary to face the fact that systematic investigation of family dynamics, even utilizing the family treatment situation, is a formidable undertaking indeed.

The biases of the present writer as to where pay dirt lies in investigating family dynamics have perhaps become more clear. It is the writer's judgment that it lies in the psychoanalytic view of deep, concealed, family relationship needs which are unconscious, infantile, and corrective of past hurts or perpetuations of past gratifications; in each family the individual motivations are a blend of the old and the new family systems. Each individual has a personal way in which he interprets that he is "loved" or in relationship. Some people get their definition of self and feel in relationship when they are abused, when they argue, when they retreat, when they are stimulated, etc., all based on the struggle with their "internal objects" (Fairbairn, 1952). Through all their lives they train real others into relating to them in a way that enables them to continue the internal relationships; they try to reduplicate original family situations in their attempts at mastery, settling of old scores or pains, or getting the love in unalloyed form without the disturbing elements. The mate such a person chooses is the one with whom he can maintain or work through the relationship with the introjects; the other person is needed to complete and complement the self, even if all that is required is confirmation of a fictional self. These marriage partners, of course, have their own scripts that they are following, and the motive systems interlock, are parallel at certain points, and conflict at other points, and, along with the children, a new gestalt is formed which we call the family dynamic system—an enormously involved network which, until the advent of long-term family treatment, had been unperceived by science. The interweaving motives of the family members are concealed behind subterfuges in the routine course of living; most of the time the motives are hidden and masked: they may apparently seek the opposite, or even seem to be seeking nothing at all. What kind of unruly data is this where nothing is as it seems, where an event not only does not follow the moment before, but may be determined by something which happened minutes, hours, or even years before, or perhaps never happened and existed only in fantasy?

The behavioral scientist, true to his tradition in studying these situations, has achieved his security by selecting the variables that were readily available, were objective and consensually observable, and could be counted and reported to his colleagues. The point need not be labored, perhaps, that clinicians always wince when an experimental psychologist delimits a clinical concept for study, operationally redefines it, creates a measuring instrument for it, and ends up measuring something that bears almost no resemblance to the original, although it does have the dubious merit of precision. (The writer is aware, too, of the discomfort of the experimentally minded psychologist at the free-wheeling nature of the clinician.) At any rate, attending only to overt, observable acts leads to relatively barren representations unless underlying attitudes, intents, strategy, and motivational formulas in the family are discovered. Questions like: "Who seeks to possess whom, and how does he go about it or disguise it?", are far more pertinent than: "Who talks to whom and how much?" But how are these depth factors to be revealed? With individuals they are disclosed in the marginal thoughts, the slips of the tongue, the blushing face, the unguarded moment, the blocking, the talking too much, the afterthoughts quickly denied, all the classical signs of resistance. With families they are seen largely in the system resistances, the reluctance to air dirty linen, the nurturing of vested interests, the loyalties, the secret alliances, the empty talk or the noisiness as a family defense. Within limits, important dimensions can be seen in even the overt behavior when over-all patterns are viewed. Because of resistance to exposure and to change, however, and because of threatened loss of relationship, the most important and meaningful information about families is the most difficult to obtain. Until the advent of family treatment, social scientists had made few attempts to study family interaction in its natural state by methods of indirection which did not interfere with spontaneity. A notable exception was Bossard's (1948, ch. 8) method of studying the family by recording, without the knowledge of the family, the table talk that occurred when the family got together at mealtime. It was not until whole families had been observed over a long period in family therapy that we began to learn the truth about what really went on in families and what the dissembled attitudes really were, that we penetrated beyond the superficial reports family members gave for public consumption or the type of casual social knowledge neighbors have about families. (How often are people shocked to hear that that "happily married" couple are getting a divorce, or to hear that a psychiatrist, "who should be able to avoid it," committed suicide or developed a mental illness because of "family problems," or to see a family known to the community as an "ideal" family produce a delinquent or schizophrenic offspring?)

We are far away from experimental manipulation of significant family life variables in their complexity and full size, although certain aspects can perhaps be brought into laboratory focus. Such transpersonal phenomena as double-bind situations, unconscious collusion, pseudomutuality, unconsciously shared fantasy systems, role complementarity, interlocking jealousy patterns, and other, admittedly conceptually loose, principles need systematic exploration. Genuine interaction research is probably also quite some distance away. Where are the instruments by which we can determine what A is really doing to B, and what B's counterstrategy is, which then makes C modify or obscure what is going on between A and B; where each response, manifestly and latently, has its reverberating, transforming, and feedback effects on all the others? We have hardly begun to approach the complexity of what is involved in studying the reciprocal processes *between* people, especially between family members who communicate with condensed phrases or gestures with a private history. Almost all of our concepts are based on individual or intrapsychic thinking. True interaction language is not yet available, although use will probably be made of such terms as *interaction, transpersonal, interdigitated, transactional, interchange, reciprocal, exchange, communion, intermingle, interposition, dovetail, interpenetrate, mutual, commingle, interdependent, interlaced, entwine, interlock, convolve, counterbalance, intertwine,* etc.

In this chapter the terms *interaction* and *transaction* have been used more or less interchangeably as if they were synonymous. Dewey and Bentley (1949) have suggested a technical distinction between the two terms, specifying interaction as occurring on the level of individuals whereby one person acts upon another; person is balanced against person in causal interconnection. Transaction, on the other hand, does not deal with individuals as such but with another suprapersonal level—with process, with abstractions, with concepts; transaction suggests the unitary nature of the phenomenon with all its circular relatedness within a situational system. If this distinction between interaction and transaction were to be used, it can be stated that none of the systematic research reported in this chapter is truly transactional in nature. On the clinical level such concepts as family loyalty systems, family homeostasis (Jackson, 1959), pseudomutuality (Wynne, Ryckoff, Day and Hirsch, 1958), family-rule systems (Haley, 1959), symbiosis (Hill, L., 1955), "undifferentiated family ego mass" (Bowen, 1960), and role equilibrium (Spiegel, 1957) would be considered to be transactional abstractions.

The foregoing, as well as concepts like Wynne's *trading of dissociations* (this volume) and Wallace and Fogelson's *identity struggle* (this volume), present quite worthwhile starting points for rigorous investigation. Wynne's trading of dissociations is defined as a deeply unconscious "deal" whereby the fixed view that each family member has of the other is exchanged for a fixed view of himself by the other (e.g., "I will see you as nonsexual if you will see me as nonmurderous"). The trading of dissociations is deeper than but related to the identity struggle, a more conscious process whereby A attempts to get B to accept A's identity for what, in B's eyes, A wishes it to be. A will try to attribute to B an identity so negative in value that B will try to satisfy A's need to be seen in this way (e.g., "I want you to see me as such-and-such a kind of person; the reason you won't is that you are a so-and-so"). When B applies the same strategy to A, in defense or in response to his own identity needs, an identity struggle emerges. The family group is usually caught up in a complex set of reciprocal identity struggles.

Scheflen (1963; in press) and Birdwhistell's (1961; in press) attempts to deal with meta levels of communication and multiple levels of linguistic, paralinguistic, kinesic, and postural behaviors during interaction, such behaviors being studied by motion picture frame analysis, promise many stimulating discoveries. Also of great interest is a concept of interpersonal defense developed by Laing.[2] The concept is tentatively labeled *alternation* and is described as

---

[2] Laing, R. D. Personal Communication. 1962.

a maneuver in which one person characterizes another's behavior in terms of the effect the behavior has on the feelings of the first person. For instance, if a child does something, the parent does not comment on what the child did; instead, what is commented on is what the action does to the parent (e.g., "You're breaking my heart"). A's behavior is defined in terms of B's feeling. When a mother says to her schizophrenic daughter, in effect, "You are getting ill; the reason I know this is that you are provoking me," the definition of illness is in terms of the effect of the daughter's behavior on the mother. When alternation is being practiced, it is very difficult to know what someone is doing except via its transactional effect upon someone else. Is there such a phenomenon as interpersonal repression? When a parent, for instance, tells his child that he (the child) cannot remember something, he is placing an injunction against reliable memory in the child. It would be a relief for the child to remember but threatening to the parent; the child's memory exists as a function of the parent's peace of mind. All sorts of possibilities present themselves for studying interpersonal defenses with these ideas in mind. A clinical symptom like jealousy is usually discussed in terms of the individual, but take a situation in which a wife suspects that her husband is being unfaithful, and the husband feeds her suspicions by frequently going out without telling her where he is going because she, too, is fanning his jealous suspicions by making secret telephone calls. The elaboration of a system of mutual projection like this is difficult to understand or treat in intrapsychic terms alone.

The essential thesis behind the transpersonal view of psychopathology is that people really do have an effect upon one another when they are in close relationship, a telling effect which is more than the resultant of two interacting intrapsychic systems. It has become a commonplace to find among Freud's germinal writings the foreshadowing of almost every development in psychiatric thinking; theoreticians are constantly being nettled when they discover that Freud not only had the idea many years before but frequently stated it better. One such notion that Freud anticipated but whose momentous implications he did not pursue is associated with the idea of cross-communication between the unconscious of one person and another. In his 1915 paper on "The Unconscious" he wrote, "It is very remarkable that the unconscious of one human being can react upon that of another, without the conscious being implicated at all. This deserves closer investigation, especially with a view to finding out whether preconscious activity can be excluded as a factor in bringing this about; but for purposes of description the fact is incontestible." (Freud, 1957, p. 194). Formal recognition of this phenomenon lay dormant for a number of years, although sensitive novelists and dramatists have portrayed it. It must also have been recognized by psychotherapists, especially those who saw the bilateral psychopathology in patients intimately related with one another. It is only in retrospect now that we can identify as another landmark in transpersonal psychopathology the pioneering article by Johnson and Szurek (1952), alerting us to the fact that a child can act out the unconscious, disowned wishes of a parent. A number of apparently incongruous human behaviors became more understandable when viewed from the standpoint of the unconscious current and identification between people: how schizophrenics in a hospital will seek each other out and cluster together; how friendships are formed between people who represent unconscious aspects of each other (e.g., a shy, demure girl becoming a close friend of a psychopathic, sexually acting-out girl); how a woman whose husband's drinking or gambling was a source of much pain and turmoil marries another gambler or alcoholic or who, after the husband dies, begins to drink or gamble herself; how, in the same family, one brother becomes a priest and another brother becomes a gangster. How do we account for the exchange of symptoms in families, or their transmission across generations? (Fisher and Mendell, 1956; Henry, 1951). The unconscious exchange frequently appears in the form of themes or recurrent problems between people who are deeply related; both parties in the interchange take a position vis-à-vis *the problem*. The problems are similar but the defenses against them are the opposite: both have a problem about, say, sexuality or hostility, and one expresses it while the other objects. The one who objects get vicarious satisfaction out of the way the other expresses it. The danger in oneself can be handled by dealing with it in the other; the other than "cooperates" by seeming to be or actually behaving dangerously, thus reinforcing the conviction on the part of both parties that all of the danger resides in the other. When this sort of thing occurs, we say that these people "have it made"; they go together like ham and eggs and really need each other. Cottrell (1942), from a sociopsychological point of view, has evinced some recognition of this idea: ". . . the reactive system [of a person] includes not only those patterns the person has manifested but also the response patterns of the others of his life situation. Thus, from this point of view, the rebellious child is also in part the authoritarian parent; the saint is part sinner; the communist is part capitalist; the southern white is part Negro psychologically . . . The more intimate the contact through time, the greater will be the tendency for the patterns to coincide" (p. 376). Psychopathology which interlocks on an unconscious level, then, is a phenomenon that has long been with us, but scientific recognition has been only peripheral until the advent of couple and family psychotherapy. It is a puzzlement why the overwhelming proportion of behavioral science research deals with reality oriented, secondary process, conscious behavior and why so few efforts have been made to study systematically the unconscious and the relationship between the levels of awareness. This may explain the triviality of most of the variables selected for the studies that fill our journals.

A final word about the future of family research of the type being discussed in this chapter. Just as the small-group field went through its stages of the speculative era, empirical fact-finding, and the testing of theoretical hypotheses, with feedback from each stage enriching the other, so the transactional study of families will probably have to undergo its own disquietudes of growth and maturity. This whole area of endeavor is still in its infancy; much broad investigation and intuitive observing are being done, as represented by the thinkers in this volume. We shall probably soon see a plethora of data-collecting of all kinds, perhaps with some techniques and methods appropriated from the small-group discipline but others being created *de novo* to meet the unique problems of this new field. Exciting findings await the family investigator. Fact collecting and theory should not go their separate ways, however; it is hoped that we will not witness again the sight of psychoanalysis and academic psychology losing touch with each other in dealing with the same phenomena. One hopes that we can avoid amassing data of the simplistic kind, that we can avoid precise measurement that does not take into account the meaningfulness of what is being measured. The observer certainly needs to be sensitively attuned to the emotional forces of the family process and not be overwhelmed by misleading trivia. One can even go so far as to say that what seems to be called for are flexible measuring sticks which extract phenomenologically dynamic units.

The field of family study, in the sense in which it is being used in this chapter, will have to be divided up into areas more meaningfully and logically developed out of intimate knowledge of the family rather than, say, leadership, decision making, status and power, group cohesiveness, and other areas borrowed from the small-group discipline. As we gain more sophistication about family dynamics, we shall probably see fewer attempts to investigate pseudo problems, like whether mother is more dominant than father and who is the sickest member of the family. The point is, those of us who do family treatment have become aware of another level of the family which has been largely untouched by prior scientific investigation because we had never before created the conditions and the special kind of microscope under which it could be revealed, namely, the system aspect of the family. Study of this exceedingly intricate complex, to which every family member contributes on multiple levels and in which each has a vital stake, represents, as this writer sees it, the ultimate challenge of the study of family dynamics. The family system has a structure of its own, which is largely underground and unconscious; it has its own myths, rituals, rules, and powerful influences. The system remains even when one person leaves it, and it absorbs and accommodates itself to whomever or whatever comes into contact with it; the effect of the community or social class on it is less than we would have thought. The system changes very slowly or not at all. In the study of the family system, emphasis has to be given to transactional wholes rather than to a collection of individual events.

One of the most pressing research questions is that, if observing the family affects the spontaneity and freedom of the behaviors, how can we really know the family in its natural state? In an ultimate sense, in order to get at the really significant variables of family life and determine and manipulate all of the conditions, the investigator would have to have the kind of life-and-death control over the family that an experimenter has in doing certain kinds of animal or physiologic research (e.g., you would have to record and film families in their homes without their knowledge—obviously an unethical procedure). The closest approximation we can make to this theoretically ideal state is the family treatment situation, where, indeed, the therapists come to be seen by the family as possessing great power over them; during the course of developing transference feelings, they reveal more of what they are really like. It is being suggested here, then, that the basic and significant variables of family dynamics will arise spontaneously while the family members' long-term interaction with each other is being observed, and that they require special therapeutic techniques of exposure; in short, that extended family treatment is the *sine qua non* medium within which to study family dynamics. Weakland (1962) has presented a few ideas along these lines in his paper, "Family Therapy as a Research Arena." If the family treatment situation is to be utilized for an understanding of family dynamics, it will be necessary, of course, to determine the effect of the therapists upon what one learns about the families.

It is true that so-called normal families will ordinarily not allow access to their privacy (the system) unless some symptom such as mental illness or delinquency in one member *which disturbs the family system* forces them to seek help. Investigation of symptom-free families in a series of exploratory sessions, dealing with the normal crises every family has to deal with, is one research project well worth doing. Family treatment itself, furthermore, presents opportunities to examine many problems heretofore unavailable for examination. For example, by seeing the family together over a long period of time, we have an unparalleled opportunity to observe at first hand part of the process that forms personality in the offspring. One of the best previous sources, individual psychotherapy or psychoanalysis, has had to rely on reconstructions from the patient's memories or fantasies. It is true that the latter have a psychic reality that make them suitable for individual treatment purposes, but, veridically, science is interested in the actual unfolding events. Evaluation of the *treatment* aspect of family therapy, both from a process and outcome point of view, is probably premature at this stage.

Anyone planning to do research on family dynamics should acquaint himself with the literature on family treatment and should observe the family in the unique family treatment situation. Otherwise, an extremely important dimension of the family will be missed. Doing family therapy has helped us become aware of certain family parameters that we did not know existed. It will be hard for anyone who has seen families under the emotional impact of treatment to ever again do family research in the traditional ways. For the first time, he will be viewing the family where it lives emotionally, and he will come away with more knowledge about the family than he would get from reading a collection of books and articles. And for the first time he will also begin to get a picture of the kinds of extravagant behaviors that go on behind closed doors, behaviors that we strongly suspect go on in some degree and form in all families. In any event, it is not of small practical relevance to examine systematically the deeper cross-currents of family life, the place where the best and the worst in man is bred.

References

ALBEE, E. (1962). *Who's afraid of Virginia Woolf?* A play. New York: Atheneum.

ARRINGTON, R. E. (1943). Time sampling in studies of social behavior: A critical review of techniques and results with research suggestions. *Psychol. Bull. 40*, 81–124.

ASCH, S. E. (1951). Effects of group pressure upon the modification and distortion of judgments. In H. Guetzkow (Ed.) *Groups, leadership, and men.* Pittsburgh: Carnegie Press, pp. 177–190.

BACHOVE, C., AND ZUBALY, B. M. (1959). Exploratory study on family interrelationships in a small sample of non-clinic families. Master's thesis, Bryn Mawr.

BACK, C. W. (1951). Influence through social communication. *J. abnorm. soc. Psychol. 46*, 9–23.

BALDWIN, A. L. (1949). Effects of home environment on nursing school behavior. *Child Develpm. 20*, 49–62.

BALES, R. F. (1950). *Interaction process analysis.* Cambridge, Mass.: Addison-Wesley.

BALES, R. F. (1951). Some statistical problems in small group research. *J. Amer. Statist. Ass. 46*, 311–322.

BALES, R. F. (1958). Task roles and social roles in problem-solving groups. In E. Maccoby, T. Newcomb, and E. Hartley (Eds.) *Readings in social psychology.* New York: Holt, pp. 437–447.

BALES, R. F., AND GERBRANDS, H. (1948). The interaction recorder—an apparatus and check list for sequential content analysis of social interaction. *Hum. Relat. 1*, 456–464.

BALES, R. F., AND SLATER, P. E. (1955). Role differentiation in small decision-making groups. In T. Parsons and R. F. Bales (Eds.) *Family, socialization and interaction process.* Glencoe, Ill.: Free Press, pp. 259–306.

BATESON, G., JACKSON, D. D., HALEY, J., AND WEAKLAND, J. H. (1956). Toward a theory of schizophrenia. *Behav. Sci. 1*, 251–264.

BATESON, G., JACKSON, D. D., HALEY, J., AND WEAKLAND, J. H. (1963). A note on the double bind, 1962. *Family Process 2*, 154–161.

BAVELAS, A. (1950). Communication patterns in task-oriented groups. *J. acoust. Soc. Amer. 22*, 725–730.

BIRDWHISTELL, R. L. (1961). Paralanguage: 25 years after Sapir. In H. W. Brosin (Ed.) *Lectures on experimental psychiatry.* Univer. Pittsburgh Press, pp. 43–63.

BIRDWHISTELL, R. L. (in press). Movement and kinesics. In G. Bateson, R. L. Birdwhistell, H. W. Brosin, C. F. Hockett, and N. A. McQuown (Eds.) *Natural history of an interview*, 3 vols. New York: Grune & Stratton.

BISHOP, B. M. (1951). Mother-child interaction and the social behavior of children. *Psychol. Monogr.* No. 11, *65*, 1–34.

BORGATTA, E. F., COTTRELL, L. S., AND MEYER, H. J. (1956). On the dimensions of group behavior. *Sociomet. 19*, 223–240.

BOSSARD, J. H. (1948). *Sociology of child development.* New York: Harper.

BOWEN, M. A. (1960). Family concept of schizophrenia. In D. D. Jackson (Ed.) *The etiology of schizophrenia.* New York: Basic Books, pp. 346–372.

BOWMAN, C. C. (1956). Research in family dynamics: A criticism and a proposal. *Soc. Forces 34*, 201–207.

BURGESS, E. (1947). The family and sociological research. *Soc. Forces 26*, 1–6.

CAPUTO, D. V. (1963). Parents of the schizophrenic. *Family Process 2*, 339–356.

CARTER, L., HAYTHORN, W., MIEROWITZ, B., AND LANZETTA, J. (1951a). The relation of categorizations and ratings in the observation of group behavior. *Hum. Relat. 3*, 239–254.

CARTER, L., HAYTHORN, W., MEIROWITZ, B., AND LANZETTA, J. (1951b). A note on a new technique of interaction recording. *J. abnorm. soc. Psychol. 46*, 258–260.

CARTWRIGHT, D., AND ZANDER, A. (1962). *Group dynamics: Research and theory.* (2nd ed.) Evanston, Ill.: Row, Peterson.

CHAMPNEY, H. The measurement of parent behavior. (1941). *Child Develpm. 12*, 131–166.

CHAPPLE, E. D. (1949). The Interaction Chronograph: Its evolution and present application. *Personnel 25*, 295–307.

CHAPPLE, E. D. (1953). The standard experimental (stress) interview as used in Interaction Chronograph investigations. *Hum. Organ. 12*, 23–32.

CHAPPLE, E. D., AND LINDEMANN, E. (1942). Clinical implications of measurements of interaction rates in psychiatric interviews. *Appl. Anthrop. 1*, 1–11.

COTTRELL, L. S. (1942). The analysis of situational fields in social psychology. *Amer. sociol. Rev. 7*, 370–382.

COTTRELL, L. S. (1948). The present status and future orientation of research on the family. *Amer. sociol. Rev. 13*, 123–136.

COUTU, W. (1949). *Emergent human nature.* New York: Knopf.

DAGER, E. Z. (1959). A review of family research in 1958. *Marr. & Fam. Liv. 21*, 287–299.

DEWEY, J., AND BENTLEY, A. F. (1949). *Knowing and the known.* Boston: Beacon Hill.

DRECHSLER, R. J., AND SHAPIRO, M. I. (1961). A procedure for direct observation of family interaction in a child guidance clinic. *Psychiatry 24*, 163–170.

DRECHSLER, R. J., AND SHAPIRO, M. I. (1963). Two methods of analysis of family diagnostic data. *Family Process 2*, 367–379.

EHRMANN, W. (1957). A review of family research in 1956. *Marr. & Fam. Liv. 19*, 279–294.

EPSTEIN, N. B., AND WESTLEY, W. A. (1959). Patterns of intra-familial communication. In D. E. Cameron and M. Greenblatt (Eds.) *Psychiatric research reports*, vol. 11, pp. 1–12.

FAIRBAIRN, W. R. D. (1952). *An object-relations theory of the personality.* New York: Basic Books.

FARINA, A. (1960). Patterns of role dominance and conflict in parents of schizophrenic patients. *J. abnorm. soc. Psychol. 61*, 31–38.

FARINA, A., AND DUNHAM, R. M. (1963). Measurement of family relationships and their effects. *Arch. gen. Psychiat. 9*, 64–73.

FERREIRA, A. J. (1963a). Decision making in normal and pathologic families. *Arch. gen. Psychiat. 8*, 68–73.

FERREIRA, A. J. (1963b). Rejection and expectancy of rejection in families. *Family Process 2*, 235–244.

FESTINGER, L., PEPITONE, A., AND NEWCOMB, T. M. (1952). Some consequences of de-individuation in a group. *J. abnorm. soc. Psychol. 47*, 382–389.

FESTINGER, L., SCHACHTER, S., AND BACK, K. W. (1950). *Social pressures in informal groups.* New York: Harper.

FISHER, S., BOYD, I., WALKER, D., AND SHEER, D. (1959). Parents of schizo-phrenics, neurotics, and normals. *Arch. gen. Psychiat. 1,* 149–166.

FISHER, S., AND MENDELL, D. (1956). The communication of neurotic patterns over two and three generations. *Psychiatry 19,* 41–46.

FOURIEZOS, N. T., HUTT, M. L., AND GUETZKOW, H. (1950). Measurement of self-oriented needs in discussion groups. *J. abnorm. soc. Psychol. 45,* 682–690.

FREEDMAN, M. B., LEARY, T. F., OSSORIO, A. B., AND COFFEY, H. S. (1951). The interpersonal dimension of personality. *J. Pers. 20,* 143–161.

FRENCH, J. R. P. (1941). The disruption and cohesion of groups. *J. abnorm. soc. Psychol. 36,* 361–377.

FREUD, S. (1957). The unconscious. In: The complete psychological works of Sigmund Freud. Standard ed., J. Strachey (ed.), vol. XIV. London: Hogarth Press, pp. 166–204. (Originally published in Zeitscrift, Bd. III, 1915)

FRIEDMAN, A. S. (1962). Family therapy as conducted in the home. *Family Process 1,* 132–140.

GARMEZY, N., FARINA, A., AND RODNICK, E. H. (1960). The structured situational test: A method for studying family interaction in schizophrenia. *Amer. J. Orthopsychiat. 30,* 445–452.

GOFFMAN, E. (1956). *The presentation of self in everyday life.* Edinburgh: Univer. of Edinburgh, Social Sciences Research Centre.

GOODRICH, D. W., AND BOOMER, D. S. (1963). Experimental assessment of modes of conflict resolution. *Family Process 2,* 15–24.

GROSS, E. (1956). Symbiosis and consensus as integrative factors in small groups. *Amer. sociol. Rev. 21,* 174–179.

GROSS, N., AND MARTIN, W. E. (1952). On group cohesiveness. *Amer. J. Sociol. 57,* 546–553.

GUETZKOW, H. (1950). Unitizing and categorizing problems in coding qualitative data. *J. clin. Psychol. 6,* 47–57.

HAEBERLE, A. (1959). Quantification of observational data in various stages of research. *Amer. J. Orthopsychiat. 29,* 583–589.

HALEY, J. (1959). The family of the schizophrenic: A model system. *J. nerv. ment. Dis. 129,* 357–374.

HALEY, J. (1962). Family experiments: A new type of experimentation. *Family Process 1,* 265–293.

HARE, A. P. (1962). *Handbook of small group research.* Glencoe, Ill.: Free Press.

HARE, A. P., BORGATTA, E. F., AND BALES, R. F. (1955). *Small groups: Studies in social interaction.* New York: Knopf.

HEMPHILL, J. K., AND WESTIE, C. M. (1950). The measurement of group dimensions. *J. Psychol. 29:*325–342.

HENRY, J. (1951). Family structure and the transmission of neurotic behavior. *Amer. J. Orthopsychiat. 21,* 800–818.

HENRY, J., AND WARSON, C. (1951). Family structure and psychic development. *Amer. J. Orthopsychiat. 21,* 59–73.

HEYNS, R. W., AND LIPPITT, R. (1954). Systematic observational techniques. In G. Lindzey (Ed.) *Handbook of social psychology,* vol. 1. Cambridge, Mass.: Addison-Wesley, pp. 370–404.

HILL, L. (1955). *Psychotherapeutic intervention in schizophrenia.* Chicago: Univer. of Chicago Press.

HILL, R. (1951). Review of current research on marriage and the family. *Amer. sociol. Rev. 16,* 694–701.

HILL, R. (1958). Sociology of marriage and family behavior, 1945–1956. *Current sociol. 7,* 1–33.

HILL, R., FOOTE, N., MANGUS, H. R., POLAK, O., AND LESLIE, G. (1957). Appraising progress in research. *Marr. & Fam. Liv. 19,* 59–108.

HILL, R., AND HANSEN, D. A. (1960). The identification of conceptual frameworks utilized in family study. *Marr. & Fam. Liv. 22,* 299–311.

HOFFMAN, L. W., AND LIPPITT, R. (1960). The measurement of family life variables. In P. Musson (Ed.) *Handbook of research methods in child development.* New York: Wiley, pp. 945–1013.

JACKSON, D. D. (1959). Family interaction, family homeostasis, and some implications for conjoint family psychotherapy. In J. Masserman (Ed.) *Science and psychoanalysis,* vol. 2. *Individual and familial dynamics.* New York: Grune & Stratton.

JANSEN, L. T. (1952). Measuring family solidarity. *Amer. sociol. Rev. 17,* 727–733.

JOEL, W., AND SHAPIRO, D. (1949). A genotypical approach to the analysis of personal interaction. *J. Psychol. 48,* 9–17.

JOHNSON, A. M., AND SZUREK, S. A. (1952). The genesis of anti-social acting out in children and adults. *Psychiat. Quart. 21,* 323–343.

KELLEY, H. H. (1951). Communication in experimentally-created hierarchies. *Hum. Relat. 4,* 39–56.

KENKEL, W. F., AND HOFFMAN, D. K. (1956). Real and conceived roles in family decision making. *Marr. & Fam. Liv. 18,* 311–316.

KILLIAN, L. M. (1952). The significance of multiple-group membership in disaster. *Amer. J. Sociol. 57,* 309–314.

LEARY, T. (1957). *Interpersonal diagnosis of personality.* New York: Ronald Press.

LEAVITT, H. J. (1951). Some effects of certain communication patterns on group performance. *J. abnorm. soc. Psychol. 46,* 38–50.

LEVINGER, G. (1959). The assessment of family relationships: A progress report. Western Reserve Univer., Cleveland, Ohio (mimeo).

LEVINGER, G. (1963). Supplementary methods in family research. *Family Process 2,* 357–366.

LIPPITT, R., AND ZANDER, A. (1943). Observation and interview methods for the Leadership Training Study. New York: Boy Scouts of America (mimeo).

LOVELAND, N. T., WYNNE, L. C., AND SINGER, M. T. (1963). The family Rorschach: A new method for studying family interaction. *Family Process 2,* 187–215.

MANGUS, A. R. (1958). Discussion of paper presented by James Titchener. In B. Pasamanick and P. H. Knapp (Eds.) *Psychiatric research reports,* vol. 10, pp. 89–99.

MARCH, J. G. (1953). Husband-wife interaction over political issues. *Publ. Opin. Quart. 17,* 461–470.

MILLS, T. M. (1953). Power relations in three-person groups. *Amer. sociol. Rev. 18,* 351–357.

MILLS, T. M. (1954). The coalition pattern in three person groups. *Amer. sociol. Rev. 19,* 657–667.

MITCHELL, H. E. (1961). Application of the Leary technique to family units: Illustrative cases. Conference on *Psychotherapy and the family.* Temple Univer. Dept. of Psychiatry, March 30.

MITCHELL, H. E. (1963). Application of the Kaiser method to marital pairs. *Family Process 2,* 265–279.

MOUSTAKAS, C. E., SIGEL, I. E., AND SCHALOCK, H. D. (1956). An objective method for the measurement and analysis of child-adult interaction. *Child Develpm. 27,* 109–134.

NIMKOFF, M. F. (1948). Trends in family research. *Amer. J. Sociol. 53,* 477–482.

NIZER, L. (1961). *My life in court.* New York: Doubleday, pp. 155–157.

NYE, F. I., AND BAYER, A. E. (1963). Some recent trends in family research. *Soc. Forces 41,* 290–301.

ORNE, M. T. (1962). On the social psychology of the psychology experiment: With particular reference to demand characteristics and their implications. *Amer. Psychologist 17,* 776–783.

OSGOOD, C. E., SUCI, G. J., AND TANNENBAUM, P. H. (1957). *The measurement of meaning.* Urbana: Univer. of Illinois Press.

PARLOFF, M. B. (1961). The family in psychotherapy. *Arch. gen. Psychiat. 4,* 445–451.

PARSONS, T. (1955). Family structure and the socialization of the child. In T. Parsons and R. F. Bales (Eds.) *Family, socialization and interaction process.* Glencoe, Ill.: Free Press, pp. 35–131.

PHILLIPS, L., KADEN, S., AND WALDMAN, M. (1959). Rorschach indices of developmental level. *J. genet. Psychol. 94,* 267–285.

RODNICK, E. H., AND GARMEZY, N. (1957). An experimental approach to the study of motivation in schizophrenia. In M. R. Jones (Ed.) *Nebraska symposium on motivation.* Lincoln: Univer. of Nebraska Press, pp. 109–184.

ROMAN, M., AND BAUMAN, G. (1960). Interaction testing: A technique for the psychological evaluation of small groups. In M. Harrower, P. Vorhaus, M. Roman, and G. Bauman (Eds.) *Creative variations in the projective techniques.* Springfield, Ill.: Thomas, pp. 93–138.

ROSEBOROUGH, M. E. (1953). Experimental studies of small groups. *Psychol. Bull. 50,* 275–303.

ROSENTHAL, D., AND COFER, C. N. (1948). The effect on group performance of an indifferent and neglectful attitude shown by one group member. *J. exp. Psychol. 38,* 568–577.

RUESCH, J., BLOCK, J., AND BENNETT, L. (1953). The assessment of communciation: I: A method on the analysis of communications. *J. Psychol. 35,* 59–80.

SCHAFFER, L., WYNNE, L. C., DAY, J., RYCKOFF, I. M., AND HALPERIN, A. (1962). On the nature and sources of the psychiatrists' experience with the family of the schizophrenic. *Psychiatry 25*, 32–45.

SCHEFLEN, A. E. (1963). Communication and regulation in psychotherapy. *Psychiatry 26*, 126–136.

SCHEFLEN, A. E., ENGLISH, O. S., HAMPE, W., AND AUERBACH, A. (in press). *Analysis of psychotherapy: Whitaker and Malone.*

SCHMIDEBERG, M. (1948). Parents as children. *Psychiat. Quart. 22*, 207–218.

SEARLES, H. F. (1959). The effort to drive the other person crazy—an element in the aetiology and psychotherapy of schizophrenia. *Brit. J. med. Psychol. 32*, 1–18.

SHERIF, M., AND CANTRIL, H. (1947). *The psychology of ego-involvements.* New York: Wiley.

SOHLER, D., HOLZBERG, J. D., FLECK, S., CORNELISON, A. R., KAY, E., AND LIDZ, T. (1957). The prediction of family interaction from a battery of projective techniques. *J. proj. Tech. 21*, 199–208.

SPIEGEL, J. P. (1957). The resolution of role conflict within the family. *Psychiatry 20*, 1–16.

STEINZOR, B. (1949). The development and evaluation of a measure of social interaction. *Hum. Relat. 2*, 103–122.

STRODTBECK, F. L. (1951). Husband-wife interaction over revealed differences. *Amer. sociol. Rev. 16*, 468–473.

STRODTBECK, F. L. (1954). The family as a three-person group. *Amer. sociol. Rev. 19*, 23–29.

STRODTBECK, F. L. (1958). Family interaction, values, and achievement. In D. C. McClelland, A. L. Baldwin, U. Bronfenbrenner, and F. L. Strodtbeck (Eds.) *Talent and society.* New York: Van Nostrand, pp. 135–194.

STRODTBECK, F. L., AND HARE, A. P. (1954). Bibliography of small group research: From 1900 through 1953. *Sociomet. 17*, 107–178.

SULLIVAN, H. S. (1947). *Conceptions of modern psychiatry.* Wash., D.C.: William Alanson White Psychiat. Found.

SWANSON, G. E. (1951). Some problems of laboratory experiments with small populations. *Amer. sociol. Rev. 16*, 349–357.

THELAN, H. A., AND WITHALL, J. (1949). Three frames of reference: The description of climate. *Hum. Relat. 2*, 159–176.

TITCHENER, J., AND EMERSON, R. (1958). Some methods for the study of family interaction in personality development. In B. Pasamanick and P. H. Knapp (Eds.) *Psychiatric research reports*, vol. 10, pp. 72–88.

TITCHENER, J., D'ZMURA, T., GOLDEN, M., AND EMERSON, R. (1963). Family transaction and derivation of individuality. *Family Process 2*, 95–119.

VIDICH, A. J. (1956). Methodological problems in the observation of husband-wife interaction. *Marr. & Fam. Liv. 18*, 234–239.

WALTERS, J. (1962). A review of family research in 1959, 1960, and 1961. *Marr. & Fam. Liv. 24*, 158–178.

462 INTENSIVE FAMILY THERAPY

WALTZLAWICK, P. (1963a). A structured family interview. Palo Alto Medical Research Foundation, Palo Alto, Calif. (mimeo).

WATZLAWICK, P. (1963b). A review of the double bind theory. *Family Process 2*, 132–153.

WEAKLAND, J. H. (1960). The "double-bind" hypothesis of schizophrenia and three-party interaction. In D. D. Jackson (Ed.) *The etiology of schizophrenia*. New York: Basic Books, pp. 373–388.

WEAKLAND, J. H. (1962). Family therapy as a research arena. *Family Process 1*, 63–68.

WYNNE, L. C. (1961). The study of intrafamilial alignments and splits in exploratory family therapy. In N. W. Ackerman, F. L. Beatman, and S. N. Sherman (Eds.) *Exploring the base for family therapy*. New York: Fam. Serv. Ass. of Amer., pp. 95–115.

WYNNE, L. C., RYCKOFF, I. M., DAY, J., AND HIRSCH, S. I. (1958). Pseudo-mutuality in the family relations of schizophrenics. *Psychiatry 21*, 205–220.

WYNNE, L. C., AND SINGER, M. T. (1963). Thought disorder and the family relations of schizophrenics: I. A research strategy. *Arch. gen. Psychiat. 9*, 191–198.

12

HAROLD F. SEARLES

The Contributions of Family Treatment to the Psychotherapy of Schizophrenia

My qualifications for writing about this subject are in some regards slender indeed: I have participated in only about forty family therapy sessions. But I have had the privilege of working as a consultant, over a period of more than two years, to a research group engaged in such family therapy at the National Institute of Mental Health; to Dr. Lyman C. Wynne, head of that project, I am indebted for this experience, as well as for the rare opportunity to engage in this actual form of treatment itself. Fourteen years of experience with the individual therapy of schizophrenic patients, at Chestnut Lodge, has inevitably involved a sufficient number of direct and indirect contacts with families—contacts occurring, in the instances of several families, over a span of ten years or more, so that I have had reason to become interested in the potentialities, as well as the difficulties, of family therapy. A two-year period of experience with group psychotherapy, at a Veterans Administration out-patient clinic prior to my coming to the Lodge, early helped me to see somewhat

This study was supported by a grant from the Ford Foundation to the Chestnut Lodge Research Institute.

beyond the dyadic frame of reference. But the primary reason for my temerity in presenting my thoughts about this subject springs from my conviction that this is an important new field which the great majority of my fellows in individual therapy have not yet tasted and in which those persons who count themselves really experienced authorities are few indeed.

Partly, I think, because of the dyadic context of our training analyses, we have been slow to recognize the importance in psychoanalysis and psychotherapy of the *family* frame of reference. It came to me as a surprise, in the course of working with my first supervised case, to detect that, for a brief portion of one analytic hour, the neurotic patient was reacting to me, not as being a single transference figure, but rather as being both parents simultaneously, as being, specifically, her mother and father in sexual intercourse with one another. I later found an example of this very phenomenon described in the psychoanalytic literature;[1] but any such forms of more-than-one-other-person transference phenomena, any such kinds of *family* transference, are rarely to be found in the literature of psychoanalysis. Somewhat later on, I found that an initially catatonic woman had come to manifest, in her transference to me, a kind of *family-wide* sense of common helplessness, a conviction that there was not a strong figure in the whole family, and a sense of helpless waiting for some strong person to come upon the family (i.e., in the transference, to come upon the analytic session) scene. This had a distinctly different quality from the kind of two-person, mutual helplessness which one encounters so frequently.

When my father died, ten years ago, many were the persons whose lives he had enriched, in the Catskill village where he had lived out his life from birth onward, who came to offer consolation to my mother and sister and me and to share with us their own sense of loss. But one woman struck a chord which none of the others, however deep and genuine their feelings, touched upon: she spoke, in a single simple sentence, of the special loss involved when, for the first time, a family loses one of its members. This disclosed in me a kind of *family*-oriented feeling which, simple and obvious though it may sound, had been evoked neither by the other visitors, nor by the several years of my nearly completed personal analysis, in the course of which there had been abundantly detailed exploration of my feelings for *each* of my parental family members.

In recent years, in the course of working on committees concerned with various matters in the local psychoanalytic society and institute, I have wondered, of course, how many of our typical problems

---

[1] I have not been able to locate this reference.

arise from the acting-out of neurotic conflicts on the part of various students and society members, conflicts which have escaped, or are escaping, resolution in their respective training analyses. After having begun to think intensively about the subject of this paper, I have come to wonder whether the problem student, for example, is simply displacing upon the class instructor some negative feeling which needs to be experienced toward his training analyst, or, rather, whether these problem situations do not arise in part because, by tradition, the training analysis relationship is accepted as being, not only in actuality but also at a fantasy level, a dyadic frame of reference, such that various of the analysand's *family*-oriented conflicts seek, for their expression, an arena—such as the analytic classroom session or the analytic society or committee meeting which is in reality more similar to the family setting in which the particular conflict had its origin.

Approximately the first half of this paper will be devoted to a topic which, as I shall try to show, is of fundamental importance in the family therapy of schizophrenia: the distinction between processes which are predominantly intrapsychic and processes which are predominantly interpersonal. In the remainder of the paper I shall deal with various manifestations of positive feelings in the family background and in the family therapy interaction and with various countertransference phenomena.

Intrapsychic Processes and Interpersonal Processes in Psychotherapy

In working 14 years ago with my first psychoanalytic patient, an obsessive-compulsive man, it came to me as a surprise to realize that I had become, for him, more the personification of the mother of his childhood than was his own biological mother herself, who was living in the same small community and with whom he was interacting almost daily. That is to say, it came to me as a surprise to see that the real mother, as a denizen of outer reality, was less central to his neurotic functioning than was the intrapsychic early-mother imago, the early-mother introject, which had become reprojected upon me in the evolution of the transference relationship.

From this similarly early era of my psychoanalytic work, I vividly recall the relief evidenced by a phobic man who had long since become aware, in treatment, of his murderous fury toward his father, when I realized, and pointed out to him, that he was dealing basically, not with urges to kill his father as a flesh-and-blood person in outer reality, but rather with a determination to rid himself of, to destroy, an unwanted and neurotically crippling *identification with* his father.

Since then I have seen many times the neurotic, or psychotic, individual's confusion of intrapsychic processes with interpersonal processes (or, in other words, confusion of narcissistic processes with true object relations). Late in my own analysis, the analyst (Dr. Ernest E. Hadley) helped me to realize that the resolution of the transference does not mean the destruction of the analyst himself.

To continue in the same vein, I was interested in the two contrasting reports I received of a vacation trip made by a paranoid man I was treating, with an older brother, a father-surrogate with whom my patient had had a symbiotic relationship. The intended vacation had soon been disrupted by a severe argument between the two men, and they returned without their differences having been patched up. Upon their return, the brother confided to the administratve psychiatrist that he had been afraid the patient, white with fury, might kill him. By contrast, the patient expressed to me no awareness of wanting, or having wanted, to kill his brother, but he repeatedly and emphatically stated to me, "He's not my father!," spoke resentfully of the brother's trying, domineeringly, to "father" him, and spoke of the brother in such a tone, in fact, as to make clear that he, the patient, had psychologically ejected this brother from the family altogether. Previously, the patient had had a symbiotic experience of his whole parental family, such that when, for example, I once asked if he were not perhaps quite angry at the other members of his family, he showed genuine astonishment and replied, "Why, no, Dr. Searles, I'm not angry at *them; they're family!*," as if to be angry at one's family were inherently impossible, like reacting to one's right hand as separable from one's self. In short, what I felt to have been transpiring, during that vacation trip, was a process of long-overdue individuation on the part of the patient (and, I would assume, to some significant degree on the part of the overtly less ill brother also), a process of resolution of their erstwhile symbiosis, an event in which neither of the two participants could clearly see both the murderous (i.e., interpersonal) and individuation (i.e., intrapsychic) dimensions simultaneously. In my subsequent work with the patient, I recurrently saw his fear, at successive steps in his individuation, lest I be destroyed by the deepening separation between us.

One not infrequently sees evidence in a schizophrenic person's parent, similarly, of his or her fear that to function as a separate individual vis-à-vis the patient would mean the latter's death. One mother, for example, described to me her reason for having retained, for several years longer than she had meant to, an overly indulgent nursemaid for her now-schizophrenic son: she said that the nurse reported, one day, that while she was walking along the street with the patient on one hand and an older brother on the other hand, the patient had suddenly let go of the nurse's hand and darted across the street. Somewhat later in the same interview, the mother was describing her sense of helplessness to go ahead and speak her mind to her son, who, it had become clear to me (largely, of course, through my own first-hand experience with the patient), characteristically reinforced his regressive demands upon his mother and other persons with implied suicidal threats. When I endeavored to find out why she kept feeling a need for prescriptions from me as to what she should say to her son, the mother explained that "If I say something wrong, Bill might *do something.*" The vagueness of this wording, and the dread in her tone, left me in no doubt that she was chronically afraid to be herself with her son, lest he commit suicide. I found abundant evidence, on many occasions in addition to this one, that the mother was struggling with repressed murderous feelings toward the patient; but my main point here is her readiness to assume that if she allowed herself to reveal to this son the degree of hurt and anger and genuine concern which she could relatively freely express to me about him, he would somehow be destroyed. It was evident, further, that he exploited her fearfulness on this score by exacting infantile gratifications from her, in their basically symbiotic relationship, to an extent which had long impeded his own maturing.

In a number of married patients who were bent on divorce, I have seen that the patient's determination to "get a separation from" the marital partner consisted basically in a striving, long unrecognized as such by the patient himself or herself, to achieve a separation at an *intra*psychic level, to achieve a genuine individuation vis-à-vis wife or husband with whom there was a symbiotic mode of relatedness. In such instances, the marital partner had been responded to, not predominantly as a real other person, but rather as the personification of the unacceptable, projected part-aspects of the patient's self, or, one might say, as the personification of his own repressed self-images. Thus, the patient does have a need, however unrecognized as such, to achieve a separation between those repressed and projected aspects of himself, on the one hand, and the marital partner as a real and separate person on the other hand. The achievement of a "separation" at *this* level is essential both for he himself becoming a whole integrated individual, as well as for the achievement of a healthy object-relatedness in his marriage. It may well be that many instances of marital separations or divorces take place on the basis of such an unformulated, unconscious effort at individuation, an effort which fails because it is not seen in its true light and which leads instead simply to a subsequent, unrecognizedly symbiotic marriage, in which the next partner is reacted to, similarly, not as a real person but as the personification of unacceptable aspects of the self. In an earlier paper (Searles, 1951), I have conjectured that some instances of murder may represent, similarly, a miscarried and unrecognized effort at individuation.

I assume that there is no relationship between persons in which true object relations hold sway to the exclusion of any ingredients of projection (and introjection), nor any relationship so symbiotic (so dominated by projection-and-introjection) that no increment of real object-relatedness has been achieved. These clinical examples are intended to point up the distinction between those relationships which are *predominantly* on a truly interpersonal basis and those which are predominantly on a symbiotic (projective-and-introjective) basis.

These considerations are relevant to the onset of the schizophrenic psychosis, which, as I have indicated elsewhere (Searles, 1961b), seems typically to occur in a setting of the rupture of an identity-sustaining symbiotic relationship with a parent or parental figure. The patient is suddenly faced, thereby, with the overwhelming realization that the parent has been responding to him, not basically as a person in his own right, but rather as an extension of the parent. One patient expressed it as a realization that "people are only interested in themselves." To paraphrase this and analogous comments I have heard, the patient who has felt heretofore that he was in the very center of the parent's concerns, suddenly is faced with overwhelming evidence that the parent is so self-absorbed, really, as to be unaware even that the son or daughter, as a separate individual, exists. Thus, the "he" which the patient has been ceases to exist in his subjective experience also (since his sense of identity has been so largely bound up with his now-severed symbiosis with the parent) and there ensues a schizophrenic experience of himself-and-the-world (dedifferentiated, jumbled up together, and distorted in additional ways which I need not elaborate here), out of which a new sense of identity must, if he is to become a new and healthy person, eventually grow.

In the individual therapy relationship, this distinction between intrapsychic processes and interpersonal processes is often difficult to detect. For example, in an hour with a paranoid man, I was listening to his description of a TV program in which Bob Hope, comedy script in hand, had had as his guest an Army sergeant who was an aspiring amateur comedian. The patient clearly implied that Hope had reacted competitively to the sergeant, and he described how, when the sergeant had asked Hope for some of the script so that he could have the chance to show his own ability as a comedian, Hope had torn off a little corner of one sheet and had given it to him. The patient spontaneously related this to our relationship, likening me to Hope and saying, in a pleading tone, "Give me a break, Dr. Searles." I had long seen abundant evidence of his competitiveness with me, and my first reaction was to think of this as a plea from him to be given a fair chance in the competition with me. But then I realized that the more pertinent striving being evidenced here was his need and desire to *identify* with me, just as, I saw in retrospect (despite his clear emphasis, not reproduced here in detail, upon the competitive features of the relationship between the two persons on the TV program), the aspiring amateur must indeed have been hungry to identify with the accomplished Bob Hope.

On innumerable occasions, in my supervisory work as well as in my own therapeutic sessions with patients, I have seen that basically identificatory strivings are being defended against by competitive strivings which are, I think, more comfortable to therapist as well as to patient than are the early ego-building identificatory needs, the gratification of which is essential for any healthy object-relatedness, including a healthy ability to compete appropriately with one's fellow men. By the same token, I have come to see that the deeply repressed cannibalistic urges, of which the schizophrenic patient becomes aware only after prolonged therapy in most instances, are expressive basically, not of a truly interpersonal destructiveness, but rather of primitive but healthy identificatory needs.

The tangibly real quality of introjects in the subjective experience of the schizophrenic patient (whether experienced as being within the confines of his own body or, in reprojected form, as attributes of the outer world) is often startling for the therapist to discover. One cannot work long in this field without realizing the great service which has been performed by Melanie Klein (1932, 1955) and her followers (irrespective of the validity, or lack of validity, of some aspects of Kleinian theory) in highlighting the significance, in psychotic personality functioning, of such internalized objects. Several years ago, for example, it dawned on me that the schizophrenic woman's fear of rape is not basically a fear lest she be raped by a man, but rather a fear lest she be raped by a phallic mother-figure—by one or another woman round about, to whom she reacts as possessing a very real and terrifying penis—the projection of the penis, which at an unconscious level, she herself possesses on the basis of identification with the mother who, during the child's upbringing, in various ways acted out her unconscious conviction that she, the mother, possessed such a penis. It is often striking, too, to sense the biological literalness with which the patient perceives the male therapist as having female breasts and a vagina. Further, two of my six schizophrenic patients currently express their experience of both their own body and of mine as being peopled with myriad persons, expressing this in such a way as to leave no doubt that they do not perceive and conceptualize this as a figurative or symbolic phenomenon, but as a quite tangibly concrete one. One woman experiences these "persons" (a changing multitude of figures from current and past years, whom she often identifies with considerable conviction), as being confined within her shoulder, or her leg, or as being distressingly active within her head just above her eyes; or one among them is struggling to get free just below one of her scapulae; and so on.

The extent to which the schizophrenic patient possesses an introjected *family*, before he is brought to us for treatment, is sometimes seen in the patient who is able fairly rapidly to reproject such internalized (and no doubt greatly distorted) family members upon a collection of real persons about him on the hospital ward, such that his childhood family milieu and typical family interactions become reproduced with a fidelity of detail which is sometimes remarkable.[2] Similarly, in the still more deeply ill patient who is less capable of forming object relations and less capable, therefore, of thus unconsciously molding his current interpersonal world on the ward into the childhood family pattern, one sometimes sees to what a remarkable extent a hallucinated family is serving to perpetuate, for him, the familiar environment of his childhood family as (distortedly, no doubt) he perceived that family. Thus, whereas in the instance of the first type of patient, the ward personnel may be able quite readily to see that one of them is perceived as mother by the patient, another as father, another as sister, and another as Cousin Jeanne, in the instance of the latter patient it may become clear to the therapist that the patient rather durably experiences his mother as being in the ceiling and his father in the radiator. Or, in some instances, there is no structural embodiment for the hallucinations which is perceivable to the therapist with any consistency.

---

[2] In my paper in 1959, "Integration and Differentiation in Schizophrenia: An Over-All View," I presented some of my observations about this point; and just before the present volume went to press I discovered that Boszormenyi-Nagy and Framo, in their paper in 1962, "Family Concept of Hospital Treatment of Schizophrenia," give a most interesting presentation of similar concepts at which they, too, have arrived.

I have been discussing this subject at such length because it is of central significance to the family therapy of schizophrenia, and yet its significance is most easily overlooked in that very setting. When, for example, the schizophrenic patient reacts in the family setting to his mother as being cold and depriving, or to his father as being maternally warm but sexually provocative, it is all too easy for us as observers to be convinced that the patient is responding realistically to the parents as real persons, for we can see them to possess these qualities; moreover, we know that these persons have been most instrumental in the childhood development of the character traits which the patient is evidencing. It is comparatively seldom that the patient's reactions are sufficiently distorted or off-key or ill-timed to reveal that his central problem lies, not in the real mother and father whom we are perceiving, but rather in an *introject*, formed many years ago, of the cold and depriving early mother and an *introject* of the maternally warm but sexually provocative father, introjects which he has been able to externalize upon the real mother and father, to whom such qualities seem so naturally to "belong," rather than perceiving these qualities as attributes, also, of himself and achieving an integration of these various qualities within his own ego.

A paranoid woman, married and the mother of three children, for several years in the course of her individual therapy maintained so tenacious and so vociferous a conviction that her husband was impotent and worthless that he finally grew unwilling to wait longer for her recovery, divorced her, and married another woman. Although I was quite aware, all along, that she was abundantly delusional, such contacts as I had with her husband coincided sufficiently with her view of him, as did her parents' expressed estimates of his worth, that I accepted her view of him as comparatively realistic. It was only later on that I felt I had erred grievously in not seeing the extent to which her view of her husband had been, all along, a sick and distorted view. Likewise, all through these years she had castigated me, very similarly, for my impotence in manifold regards; my own sense of helplessness in face of her massive pathology was sufficiently intense that I inwardly accepted her view of both me and her husband as being less than real men. It was only after several years of therapy, and after her husband had divorced her, that the therapeutic investigation had proceeded sufficiently deeply to reveal the extent to which she had been projecting upon both him and me (as well as upon many other persons round about) an unconscious, castrated-male image of herself. Significantly, as this image became resolved, she came to realize for the first time in all our work that she (who had continually been sexually misidentifying herself and other persons) was a woman and that I a man. But, when she was psychologically ready to relate herself to the real man (whatever his weaknesses) in her former husband, and to respond to this real man affirmatively rather than castratively, it was too late.

In an experience I had, in company with another therapist, with one schizophrenic young woman and her parents, it was striking to discover to what a degree various interactions in which strongly oedipal ingredients were readily apparent were, at a deeper level, being determined by pre-oedipal processes, processes of a symbiotic, early ego formation nature. For example, the father, although at one level greatly concerned to establish his dominance as father and leader in the total group situation, at a deeper level was concerned with conflicts relevant to the matter of ego boundaries: specifically, his deep need for masculine identification with the cotherapists, versus his anxiety lest such identification lead to the loss of his symbosis with his daughter, reacted to by him, at this deep level, as the Good Mother. When I endeavored to help him recognize the erotic components in his feelings toward his daughter, components which I described as natural to any father's feelings toward his daughter and which I readily acknowledged as part of my feelings for my own daughter, he was horrified, reacted to me as something untouchably alien and inhuman, and declared, in a voice shaking with feeling, "If you know she's your flesh and blood, nothing like that pops into your mind!" and, emphasizing the unbridgeable gulf between himself and me, shouted, "That's *my* name, *Davis*, not *Searles!*" This was only the culmination of a series of incidents pointing up his anxiety lest he lose his sense of union with the Good Mother image which he attributed to his daughter and become fused instead with the horrifyingly evil parent image which he externalized upon me, upon his wife, or, at times, upon both of the therapists.

It is especially because the family members themselves are so unaware of this realm of projected (and introjected) intrapsychic content, so unaware of any boundaries between intrapsychic and genuinely interpersonal realms, so unaware that they are not reacting primarily to the other persons in the room as flesh-and-blood persons in outer reality but primarily as the personifications of repressed and projected self-images, that the therapist himself must be alert to these separate, or potentially separate, realms.

A number of writers have emphasized the importance of distinguishing between these realms of experience. Warren M. Brodey's (1959, 1961) stimulating concepts, derived from the family therapy of schizophrenia, concerning the distinctions among what he calls

image, object, and narcissistic relationships, are of the most fundamental value in this connection. Rather than attempting to paraphrase his views, which are rich indeed, I shall give only two brief
quotes to point up the relevance of his work to the present paper:

> . . . *In the image relationship,* the inner image of the other person takes
> precedence: the emphasis is on *changing reality to fit with expectation*
> rather than expectation to fit reality . . . . . . the *narcissistic rela-
> tionship* is . . . descriptive of two people *each making an image rela-
> tionship to the other and each acting within this relationship so as to
> validate the image-derived expectation* of the other . . . . [Brodey,
> 1961][3]

Arieti (1961), in discussing the question of whether or when
a nonhospitalized schizophrenic patient should leave his family to
live by himself, asks,

> First of all, is it advisable? On the one hand we may think that it is in
> the family that the troubles of the patient started, and there, probably,
> that they are maintained. On the other hand, we may feel that to remove
> the patient from his family would not really be helpful because *this
> would be merely a removal from the external situation, not from the
> introjected conflicts.* As a matter of fact, one might even think that this
> separation might re-exacerbate the symptoms. We remember, for in-
> stance, Geraldine, who started to hallucinate again when she was
> separated from her mother.[4]

Lidz and Fleck (1960) report that, among the traits which recur
frequently among the mothers of schizophrenic patients, is a tendency on the mother's part to confuse the child's needs with her
own needs projected upon the child, a failure to recognize ego boundaries between herself and the child. Bowen (1960), from his experience with the family therapy of schizophrenia, describes it thus:

> . . . the subjects of the mother's overconcerns about the patients and the
> focus of their 'picking on the patients' are the same as their own feelings
> of inadequacy about themselves. This point is so accurate on a clinical
> level that almost any point in the mothers' list of complaints about the
> patient can be regarded as an externalization of the mother's own in-
> adequacies.

A number of writers have described the parents in these families
as being so much a part, still, of their own parental families that
they are not really psychologically a part of their marital family.

---

[3] Italics mine.
[4] Italics mine.

Lidz, Cornelison, Fleck, and Terry (1957), reporting data from 16 families of schizophrenic patients studied by them over a period of several years, state that in five of these families, the parents' loyalties remained in their respective parental homes, preventing the formation of a nuclear family in the marital home. The cardinal emotional attachment and dependency of one or both partners in these five families, the authors found, remained fixed to a parental figure and could not be transferred to the spouse. Wynne, Ryckoff, Day, and Hirsch (1958) point out that:

. . . going into the Army, moving to another city, even getting married and having children of one's own, may in some cases mean going through the motions of following social conventions as part of familial expectations, without a genuine sense of identity apart from the (parental) family system.

It is worth noting that such an attachment to the parental family is, basically, but one form of an emotional investment in *internal objects* which I have been describing as so necessary to distinguish from an investment predominantly in genuine interpersonal relationships. A paper by Towne, Sampson, and Messinger (1961) helps to highlight the importance of this intrapsychic realm. Reporting upon a group of 17 young women who had become schizophrenic within a relatively few years after marriage, they suggest that:

. . . these women foundered upon two broad tasks presented by participation in the marital family: detaching themselves from the claims of parental ties, and synthesizing conflicting childhood identifications within a workable adult identity . . .

Thus, in the crisis preceding hospitalization, Mrs. White (for example) was confronted with various identification fragments (and defenses against them) which had previously remained in partial dissociation. These images of herself—as a confused little girl in possession of secret and terrible information; as a long-suffering, neglected and betrayed wife and mother; as a frustrated, masculine careerist; as an oedipally victorious daughter, and as a promiscuous philanderer—were related to earlier identifications formed in relation to a frustrating and martyred mother, a prepossessing male mother-substitute, and a seductive, jealous, oedipal father.

What I have been trying to bring out is the fact that, in the family therapy of schizophrenia session, the patient (as well as the other family members) is often successful in externalizing (unconsciously) upon one or another of the others in the room such repressed self-images as Towne *et al.* (1961) describe, that it is extraordinarily difficult, however essential, for the therapist to keep clear that it is not basically the mother or father, for example, who is central to the patient's illness, but rather the patient's introject, distorted and unintegrated into his ego, of that parent. I am putting this in extremely oversimplified terms, of course, simply to highlight this principle.

I have wondered whether it is possible that, just as an individual family member has what one might call "unconscious selves" or unconscious self-images, there may perhaps be, in the family, a *somewhat* integrated "unconscious family" which is determining, far more than meets the eye, what transpires in the family therapy interaction. My experience with the ward group relatedness, as well as with the parental and marital family relatedness, of patients with whom I have worked in individual therapy suggests that there are indeed such "unconscious families," however poorly integrated and shifting, and that it may therefore be crucial, in doing family therapy, to try to determine who, at the moment, is really (at an unconscious level in the family) being the father, who the mother, who the son, and so on, quite irrespective of the sociologic and biologic realities of the situation. A comparatively simple example comes from the marital family situation of a paranoid woman with whom I worked for several years. Among herself, her husband, and her teen-age daughter, it was evidently *generally* agreed upon, though at an unconscious level in all three (until this came more into the open in the patient's "delusional" material), that the husband occupied the role of wife and mother in the family and that the daughter had succeeded in displacing the patient from the husband and father role. It is, I believe, toward the derepression of such "unconscious family" modes of relatedness that one's family therapy efforts must be directed.

When one considers that projection and introjection must be among the basic psychodynamic processes by means of which object-relatedness is achieved in the normal development of the child, it is striking to see the extent to which the products of such processes, occurring among the members of the schizophrenic patient's family, are *in competition with* genuine object-relatedness. The real mother in the room, for example, must carry on a quite real competition with her own, and with the father's, introjects of the Good Mothers of their respective childhoods, and the schizophrenic son or daughter who is present is reacted to as living evidence of the mother's failure in that competition. That is, the fact that this son or daughter, sitting there is afflicted with schizophrenia, is testimony of the mother's having failed to fulfill the mothering role in the way in which these idealized and internalized Good Mothers presumably would have done.

One of my schizophrenic patients said to me during an individual therapy session, "I want you to know that I don't come here because I'm interested in seeing *you*; I just like to hear myself talk." This reminded me of an incident when I was talking with her father in a corridor of the sanitarium at the time of her admission. As we talked, he showed no interest in me at all, but was admiring himself in a mirror which happened to be located above my shoulder.

Dr. Leslie Schaffer has commented, ironically but very perceptively, after observing a family therapy session through a one-way screen, "I had a thought that if someone were standing sufficiently far out, it might look as if these people were talking with each other." The spuriousness of the "object-relatedness" in these families consists, I believe, in the fact that, taken as a whole, they are defensive and premature. Specifically, they are defensive against the threat of symbiotic undifferentiatedness, and they are premature because such undifferentiatedness needs to hold sway, at a deep level, between any two persons, needs to hold sway and be faced and accepted before genuine object-relatedness can mature from this undifferentiatedness.

I have been helped, in reaching the above concept, by a statement made by Hendrick (1931):

We are suggesting that cannibalization (ingestion, introjection, scotomization) is not the skeletal mechanism of autism, but that the refusal of the primitive ego to perform this function is. Renunciation of the outer world appears actually to be equivalent to "vomiting" instead of normal ingestion, to ejection of the tentatively introjected object.

Of additional illumination has been a comment by Havens (1961) in a paper which I had the pleasure of discussing. In describing the maternal relationships of hallucinated schizophrenic patients, Havens (in support of the above-quoted statement by Hendrick, which is included in Havens' paper) reports that

. . . The mother is neither differentiated from the patient nor completely absorbed. The relationship appears to have been one not of symbiosis but of *seige* and the state of seige represented by the object's (i.e., the mother-hallucination's) distance from the patient is the extension into imaginary life of the long-term family condition. When this is true, the hallucination does not represent the externalization of a previously "absorbed" mother-figure but the substitution of an imaginary object for a real one that was never identified with.

A healthy family may be thought of as being, at an unconscious level of participation, a fermenting mixture of projected and introjected part-aspects of the personalities of the various participants, out of which the children in the family develop individual beings, and out of which the parents, as well, achieve a deepening and refashioning of the selves which were established during their respective childhoods. The family which includes a schizophrenic member may be likened more, in this regard, to a seething cauldron, in which such pseudo object-relatedness as one observes is largely defensive against the inordinately great, primitive identification needs of a collection of persons none of whom has successfully traversed this era of early ego-formation and in all of whom there is a basically healthy need, therefore, for undifferentiated (or, at a somewhat later developmental level, incorporative) relatedness but a correspondingly great anxiety lest their tenuous object-relatedness, which is so largely spurious and ill-established, be dissolved into such primitive undifferentiatedness. It can be seen that the striving toward symbiosis, here, is not merely a striving to complete an interrupted developmental phase in the past, but is also a striving to overcome the gulf which, as the participants must at some deep level be painfully aware, separates them from one another, despite their ostensible object-relatedness (or, in the phrase of Wynne et al., their pseudomutuality). It is the intensity of this conflict between the more primitive versus the more adult modes of relatedness which is, I believe, pathognomonic of the family of which the schizophrenic person is a member.

Bowen is one of the persons who has pioneered, not only in the development of the family therapy of schizophrenia, but also in highlighting the importance of symbiotic relatedness in these families. In an article (1960) tracing the development of his orientation to this mode of therapy of schizophrenia, he emphasized that: "The family unit is regarded as a single organism and the patient is seen as that part of the family organism through which the overt symptoms of psychosis are expressed." Wynne et al. (1958) use comparable phraseology in describing their approach to the family therapy of schizophrenia: "In this program a case is regarded as consisting of an entire family unit, including both parents and offspring."

The more deeply one comes to perceive the psychodynamic processes which hold sway in these families, the more startled one is to discover to what an extent the family is not truly a family at all, in the sense of a group of individuals, but comprises in aggregate what might be thought of as one symbiotic individual. Wynne et al. (1958) have described perceptively and in vivid terms a kind of "rubber fence" which one discovers in these families, which serves to provide the family with a sense, however false, of mutuality and complementarity in their relationships with one another:

> The shared, familial efforts to exclude from open recognition any evidence of noncomplementarity within the pseudomutual relation become group mechanisms that help perpetuate the pseudomutuality. In the families of schizophrenics these mechanisms act at a primitive level in preventing the articulation and selection of any meanings that might enable the individual family member to differentiate himself either within or outside of the family role structure. Family boundaries thus obscured are continuous but unstable, stretching, like a rubber fence, to include that which can be interpreted as complementary and contracting to extrude that which is interpreted as noncomplementary.

I think of this "rubber fence" as serving basically to preserve, for the family, what might be thought of as a family-wide, symbiotic ego. Individuation poses such a great threat, because, were individuation to occur in a family where so little ego structure has become established in any of the individuals and where there is so great a dependency upon a family-wide, shared or symbiotic ego, this would be tantamount to ego fragmentation. Thus, the rubber fence, hypocritical though its manifestations appear to the therapist who works with the family, represents the family members' largely unconscious attempt to cope with, and conceal, their pathetically genuine lack of collective ego structures.

It is notable, in this same connection, that this rubber fence forces each family member toward greater *freedom*, in their behavior toward one another, than the extrafamilial culture will allow. Specifically, the danger of incest is heightened in a family where a potential incest partner cannot be renounced for fear of renunciation of the so-necessary underlying symbiotic attachment to that person. The rubber fence forces the family member to turn his emotional needs toward tabooed goals, toward sexual involvement with, and aggression against, the very persons whom the extrafamilial culture (with which the family member is in some degree of contact) decrees it most forbidden to have such impulses: the parents and siblings. Another way of putting it is that the need of the family members to serve as partial egos for one another, as part-objects for one another, intensifies the incest and murder threat attaching to such rudimentary object relationships as are getting formed within, by decree of the family-symbiosis, the family itself.

But, while any developing genuine person-to-person closeness within the family involves such intense taboos from the extrafamilial culture, any genuine moving apart involves, as I have noted, a comparably intense threat of collective ego fragmentation. Wynne *et al.* (1958) comment that:

. . . both parents have frequently emphasized their vulnerability to cardiovascular disaster if they should become upset . . .

. . . The social organization in these families is shaped by a pervasive familial subculture of myths, legends, and ideology which stresses the dire consequences of openly recognized divergence from a relatively limited number of fixed, engulfing family roles.

The longer I have worked with schizophrenic patients, the more I have come to respect the intensity of the anxiety, so apt indeed to produce ego fragmentation and/or psychosomatic disaster, which is represented by such "myths, legends, and ideology." A schizophrenic man with whom I once worked for a prolonged time had a history in which each of his parents had died of coronary occlusion at times when the patient's symbiotic attachment to them was in danger of resolution; an older sister had a severe though nonfatal coronary occlusion precisely at a point when the patient's symbiosis with her had started to shift markedly; the patient lingered almost at death's door for several months in reaction to severe threats to his own symbiotic attachments; and for my part, I had, on more than one occasion, "countertransference" reactions which I had never felt before in my work with anyone: acute anxiety lest I drop dead, occurring during phases of intensified growth on the patient's part, and evoked by his anxiety, based on repeated past experiences in his family, lest this indeed happen to me. I am citing, here, only the most striking one among many hardly less sobering experiences from my work and from colleagues' reports of their work here at Chestnut Lodge.

From this viewpoint, then, the rubber fence can be looked upon as the family's collective, and unconscious, dynamic equilibrium between their intense need, on the one hand, to maintain a collective ego, the only at all reliable ego there is in the family, and, on the other hand, their ceaseless strivings, respectively, for individuality. The emergence of psychosis in the patient represents, therefore, not only his own heretofore-thwarted striving toward individuality, but also the vicariously expressed strivings of a similar nature on the part of the other family members. It is probably more adequate to conceptualize this advent of psychosis as a shift in the total family's mode of dealing with their unresolved, conflicting needs for symbiosis and individuation.

Positive Feelings

As I have reported elsewhere, I have become deeply impressed with the intensity of the schizophrenic patient's positive feelings

(Searles, 1958, 1961a), and I believe that many of the therapists who are exploring this comparatively new field of the family therapy of schizophrenia are underestimating, perhaps out of their eagerness to demonstrate the other family members' contribution to the patient's illness, the real and deeply significant role of positive feelings in the family interaction as a whole. A number of my patients, after several years of individual therapy, have become able to reveal the warm delight which they, and the family as a whole, find in just such kinds of family craziness as are portrayed in the literature in this field as bearing an exclusively malignant connotation. A number of my women patients came to express anguish at their childless state, anguish related in part to their inability to perpetuate the family name; such communications have been filled in each instance with a sense of deeply human tragedy. In the instance of a schizophrenic man with whom I have worked, intensively, for thirteen years, I have come to realize that his parents' devotion to this long treatment endeavor has not been based primarily, as I long thought, upon guilt but rather upon affection—or, to put it more bluntly, love—of a degree of intensity which I have found both moving and humbling to behold. Their hatred for their son, of which I long ago saw much solid evidence, was in a way easier for me to discover than was this underlying love, which only the passage of the years has brought before me in such a way that I can no longer ignore or minimize it.

It is essential for us to realize that the kind of family loyalty which one finds in these families has, for all its constrictingly pathologic aspects, a nucleus of genuinely positive feeling which is, for the family members, including the patient, most cherished indeed. However tragically warped and turned in upon itself, there is locked up here one of the highest aspirations of the human spirit. On occasion, when I have seen the anguish experienced by a schizophrenic patient at finding himself torn between his newly developing self, on the one hand, and his family loyalty on the other hand, I have been reminded of the words of the Psalmist: "If I forget thee, O Jerusalem, let my right hand forget her cunning."[5]

Even the brief experience which I have had with the family therapy of schizophrenia has been replete with evidence of positive feeling, though this is often less dramatically evident than are the many manifestations of real and pervasive hatred. I have been greatly struck by the degree of trust implied in a father's exposing not only himself but his whole family to the efforts of the family therapist. I have seen something of how hungry are the family

---

[5] Psalms 137:5

members for more of real family relatedness, for more of the real interpersonal closeness which they are at some level aware of missing; the power of this striving to become genuinely a family is, I think, of a piece with every neurotic or psychotic human being's striving toward health as an individual.

In evaluating a family's potential strength and capacity for growth as a family, it is well to keep in mind that we are working with a family which has decompensated, which has become disorganized and is not functioning at the level at which it was functioning in earlier and better years. That is, just as regression is one feature of the psychosis which has become overt in the patient himself, at least some significant degree of regression has occurred in the over-all family relatedness; so, not merely the patient himself, but all these persons may possess more maturity, collectively and as a family, than is apparent in the present state of decompensation, or regression, in their family life. A paper by Lidz and Fleck (1960), describing the serious disorganizations which occur in the families of schizophrenic patients, has helped me to see this aspect of the family therapy situation.

Along the same line, if the mother, for example, as we currently see her in family therapy, is significantly different from the *early* mother (the mother of the patient's early childhood), and still more widely different from the patient's distorted and introjected early mother-*images*, then this has some important implications. Part of the mother's ego identity must be having to remain at this earlier level to meet the primitive needs of her psychotic son or daughter. It would follow that part of her resentment toward the offspring is related to this thwarting of her own maturation and that among the beneficial results of family therapy will be her becoming freer to be her more mature self. Benedek's (1959) paper, "Parenthood as a Developmental Phase," helps us to realize that not only childhood and adolescence, but also adulthood, is a time of continuously unfolding development; so we can surmise, in approaching the family therapy of schizophrenia, that not only was the patient's childhood development thwarted by the mother, but also the mother's development as a mother is being thwarted by the schizophrenic offspring.

In the first family therapy session in which I participated, I found myself enjoying greatly the interaction in which I was taking part, and I realized that I very much wanted it not to change; this gave me a firsthand sample of the positive gratifications which the family members themselves may be deriving from the status quo. It stands to reason that the family must be harboring much more of positive feeling toward one another than they reveal at all openly and early in treatment; if not, in light of the severity of the clashes which occur among them during the sessions, they would kill one another, or otherwise destroy their ties to one another, in the intervals between the therapy sessions. The fact that they do not thus act upon, between sessions, such feelings as they have verbalized during the therapeutic interaction may be taken as a very significant, though nonverbal, acknowledgment by all of them as to the important role of transference, projection, introjection, and other distortions in their therapeutic-session reactions to one another.

It is essential for therapy that we make contact with the positive strivings in the family, for without an awareness of these we cannot understand the historical development of psychosis in the patient and disorganization in the family as a whole; in this development the factor of unassimilated grief (over the loss of cherished relationships) has a fundamental role. Furthermore, without an appreciation of the strength of the love feelings, no matter how repressed, we cannot appreciate the absolutely key role of *ambivalence* in the pathology with which we are trying to cope. I have reported earlier my finding that schizophrenic regression is a defense not against aggression alone, as is stated by Bak (1954) and others, but against, rather, ambivalence; against, that is, intensities of both hatred and love which, without the benefit of psychotherapy, tear apart the individual's attempt at more mature ego integration (Searles, 1961a). Those writings which detail only the hateful aspects of the relatedness among the members of the schizophrenic patient's family bypass altogether the central tragedy in these families: the extent to which the family members are being crippled and paralyzed by their inability to face the fact that they *both* intensely hate *and* deeply love one another. Only insofar as the therapist can help them to face both their love and their hatred can they relinquish the symbiotic mode of relatedness which is serving as their family-wide unconscious defense against this ambivalence, but which is thwarting, by the very nature of this relatedness, their development of ego maturity and genuine object-relatedness with one another.

I wish to make a few more comments concerning the family etiology of schizophrenia in the patient, beyond this matter of positive feelings, before turning to the topic of countertransference.

Loss, or the Threat of Loss, of Membership in the Family

It is to be noted that, in these particular families, the matter of membership in the family is, for each member, not something biologically given, but is to be maintained only through participation in the family symbiosis. The patient, as a child, has had only two choices: (1) to be part of the family symbiosis, or (2) to be reacted to as a nonmember of the family, and, by the same token, as "crazy." Ironically, since one must have a successful experience with the symbiotic phase of ego maturation in order to avoid autism (craziness), and since the family offers the patient his only *available* chance for symbiotic experience (unless a therapist comes along and offers him such an experience), it is tragically true that, for him, nonmembership in the family indeed is tantamount to craziness. Long before the onset of his psychosis, the patient has labored under the chronic threat of psychological banishment from the family should he fail to fulfill his role as the personification of the warded-off part-aspects of his parents', and other family members', personalities. It is significant, too, that when and if he eventually recovers from his schizophrenia, he may find that the rest of the family presents a closed-corporation aspect to him; they have no place, here, for a whole person.

During the prodromal phase of the patient's schizophrenia, his progressive withdrawal from the other members of his family is so conspicuous that we may underestimate the mutuality of this withdrawal, the extent to which the other family-members have lost interest in him and have barred him, progressively, from functional membership in the family. The observations by Schwartz and Will (1953) concerning the degree to which ward-personnel participate in, and contribute to, the therefore mutual withdrawal involving the progressively-withdrawing schizophrenic patient, help one to realize what the patient has experienced, prior to his hospitalization, vis-à-vis the members of his family.

In many of these families, the ego state of *not knowing*, of seeking for clarification, is considered equivalent to being crazy, which in turn means being considered hopelessly apart and ineligible for membership in the family. The child has long ago learned not to question seriously the blandly pointless and discoordinated discussions which are so typical of these families. None of the members dares to question these, for to feel, and reveal, confusion is to run the risk of being considered crazy for questioning that which is tacitly agreed to be obvious and unquestionable. The previously mentioned paper by Wynne *et al.* (1958) deals perceptively with matters relevant to this point. Particularly with each of the paranoid schizophrenic patients I have treated, it has been a most welcome and hard-won development for the patient to become able to reveal his deep and previously repressed confusion; growth is possible only to the extent that one can endure confusion and uncertainty.

The patient has been reacted to conflictually, in the family, by the various others not simply as a whole person but, even more ego disruptively, as a part-object for the maintenance of their respective psychic economics. One of my patients expressed this in somatic terms, saying that one "faction" always controlled her lungs, another her stomach, another her heart, and so on. Normally, I presume, a mother protects the little child, mainly through her own comparatively unambivalent symbiosis with him, from such complex and conflictual "usage" by the various family members.

One of my paranoid patients, telling how in high school his brother had condemned him as being a "force of evil," gave me some glimpse of how devastating it must be, for a child who has no solid whole-person relationships to which to cling, to be thus reacted to as part-object—as, in this instance, the embodiment of the brother's repressed and projected hostility.

The increasingly formidable impact, upon the other family members, of the progressively anxious and hostile child who is on the way to schizophrenia is itself an etiologic factor of great importance. Whereas I used to feel scorn for those parents who are always seeking prescriptions as to "what to say" to their schizophrenic son or daughter, I have come to realize that the patient, with his deeply hurtful and anxiety-provoking verbal and nonverbal behavior, stirs up such powerful and conflictual feelings in the parents that it would be difficult for any one, under these circumstances, to be able unaided to find words to express the welter of hurt, grief, rage, and so on, which, as the therapist learns at first hand, is evoked. Because the parents cannot integrate such deeply ambivalent feelings in reaction to the patient's communications, their front of bland denial-of-feeling tends to become intensified. So the patient finds himself progressively deprived of any real and accessible person to whom to relate; this in turn throws him more and more back upon functioning, toward the other family members, as a projected part-object.

In general, the nature of the family symbiosis, with its spurious (though defensively so essential) atmosphere of "family oneness," places a taboo upon any meaningful one-to-one relationships within (or outside) the family. But one-to-one relationships represent the highest order of interpersonal complexity which the young child (or the adult schizophrenic patient) can integrate successfully and are utterly essential to the formation of healthy identifications and the healthy emergence from (in contrast to an autistic flight from) symbiotic relatedness.

Countertransference

In approaching the subject of countertransference, we should take the full measure, first, of the emotional burdens which are *inherent* in the family therapy of schizophrenia and which will evoke deeply conflictual feelings, and anxiety of oftentimes severe degree, in any therapist no matter how well analyzed he may have been. He inevitably will experience much conflict and anxiety with respect to his role in relationship to the family group, as a reflection, or sample, of the anxiety and ambivalence which was aroused in the patient himself, in earlier years, with regard to the matter of membership or nonmembership in the family. The acute sense of isolation which I at times have experienced in this situation, when I felt shut out by all others in the room, was reminiscent to me of one of the most severe kinds of pressure which one encounters in the individual therapy of a hospitalized schizophrenic patient: the sense of deeply anxious isolation one experiences upon occasions when one feels that the patient, the ward personnel, the psychiatric administrator, and others all share a completely harmonious view as to one's own malignant unacceptability.

When, on the other hand, the therapist is feeling himself to be part of the family, he experiences a different kind of pressure, which is again, I believe, a sample of that to which the patient himself has long been exposed in the family, namely, a feeling of acute conflict as to which of the family members is most in need of support at the moment. In earlier papers, I have reported evidence of the patient's basically therapeutic efforts on behalf of his mother (Searles, 1958, 1961a), and this therapeutic attitude is, I believe, his most basic attitude toward the family members collectively.

Following one family therapy session, it occurred to me that I had had, during the session, some goals in mind with reference to each of the family members but that it had been impossible to think in terms of a goal for the family as a whole. This was presumably a reaction, on my part, to the discoordination which holds sway in these families behind the pseudomutuality which has been described by Wynne *et al.* (1958). Such a reaction gives one a clue to the extent to which this "family" is not really a family in the sociodynamic sense, but rather a group symbiosis in which the part-object roles of the various participants are shifting constantly. This is to say, one reacts emotionally less to the rigid outward structure in the family than to the underlying fluidity of ego boundaries, such that, characteristically, there is no one in the room with whom one feels a continuing sense of reliable contact.

The rapidly changing transference patterns which I encountered in this therapeutic situation were in marked contrast to my experience in doing group therapy with a group of out-patients comprised largely of neurotic individuals, with a relatively few schizoid or borderline schizophrenic indivduals; there, the transference patterns were comparatively easy to trace as they unfolded week after week and month after month. In the family therapy of schizophrenia, not only the sense of emotional relatedness but also that of meaning is, of course, markedly disrupted and discoordinate, such that it is difficult or impossible to find any one thread of meaning running throughout the typical session.

Bowen (1960), after describing the early difficulties which therapists and ward personnel encountered in terms of becoming embroiled in the various family members' different emotional points of view, reports that:

. . . When it was possible to attain a workable level of interested detachment, it was then possible to begin to defocus the individual and to focus on the entire family at once . . . Once it was possible to focus on the family as a unit, it was like shifting a microscope from the oil immersion to the low-power lens, or like moving from the playing field to the top of the stadium to watch a football game. Broad patterns of form and movement that had been obscured in the close-up view became clear. The close-up view could then become more meaningful once the distant view was also possible.

It would seem that both the close-up and the distant views are equally essential and that the family therapist needs to become able to shift from one mode of participation to the other, as the needs of the moment require. It is just such an integration of these different vantage points, such a ready communicability between them, which the patient himself (and to a significant degree the other family members also) has not been able to acquire. For him, closeness (or participation) with the other family members has meant enmeshment in a conflictual symbiotic relatedness, and extrication from this state has meant isolation and unrelatedness.

It should be seen how intensely and basically ambivalent is the reaction of the family (including the patient) to the therapist as a representative of threatening extrafamilial reality. The family members all strive unconsciously either to render him nonexistent, psychologically, or to mold him into one or another (constantly changing) part-object role (that is to say, into the personification of one or another of their repressed self-images). If they cannot succeed in so molding him or obliterating him, the family members collectively lose their fantasied omnipotence. I have described this molding as representative of a basically healthy need to ingest—to primitively identify with—a healthy mother-object; but here this basically healthy need is being expressed—until such time as a predominantly hateful orientation has given place to a predominantly loving one—in the service of maintaining the infantile fantasy of grandiosity, the fantasy that there is no durable external world which will be other than plasticine in the hands of one's own needs and desires. Yet, on the other hand, the family members desperately need for the therapist to remain solid and whole, for otherwise they cannot become well and mature. So the therapist is inescapably buffeted by the family's ambivalence toward him.

Apart from such difficulties which are inherent in family therapy, there is a truly countertransference factor of the therapist's not having adequately worked through, in his own analysis, those personal conflicts upon which this kind of therapy specifically impinges. As I intimated at the outset, our dyadically oriented training analysis leaves us, typically, with a realm of comparatively unexplored (repressed) *family*-oriented feeling which tends to emerge in the form of countertransference reactions when we attempt to do family therapy. Some papers on family therapy seem to be written in a spirit largely of childish glee at the writer's having "gotten something on" the family of the patient; there is a close similarity between this emotional tone and that of the analytic student who, too early in his analysis to have come face to face with his feelings of love and grief with respect to his mother and father, eagerly volunteers the evidence of their blameworthiness for his personal psychopathology. I surmise that the derepression of our feelings, especially those of love and grief, about our *families* has lagged behind our grasp of the feelings which have been formed within the two-person context with our mother or with our father. The defensively symbiotic front of "harmony" which prevails in the family of the schizophrenic patient tends so powerfully to obscure the participants' own feelings of genuinely human loyalty, tragedy, nobility, and other basically positive feelings that this makes it extraordinarily difficult for the therapist, also, to perceive such emotional ingredients in the family interactions; thus, it is all the more incumbent upon him not to be content with a cataloguing of the negative aspects of the family-relatedness, a cataloguing of, that is, their psychopathology. It becomes incumbent upon him to try to perceive the basically human family struggles and tragedies against which their psychopathology is defending these family-members.

One is tempted to sneer at the so-hypocrisy-laden loyalty, for example, which we find in these families; but this suggests that we have not worked through our own feelings of early loss of the

Good Objects with whom we were once so deeply and symbiotically affiliated. In general, I believe, as I have devoted the whole first third of this paper to showing, we tend to overestimate the degree of true object-relatedness which is transpiring in the family, out of our need to keep from realizing the degree to which part-object (symbiotic) relatedness held sway in our own parental family during our childhood, and the degree to which part-object introjects hold sway within us still. That is, it would be deflating to us to realize to what an extent our family members as a whole reacted to us, not as a person in our own right, but rather as the externalization of their own Good or Bad Objects; and to what an extent our own reactions to them have been comparably intrapsychic in nature. There is such a degree of genuine loss attached to this realization that we tend unconsciously to perpetuate this symbiotic parental family of ours in the realm of our repressed introjects. It is to be emphasized here that it is not the loss of our parental family members as separate and whole objects against which we are thus defending ourselves, but rather the loss of the symbiotic Family Oneness, so boundariless that all are felt to be, literally, of one heart and mind and soul.

The nature of the family therapy setting tends to evoke, then, in us, these unintegrated introjects which have thus far escaped detection in our dyadic training analysis. But I cannot overemphasize how effectively this family therapy setting tends not only to evoke the therapist's countertransference reactions, but also to keep obscured their nature *as* countertransference, rather than predominantly reality, reactions. The therapist's unconscious feelings can find vicarious expression, on the part of one or another of the family members, all too readily, because it is in such a symbiotic fashion that these persons customarily enter into, and maintain, "interpersonal" relatedness. The subtle role of the therapist's unconscious hostility or reproachfulness, for example, toward one or another of the participants in the family drama is all too apt to be overshadowed by the blatant reality of the hostility which is personified by the mother or father and by the reproachfulness which is being manifested by the patient toward them.

I wonder whether, in a setting where there is not only so ready but even eager a set of "targets" for the therapist's introjects, he may not feel threatened lest he lose his introjects, and become thus helplessly apart from what is going on in the session? And, although introjects are subjectively experienced as being in opposition to, rather than as contributing to, ego identity, they do contain significant increments of potential, or latent, ego identity; thus, I surmise that this sense of threat may become experienced as a fear lest one lose one's self, one's identity. Such thoughts, admittedly highly speculative, seem permissible when one considers how acute is the sense of isolation and anxiety which the therapist at times experiences here.

It is well to explore the personal sources of one's own interest in doing therapy in this field, for any unrecognized and acted-out personal needs must have a great influence upon our "technique." If, for example, the therapist is unaware of how hungry he is for participation in parental family life, he will find it difficult to disengage himself from a deeply participative role and move into a more detached observer position at moments when this is indicated By the same token, he will have unconscious resistance to the family's developing an increasingly healthy relatedness among themselves, a relatedness which he can not biologically share, analogous to the individual therapist's resistance to the patient's becoming well and thereby lost to him.

The literature in this field is liberally sprinkled with examples of the therapist's assuming the task of rescuing or protecting the patient from one or both parents, on the basis of an unconscious avoidance of the transference role, vis-à-vis the patient or parents or both, of the personifier of these family members' "bad introjects." A genuine working-through of the patient's, and other family members', difficulties would involve the therapist's being able to endure, for whatever period of time required for such working-through, his own being regarded by these persons as the embodiment of Bad Mother or Bad Father malevolence. But it is deceptively easy to regard oneself as a potential savior, by definition devoid of hostility, and to regard the patient as an equally unhating victim of parental hostility. Also, the active gratifications of the Good Parent (or Good Child, for that matter) role, if only we can sustain it, are great indeed. When, for example, a paranoid father who usually regarded me in the family group as being the personification of evil, saw me for a time in an utterly contrasting light and said to me, smiling benignly, "If you're innocent, you're innocent," I felt quite simply blessed, with a sense of purity and goodness which I sensed to have been one of the feeling experiences of an early childhood now lost beyond remembering.

The dramatic "interpersonal" confrontations which family therapy promotes are very apt to keep obscured the central role of such introjects. Burton (1961), reporting his therapy of a schizophrenic woman, says that:

. . . Her improvement was not matched by the growth of her family, who had considerable unconscious investment in the maintenance of her illness. In family therapy she was able, for the first time, to confront her father and husband with her needs as a person and to point out logically the part they themselves played in her illness. At this point the husband told of his ambivalence about resuming his life with her outside the hospital and began drinking again . . .

In a similar vein, Jackson (1961) observes that:

. . . Perhaps the most important aspect of family psychotherapy is that the patient has to see his parents as real people . . .

My point, here, is that we are all too apt to accept such confrontations as being genuinely and exclusively interpersonal events, and to miss the centrally significant etiologic role of the patient's own pathogenic introjects, projected here upon spouse or parents.

It seems evident that, in order for the therapist to work effectively in the family therapy of schizophrenia, his identity as a parent must be as acceptable to him, as well-elaborated and established, as is his identity as a child, for otherwise he will tend unduly much to identify with the patient-as-child and unconsciously to wreak revenge (for his own childhood grievances) upon the patient's parents. It would seem that, to meet the therapeutic needs of the family, as these needs shift moment by moment, he must be able to shift his identification, in a ready and fluid way, from child to parent and vice versa. One senses here that, no matter how limited as a therapeutic method this form of therapy may eventually prove to be, one of its enduring values will spring from the maturity which it requires, and therefore fosters, in the therapist, a maturity which can only enhance his therapeutic results in individual psychotherapy also.

Concluding Remarks

In our enthusiasm about this promising new therapeutic approach to schizophrenia, we should not forget that the patient himself is typically, no matter how great the other family members' etiologic contributions, the most deeply ill individual in the family.[6] Thus,

---

[6] This statement is an accurate summation of my own clinical experience which is, as I acknowledged at the outset, heavily weighted on the side of individual therapy with—I should explain further—chronically schizophrenic patients. When I term the patient himself typically "the most deeply ill individual in the family," I refer to the various family members' respective ego-functioning as individuals.

The validity of the above statement has been challenged by persons with vastly more experience than I in the family therapy of schizophrenia. I respect their differing and, in this regard, much greater experience, and it is not difficult for me to believe that if one has the opportunity to work with a number of families containing at the outset of treatment a young person who has only

while this new field is eminently deserving of vigorous exploration, we should not enter into it in a spirit of flight from facing the full depth of the patient's own psychopathology, from facing, for example, the awesome depth of his hostility, his despair, his grief, and his need to give and receive love; and the no less, awesome depth of, for instance, one's own ambivalent love and hatred, and therefore despair, concerning him. It is all too easy to become convinced, with him, that his own illness is now effectively resolved and his only remaining difficulty consists in his being afflicted with a malignant wife or mother or father, so that, if only these can be dragged into the therapeutic situation and the extent of their destructive contributions revealed for all to see, this basically well and loving patient can then function as such.

It is especially important for us to realize that these family-oriented problems can be worked through in the individual therapeutic relationship, and need to be worked through there in order for the patient to achieve the deepest possible level of personal integration. It is quite possible that we shall come to view family therapy as a most worthy companion to such individual therapy; but I doubt that it can ever come to replace, in integrative value, the patient's working through, in the transference-relationship to the individual therapist—no matter that this relationship is *ostensibly* a dyadic one—of his intrapsychic conflicts referable not merely to single other persons but to all family-members simultaneously. That is, just as we have learned that a patient can form an adequate mother-transference to a male therapist, and an adequate father-transference to a female therapist—without, that is, requiring for this stage of the therapy a transfer to another therapist of the opposite sex—so, my experience suggests, the transference can find the necessary *multiplicity* also as directed toward the individual therapist, even though at a biological level he is but one person. The patient who can find mother and father and siblings in the therapist, simultaneously, and who can, through identification with this therapist, make these projected internal images into truly integrated parts of himself becomes thereby, I believe, a more deeply integrated single individual than does the patient whose transference relationship is diverted and dispersed upon the various real members of the parental family in an exclusively family therapy approach.

---

recently come to manifest an acute schizophrenia, and with one or another parent evidencing, say, a long-existing ambulatory schizophrenia, one may come to the conclusion that it is the parent, as often as the "schizophrenic one," the son or daughter who in the individual therapist's viewpoint wears the label of patient, who is, all things considered, really the more heavily burdened with psychopathology.

Space will not allow me to detail more than a few examples of the "family transference" which I have come to see in individual treatment relationships and which have convinced me that individual therapy can and should be extended down into this realm, which have made me believe that the family *in toto* comes upon the individual therapy scene and should not bodily be brought into it as more than an adjunct to our focus upon the individual himself. A paranoid woman, complaining to a nurse about me, demanded, "Who the hell does he think he is? He's not my mother and father!" Later on in her treatment, during the course of one session she said, "You—Edgar and Dad and Louise . . ." Edgar and Louise were the names of two of her siblings; at this stage of the therapy she saw all other persons, including me, as multiple persons, and on innumerable occasions I was, to her, several members of her parental family simultaneously. She had not been visited for years by any of her three children and steadfastly disclaimed that she had any children. I felt baffled and despairing as to how this great real-life gulf could possibly be bridged; but my concern lessened as I began to see to what a degree she was able to perceive me, in the transference, as being one or another of her children, and to work through in this setting her anxiety, hostility, grief, and so on, with respect to her five-year-old daughter, or her seven-year-old daughter, or her three-year-old son—now, in actuality, several years older than that. Such transference developments helped greatly to pave the way for the real-life resumption of her relationships with her children.

A hebephrenic man lived, for years, in a predominantly hallucinatory world. Gradually, the chaotic, discoordinate quality of this "interpersonal" world in which he lived assumed, more and more consistently, the identity of his parental family; but I was still reacted to, by him, as having much less of a flesh-and-blood substantiality than did these hallucinatory family members. As the treatment progressed still further, I felt myself to be no longer an onlooker in this family scene; I was now on a par with these hallucinatory figures toward "whom" I had more than once felt jealousy, because of the liveliness of the patient's interactions with them and the sparsity of the crumbs of emotional responsiveness which had come my way. Still later on, he gave me to know that I was now more important to him than these hallucinations, the appearances of which, in his world, could now more and more readily be traced to the vicissitudes of the real and identifiable relationship between him and me. One time when I was trying to understand how he viewed me, he explained, in a compassionate tone, "I look at you as a father. They've all gone. Martin (the patient's own name) has gone, and Leonard (a brother who was killed in Korea) has gone, and Ethel (a sister who had long ago moved to a distant foreign country) has gone, and you're the only one who's left." I cannot adequately convey the depth and vividness of the feeling of *family* which was conveyed in his words, in his transference to me as the personification of his lonely and aged father, of whom this view was indeed so true.

A hebephrenic woman with whom I am currently working experiences both herself, and me, as respective *crowds*, and I expect that it may be a long time yet before her ego integration proceeds sufficiently far for the comparatively simple and identifiable family transference to emerge, with some consistency, as it did in my work with the above-described man. Such multiple transferences tend, of course, to be stressful for the therapist, because they threaten him with ego fragmentation (Searles, 1959b).

An exploration of the family therapy of schizophrenia enriches and enlivens one's concept of the healthy family also. It suggests that, just as in *individual* ego development there is normally a symbiotic phase which gives place, later, to individuation, there is a family symbiotic phase in the existence of the healthy family, a phase which, if the family is to live out its healthy destiny and be psychologically successful as a family, must give place to the achieved (or, in the instances of the adults, the deepened) individuation of the several participants. That is, the very conspicuous symbiotic, projected and introjected part-object phenomena which one sees in the family of the schizophrenic patient have less conflict-laden counterparts in healthy family development. As seen at any one moment in time, a family is a *group of persons;* but as viewed over the years of the family's evolution, a family is a *process of individuation out of symbiosis.*

It may well be that the most mature form of interrelatedness among the healthy person's introjects can be characterized best by the term "family of introjects," or family-relatedness among his introjects. It is notable that the schizophrenic family as a whole, like the schizophrenic patient himself, is barred by its isolation, vis-à-vis other families, from learning more healthy family relationships; and it hardly seems feasible to employ a healthy family in the service of meeting this troubled family's identificatory needs. But in those fortunate instances in which the family therapist has matured sufficiently so that there has been achieved a family interrelatedness among his introjects, the family can find *in him* the healthy family with whom they hunger to identify. In this sense he can constitute a bridge for them to traverse, out of their family isolation and into the world of the healthier families about them.

494 INTENSIVE FAMILY THERAPY

References

ARIETI, S. (1961). Introductory notes on the psychoanalytic therapy of schizophrenics. In A. Burton (Ed.) *Psychotherapy of the psychoses.* New York: Basic Books, pp. 69–89.

BAK, R. C. (1954). The schizophrenic defence against aggression. *Int. J. Psychoanal. 35,* 129–134.

BENEDEK, T. (1959). Parenthood as a developmental phase: a contribution to the libido theory. *J. Amer. Psychoanal. Ass. 7,* 389–417.

BOSZORMENYI-NAGY, I., AND FRAMO, J. L. (1962). Family concept of hospital treatment of schizophrenia. In J. Masserman (Ed.) *Current psychiatric therapies,* vol. II. New York: Grune & Stratton, pp. 159–166.

BOWEN, M. (1960). A family concept of schizophrenia. In D. D. Jackson (Ed.) *Etiology of schizophrenia.* New York: Basic Books, pp. 346–372.

BRODEY, W. M. (1959). Some family operations and schizophrenia: a study of five hospitalized families each with a schizophrenic member. *A.M.A. Arch. gen. Psychiat. 1,* 379–402.

BRODEY, W. M. (1961). The family as the unit of study and treatment—workshop, 1959: 3, image, object and narcissistic relationships. *Amer. J. Orthopsychiat. 31,* 69–73.

BURTON, A. (1961). The quest for the golden mean: a study in schizophrenia. In A. Burton (Ed.) *Psychotherapy of the psychoses.* New York: Basic Books, pp. 172–207.

HAVENS, L. L. (1962). The placement and movement of hallucinations in space: phenomenology and theory. *Int. J. Psychoanal. 18,* 426–435.

HENDRICK, I. (1931). Ego defense and the mechanism of oral ejection in schizophrenia. *Int. J. Psychoanal. 12,* 298–325.

JACKSON, D. D. (1961). The monad, the dyad, and the family therapy of schizophrenics. In A. Burton (Ed.) *Psychotherapy of the psychoses.* New York: Basic Books, pp. 318–328.

KLEIN, M. (1932). *The psycho-analysis of children.* London: Hogarth Press and Inst. of Psychoanal.

KLEIN, M., HEIMANN, P., AND MONEY-KYRLE, R. (Eds.) (1955). *New directions in psycho-analysis.* New York: Basic Books.

LIDZ, T., CORNELISON, A. R., FLECK, S., AND TERRY, D. (1957). The intrafamilial environment of schizophrenic patients: II. marital schism and marital skew. *Amer. J. Psychiat. 114,* 241–248.

LIDZ, T., AND FLECK, S. (1960). Schizophrenia, human integration, and the role of the family. In D. D. Jackson (Ed.) *Etiology of schizophrenia.* New York: Basic Books, pp. 323–345.

SCHWARTZ, M. S., AND WILL, G. T. (1953). Low morale and mutual withdrawal on a mental hospital ward. *Psychiatry, 16,* 337–353.

SEARLES, H. F. (1951). Data concerning certain manifestations of incorporation. *Psychiatry 14,* 397–413.

SEARLES, H. F. (1958). Positive feelings in the relationship between the schizophrenic and his mother. *Int. J. Psychoanal. 39*, 569–586 (Reprinted under the title, "Positive Gefuhle in der Beziehung zwischen dem Schizophrenen und seiner Mutter," in *Psyche*, 1960, *14*, 165–203).

SEARLES, H. F. (1959a). The effort to drive the other person crazy—an element in the aetiology and psychotherapy of schizophrenia. *Brit. J. med. Psychol. 32*, 1–18.

SEARLES, H. F. (1959b). Integration and differentiation in schizophrenia: an over-all view. *Brit. J. med. Psychol. 32*, 261–281.

SEARLES, H. F. (1961a). Evolution of the mother transference in psychotherapy with the schizophrenic patient. In A. Burton (Ed.) *Psychotherapy of the psychoses*. New York: Basic Books, pp. 256–284.

SEARLES, H. F. (1961b). Sexual processes in schizophrenia. *Psychiatry 24*, 87–95.

TOWNE, R. D., SAMPSON, H., AND MESSINGER, S. L. (1961). Schizophrenia and the marital family: identification crises. *J. nerv. ment. Dis. 133*, 423–429.

WYNNE, L. C., RYCKOFF, I. M., DAY, J., AND HIRSCH, S. I. (1958). Pseudomutuality in the family relations of schizophrenics. *Psychiatry 21*, 205–220.

Name Index

Abraham, K., 53, 74
Abrahams, J., 5
Abrahams, R., 395
Ackerman, N. W., 21, 148, *245–287*, 365n.
Alanen, Y. O., 191
Albee, E., 436
Arieti, S., 473
Arrington, R. E., 442
Asch, S. E., 419
Auerbach, A. H., 324, 415

Bach, G., 42
Bachove, C., 427
Back, K. W., 417
Bak, R. C., 482
Baldwin, A. L., 422
Bales, R. F., 23, 298, 305, 309, 411, 412, 416, 423, 424, 426, 427, 430, 437, 438, 439, 440, 441, 442, 443
Balint, M., 34
Balis, N., 365n.
Basamania, B., 213
Bateson, G., 15, 62, 63, 353, 385, 421
Bauer, I. L., 5
Bauman, G., 445
Bavelas, A., 419
Bayer, A. E., 409
Beckett, P. G. S., 4
Bell, J. E., 3, 7, 21, 22, 148, 183
Benedek, T., 481
Bennett, L., 419
Bentley, A. F., 450
Berlin, I. N., 5
Berne, E., 128
Bion, W., 298, 327

Birdwhistell, R. L., 415, 450
Bishop, B. M., 422
Blake, R. R., 401n.
Block, J., 419
Boomer, D. S., 431
Borgatta, E. F., 411, 412
Bosanquet, M., 344
Bossard, J. H., 449
Boszormenyi-Nagy, I., 17, 18, 20, *33–86*, *87–142*, 143n., 157, 365, 367, 392
Bowen, M., 8, 9, 10, 17, 19, 110, 148, 180, *213–243*, 450, 473, 477, 486
Bowlby, J., 54
Bowman, C. C., 410
Boyd, I., 429
Bray, D., 4
Brodey, W. M., 10, 11, 49, 298, 345, 472, 473
Brody, M. W., 95, 213
Buber, M., 50, 56, 57, 58, 61
Buhler, C., 42, 141
Burgess, E., 409
Burridge, K. O. L., 389
Burton, A., 489
Bychowski, G., 5

Cantril, H., 419
Caputo, D. V., 426
Carroll, E. J., 20, 188
Carter, L., 437, 442, 443
Cartwright, D., 411, 413, 417
Champney, H., 422
Chance, E., 23
Chapple, E. D., 437, 438, 443
Chayevsky, P., 185
Clausen, J. A., 23, 28

Page numbers in italic type designate the author's chapter.

Subject Index

501

73 74 75 76   9 8 7 6 5